Routledge Handbook of Psychiatry in Asia

Geographically and demographically Asia is a huge region with a large number of societies and cultures, each affected by their own unique problems including over-population, major natural disasters, poverty and changing social and economic factors. Inevitably this means that different mental health needs have developed across the region. Colonialism, globalization, industrialization and urbanization have brought major demographic and cultural shifts in the region but clinical mental health practices and services, and societal attitudes to mental health issues vary enormously.

This Handbook surveys the state of the current psychiatric care field across the whole Asia-Pacific region. Focusing on individual countries, each chapter includes:

- A summary of factors affecting the practice and provision of psychiatric care, including cultural attitudes to mental health issues.
- Coverage of the conceptualization, causation and prevalence of mental health issues in society.
- An overview of mental health care services and systems available and workforce training.
- Coverage of country-specific innovative practices and folk therapies.

As the first major reference work on psychiatric care in Asia this book is an essential resource for scholars and students researching mental health in Asia as well as for psychiatrists and other mental health professionals working in the region.

Dinesh Bhugra, CBE, is President of the World Psychiatric Association. He is Emeritus Professor of Mental Health and Cultural Diversity at the Institute of Psychiatry, King's College London.

Samson Tse is Associate Dean (Undergraduate Education) of the Faculty of Social Sciences, Professor of Mental Health and Director of the Master of Social Sciences in Counselling Programme at the Department of Social Work and Social Administration, The University of Hong Kong.

Roger Ng is Consultant Psychiatrist and Chief of Service of the Department of Psychiatry of Kowloon Hospital, Hong Kong.

Nori Takei is Professor of Neuropsychological Development and Health Sciences at the United Graduate School of Child Development (Osaka University, Kanazawa University, Hamamatsu University School of Medicine, Chiba University and Fukui University), Hamamatsu University School of Medicine.

Routledge Handbook of Psychiatry in Asia

Edited by
Dinesh Bhugra, Samson Tse,
Roger Ng and Nori Takei

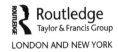

LONDON AND NEW YORK

First published 2016
by Routledge
2 Park Square, Milton Park, Abingdon, Oxon, OX14 4RN

and by Routledge
52 Vanderbilt Avenue, New York, NY 10017

First issued in paperback 2020

Routledge is an imprint of the Taylor & Francis Group, an informa business

British Library Cataloguing in Publication Data
A catalogue record for this book is available from the British Library

Library of Congress Cataloging in Publication Data
Routledge handbook of psychiatry in Asia/edited by Dinesh Bhugra,

  Samson Tse, Roger Ng, and Nori Takei.
  p. ; cm.
  Handbook of psychiatry in Asia
  Includes bibliographical references and index.
  I. Bhugra, Dinesh, editor. II. Tse, Samson, editor. III. Ng, Roger,
  editor. IV. Takei, Nori, editor. V. Title: Handbook of psychiatry
  in Asia.
  [DNLM: 1. Mental Disorders – Asia – Handbooks. 2. Cultural
  Characteristics – Asia – Handbooks. 3. Health Status – Asia –
  Handbooks. 4. Mental Health Services – Asia – Handbooks. WM 34]
  RC451.C4
  362.196890095--dc23
  2014023901

ISBN 13: 978–0–367–58173–2 (pbk)
ISBN 13: 978–0–415–71131–9 (hbk)

Typeset in Bembo and Stone Sans
by Florence Production Ltd, Stoodleigh, Devon, UK

Contents

Figures

Tables

Tables

Contributors

Helal Uddin Ahmed is Assistant Professor, Child Adolescent and Family Psychiatry, National Institute of Mental Health (NIMH), Dhaka, Bangladesh.

Marat Assimov is Professor of Psychiatry, Kazakh National Medical University, S.D. Asfendiyarov, Republic of Kazakhstan.

Dinesh Bhugra, CBE, is President of the World Psychiatric Association. He is Emeritus Professor of Mental Health and Cultural Diversity at the Institute of Psychiatry, King's College London.

Nikolay Bokhan is Professor and corresponding Member of Russian Academy of Medical Sciences (RAMSci); Director of Mental Health Research Institute SB RAMSci; and Head of Addictive States Department of Mental Health Research Institute SB RAMSci, Tomsk, Russian Federation.

Lai-Fong Chan is Senior Lecturer in Psychiatry at the National University of Malaysia (UKM) Medical Centre, Kuala Lumpur, Malaysia.

Santosh K. Chaturvedi is Professor of Psychiatry and Head of Psychiatric Rehabilitation Services, National Institute of Mental Health and Neuro Sciences (NIMHANS), Bangalore, India.

Cheng-Chung Chen is Superintendent, Kaohsiung Municipal Kai Syuan Psychiatric Hospital; and Associate Professor, Department of Psychiatry, School of Medicine, Faculty of Medicine, Kaohsiung Medical University, Kaohsiung, Taiwan.

Kai-Da Cheng is Attending Psychiatrist, Department of Community Psychiatry, Kaohsiung Municipal Kai Syuan Psychiatric Hospital; and Master's Candidate, Department of Neurosciences, School of Medicine, Faculty of Medicine, Kaohsiung Medical University, Kaohsiung, Taiwan.

Leslie Lim Eng Choon is Senior Consultant Psychiatrist, Singapore General Hospital; Clinical Associate Professor, Yong Loo Lin School of Medicine, National University of Singapore (NUS); Adjunct Associate Professor, Duke–NUS Graduate Medical School; and Visiting Consultant, Department of Palliative Medicine, National Cancer Centre, Singapore.

Chantharavady Choulamany is a Psychiatrist and Programme Manager of BasicNeeds–Lao, Vientiane, Lao People's Democratic Republic (PDR).

Victoria Patricia C. De la Llana, is Consultation-Liaison Fellow-in-Training, Department of Psychiatry, University of the Philippines, Philippine General Hospital, Philippines.

Geetha Desai is Associate Professor, Department of Psychiatry, National Institute of Mental Health and Neuro Sciences (NIMHANS), Bangalore, India.

Hervita Diatri is Lecturer at the Department of Psychiatry and Chair of Community Psychiatry Division, Faculty of Medicine University of Indonesia/Ciptomangunkusumo General Hospital, Jakarta, Indonesia.

Tatiana Galako is Associate Professor and Chair of Psychiatry, Medical Psychology and Drug Abuse, Department of Medicicine, State Academy of Kyrgyz Republic; and Associate Professor, Slavonic University in Kyrgyzstan. She also serves as the President of the Kyrgyz Psychiatric Association.

Harischandra Gambheera is Professor in Psychiatry, Consultant Psychiatrist and Clinical Director, National Institute of Mental Health, Angoda, Sri Lanka.

Shree Ram Ghimire is Third Year Resident, Department of Psychiatry, National Medical College, Birgunj, Nepal.

Bharat Kumar Goit is Associate Professor, Department of Psychiatry, National Medical College, Birgunj, Nepal.

Yueqin Huang is Professor of Psychiatric Epidemiology; Director, Division of Social Psychiatry and Behavioural Medicine, Institute of Mental Health, Peking University, PR China; Director, National Centre for Mental Health, Chinese Centre for Disease Control and Prevention; President, Chinese Mental Health Journal; and Vice-president, China Disabled Persons' Federation.

Arun Kandasamy is Assistant Professor, Centre for Addiction Medicine, Department of Psychiatry, National Institute of Mental Health and Neuro Sciences (NIMHANS), Bangalore, India.

Grigoriy Kharabara is Head of the Republican Organizational and Methodological Advisory Department of Psychiatry, Republican Psychiatric Hospital of the Ministry of Health of the Republic of Uzbekistan.

Nargiza Khodjaeva is World Health Organization Expert on Mental Health of Central Asian countries, and Director of the Republican Centre of Suicidology, Uzbekistan.

Elena Kim is Assistant Professor and Chair of Psychology Department, American University in Central Asia, Kyrgyz Republic.

Seog Ju Kim is Associate Professor at the Centre for Medicine and Korean Reunification, Seoul National University College of Medicine, South Korea.

Valery Krasnov is Director of the Moscow Research Institute of Psychiatry, Vice-president of the Russian Society of Psychiatrists.

Linda C. W. Lam is Professor and Chairperson of Department of Psychiatry, Faculty of Medicine, The Chinese University of Hong Kong, China.

Min-Soo Lee is Chairman, Professor, Department of Psychiatry, Korea University College of Medicine, Seoul, Republic of Korea.

Paul V. Lee is Associate Professor of Psychiatry, College of Medicine, University of the Philippines; and Chair, Department of Psychiatry, Quezon City General Hospital, Philippines.

Yu-Chen Lin is Nurse Specialist, Department of Community Psychiatry, Kaohsiung Municipal Kai Syuan Psychiatric Hospital, Kaohsiung, Taiwan.

Zhaorui Liu is Associate Professor of Psychiatric Epidemiology, Deputy Director, Division of Social Psychiatry and Behavioural Medicine, Institute of Mental Health, Peking University, Beijing, PR China.

Thambu Maniam is Professor and Senior Consultant Psychiatrist at the National University of Malaysia (UKM) Medical Centre, Kuala Lumpur, Malaysia.

Albert Maramis is Mental Health Consultant, WHO Country Office for the Philippines, Manila, Philippines.

Soe Min is a Senior Consultant Psychiatrist and is currently the General Secretary of the Mental Health Society, Myanmar. He formerly served as Consultant/Lecturer at the Department of Mental Health, University of Medicine, Yangon, Myanmar.

Sydney Moirangthem is Assistant Professor, Community Mental Health Unit, Department of Psychiatry, National Institute of Mental Health and Neuro Sciences (NIMHANS), Bangalore, India.

Elena Molchanova is Associate Professor, American University in Central Asia, Slavonic University, Kyrgyz Republic; and Research Fellow, Consortium for Multicultural Psychology Research of Michigan State University, USA.

Win Aung Myint is the Head and Professor of the Department of Mental Health, University of Medicine, Yangon/Mental Health Hospital Yangon, Ministry of Health; President of the Mental Health Society, Myanmar and the Programme Manager for the Mental Health Project, Myanmar.

Mahendra Nepal is Professor and Consultant Psychiatrist, Department of Psychiatry, National Medical College, Birgunj, Nepal; Foundation Professor and Former Head of Department, Institute of Medicine, Tribhuvan University Teaching Hospital, Kathmandu; and Consultant Psychiatrist, Tamworth, New South Wales, Australia.

Smriti Nepal, is an MPH student, James Cook University, Townsville, Queensland, Australia.

Roger M. K. Ng is Consultant Psychiatrist and Chief of Service (Psychiatry) and Consultant Psychiatrist, Department of Psychiatry, Kowloon Hospital, Hong Kong, China.

Saya Nurmagambetova is Professor of Psychiatry, Kazakh National Medical University, Asfendiyarov, Republic of Kazakhstan.

Seon-Cheol Park is Clinical Psychiatrist and Researcher, Department of Psychiatry, Yong-In Mental Hospital, Yongin, Republic of Korea.

Yong Chon Park is Professor, Department of Neuropsychiatry, College of Medicine, Hanyang University, Seoul, Republic of Korea.

Shi-Hooi Poon is Registrar Psychiatrist, Department of Psychiatry, Singapore General Hospital, Singapore.

Golam Rabbani is Professor of Psychiatry, Popular Medical College, Dhaka, Bangladesh; Former Director-cum-Professor, National Institute of Mental Health (NIMH), Dhaka; and President, Bangladesh Association of Psychiatrists.

Kim Savuon is President, Mental Health Association of Cambodia, Phnom Penh, Cambodia.

Winston W. Shen is Attending Psychiatrist and Chief Emeritus, Department of Psychiatry, Wan Fang Medical Centre; and Professor and Chairman Emeritus, Department of Psychiatry, School of Medicine, College of Medicine, Taipei Medical University, Taipei, Taiwan.

Pooja H. Shetty is Post-Doctoral Fellow and Senior Resident, Community Mental Health Unit, Department of Psychiatry, National Institute of Mental Health and Neuro Sciences (NIMHANS), Bangalore, India.

T. Sivakumar is Assistant Professor of Psychiatric and Neurological Rehabilitation, Psychiatric Rehabilitation Services, Department of Psychiatry, National Institute of Mental Health and Neuro Sciences (NIMHANS), Bangalore, India.

Keo Sothy is an Officer, Bureau of Mental Health, Department of Hospital Services, Ministry of Health, Phnom Penh, Cambodia.

Manit Srisurapanont is Professor of Psychiatry at the Department of Psychiatry, Faculty of Medicine, Chiangmai University, Thailand.

Shiro Suda is Lecturer, Department of Psychiatry, Jichi Medical University, Japan.

Genichi Sugihara is Assistant Professor, Department of Psychiatry, Kyoto University Hospital, Japan.

Thiha Swe is Assistant Lecturer, Department of Mental Health, University of Medicine, Mandalay/Mental Health Hospital Mandalay, Ministry of Health, Myanmar. He is a Psychiatrist and the Associate Secretary (Mandalay) of the Mental Health Society, Myanmar.

Rizwan Taj is Chairman, Department of Psychiatry, Pakistan Institute of Medical Sciences, Shaheed Zulfiqar Bhutto University; and Focal Person Mental Health, Ministry of Health Services and Regulations, Islamabad, Pakistan.

Nori Takei is Professor of Neuropsychological Development and Health Sciences at the United Graduate School of Child Development (Osaka University, Kanazawa University, Hamamatsu

University School of Medicine, Chiba University and Fukui University), Hamamatsu University School of Medicine, Japan; and Visiting Professor, the Department of Psychosis Studies, Institute of Psychiatry, London, United Kingdom.

Tran Thi Hong Thu is Head of Clinical Department, Mai Hương Psychiatric Hospital, Hanoi, Vietnam.

Samson Tse is Associate Dean (Experiential Learning) of the Faculty of Social Sciences, Professor of Mental Health and Director of the Master of Social Science in Counselling Programme at the Department of Social Work and Social Administration, The University of Hong Kong, China.

Pichet Udomratn is Professor of Psychiatry, Department of Psychiatry, Faculty of Medicine, Prince of Songkla University, Thailand. He is currently President of the Asian Federation of Psychiatric Associations (AFPA) and Chairperson of the Asian Network of Bipolar Disorder (ANBD). He formerly served as President of the Psychiatric Association of Thailand for two consecutive terms.

Salvador Benjamin D. Vista is Associate Professor of Psychiatry, College of Medicine, University of the Philippines; and Chair, Department of Psychiatry, Asian Hospital and Medical Centre, Philippines.

Hong Wang is Associate Professor of Epidemiology and Biostatistics, Department of Epidemiology and Biostatistics, School of Public Health, Peking University, Beijing, PR China.

Preface

Dinesh Bhugra, Samson Tse,
Roger Ng and Nori Takei

Introduction

Asia is the largest geographical region of the world with nearly one third of the land mass and 8.8 per cent of whole area. Over 4.4 billion people live in the geographical area in 49 countries, six countries' dependencies and another six countries which are partly or completely unrecognized. The boundaries of Asia have often shifted historically depending upon the boundaries of the Russian Federation. Two countries – Turkey and Russia – are often counted as both in Europe and Asia. Traditionally, Asia is split into six regions: Central Asia, Western Asia, Southern Asia, Eastern Asia and Southeastern Asia.

Central Asia geographically includes countries such as Kazakhstan, Uzbekistan, Tajikistan, Turkmenistan, Kyrgyzstan and Mongolia. Western Asia (otherwise known as the Middle East) consists of Bahrain, Iraq, Israel, Jordan, Kuwait, Lebanon, the Palestinian Territories, Oman, Qatar, Saudi Arabia, Syria, the United Arab Emirates and Yemen. Southern Asia (often called South East Asia) contains Afghanistan, Pakistan, India, Maldives, Sri Lanka, Nepal, Bhutan, Bangladesh and Iraq. Eastern Asia is made up of China, Hong Kong, Macao, North Korea, South Korea, Japan and Taiwan. Southeastern Asia includes countries such as Myanmar (Burma), Thailand, Laos, Cambodia, Vietnam, Malaysia, Brunei, the Philippines, Singapore, Indonesia and Timor-Leste.

In addition to geographical variation, Asia is a diverse region with geographical and linguistic diversity, and diversity in resources and religions. Most of major religions of the world – Christianity, Judaism, Islam, Hinduism, Buddhism, Jainism – originated in Asia and are still followed. These variations lead to a number of major issues in understanding psychiatric illness, help-seeking and resources provided. Cultures define what is abnormal and what resources are needed to provide healthcare. The proportion of GDP devoted to health care is often very low.

Practice of psychiatry in Asia

There are specific issues related to psychiatry, its role and its practice in Asia. Ancient texts have described psychiatric illnesses; and in many non-allopathic systems of medicine the models of illness are much more holistic, where mind and body interact with each other and are influenced by external factors such as diet, taboos, environment, weather and external influences, which makes the understanding of patients' explanatory models critical so that therapeutic alliances can be forged. Patients will often choose non-medical resources as the first port of call.

This may reflect explanatory models but also accessibility of services. As vast numbers of people live in rural areas and the majority of services are set up in urban areas it is inevitable that there will be a discrepancy between need and supply. An additional complication arises, which is to do with specialist services. Many countries may have limited numbers of general adult psychiatrists, but specialist access to, say, psychiatrists dealing with intellectual disability or psychiatry of the elderly may be even more difficult. Limited human and financial resources mean that alternative models of health care delivery have to be explored, developed and evaluated. Integration with primary health care, and increasing exposure to psychiatric health care training at undergraduate and post-graduate levels across all medical and surgical specialties can only benefit patients, and also lead to better engagement with families of patients, and thus improve outcomes.

Psychiatry has not been top of the agenda for many countries in Asia for a number of reasons. However, changes related to emigration and immigration from Asian countries to elsewhere in the world, and within the countries from rural to urban areas, bring with them specific impacts on migrants' mental health. In the past few decades the practice of clinical psychiatry in Asia has advanced a great deal, again due to increasing awareness of the potential for treatments.

In countries of the Indian subcontinent, such as Bangladesh, Bhutan, India, Nepal, Pakistan and Sri Lanka, interesting epidemiological data have been collected looking at various psychiatric disorders. The section on the subcontinent provides an overview of not only data on prevalence and incidence but also on specific issues related to delivery of mental health services and mental health legislation. It is interesting to note that in many countries around Asia similar issues continue to emerge. The role of traditional healers and traditional health care systems is also explored, to ensure that clinicians are aware of where their patients may have been and where they ought to be heading. Even within the six countries forming the geographical Indian subcontinent several common themes start to emerge. Paucity of resources, increasing demand, increasing longevity, cultures-in-transition, varying degrees of political stability, a degree of internal conflict, natural or man-made disasters and urbanization, all contributing to increasing psychopathology along with the changes in family structures, raise major challenges in health care delivery.

Mental health is a neglected field in all the countries of Asia – more in some countries than others – but the situation is beginning to change in many of them. Often there is increased emphasis on managing and controlling infectious diseases and nutritional deficiencies. Conditions such as depression are sometimes seen as life's ups and downs and so not even needing treatment or intervention by policymakers. Suicidal acts are still illegal in many countries, dating back to British colonial rule, thus making it extremely difficult to get an accurate picture of rates of self-harm and suicidal acts and the requirements for managing them. Undoubtedly, in many countries mental health services are gradually evolving, but the demand is nowhere near being met and the treatment gap is massive. In several countries psychiatric asylums are giving way to community- or district-based programmes and district-hospital-based psychiatry. Yet specialist needs, as mentioned earlier, such as the needs of the elderly or intellectually disabled individuals, are nowhere near being met. Interestingly, some of the slack is being picked up by NGOs in the face of a dearth of psychiatrists, psychologists and psychiatric nurses, not to mention other mental health professionals such as occupational therapists and social workers. The quality of training of psychiatrists is extremely variable and there is a shortage of jobs, encouraging individuals to go into private practice and raising issues about equity of care. In addition, the training often relies on Western models of psychiatry, making its broad applicability questionable in some circumstances. Local idioms of distress will reflect abnormal illness behaviour among persons with mental health problems. A lack of understanding of local cultural aspects of mental illness presentations, models of explanation and help-seeking behaviours, together with availability and use of indigenous practices, may make clinical practice inadequate in meeting the needs of patients and their carers and families. Migration of trained professionals to the West brings with it specific ethical issues, such as low-income countries subsidizing high-income countries. Many countries have been denuded of their health professionals by higher salaries, greater prestige and better educational opportunities in the West.

Mental health policy

The mental health policy and legislation in many countries also date back to colonial rule, although attempts are being made to bring them into the twenty-first century. The specific impact of human rights has often been seen as a Western imperialist tradition and so ignored. However, human rights also carry with them a huge degree of variation related to children's rights, gender-based parity and LGBT (lesbian, gay, bisexual, transgender) rights, highlighting the urgency of social justice. Other factors which influence the therapeutic alliance and engagement with and treatment of mental disorders include stigma, prejudice, discrimination and misconceptions about mental disorders. These must be considered when developing psychiatric services. Traditional medicine is popular in most countries and sometimes patients will use both traditional and medical models of treatment, occasionally leading to an accumulation of side effects and drug interactions. Patients may also prefer complementary and alternative treatments because they are easily accessible and relatively low cost. Diversity within cultures must be emphasized and taken into account. Even within India, there are 22 languages recognized in the constitution with over 500 dialects, highlighting the diverse nature of the people and making it imperative that psychiatry and psychiatrists are aware of these variations and their implications.

In the region of Southeast Asia, while there are similarities of religion and development, there are varied issues too. As Maniam highlights in his introduction to the section, although there are historical similarities across countries, their colonial exposures and experiences have been very variable.

Although their colonial masters were different, the experiences and development of psychiatric services were heavily influenced by those masters. Malaysia and Singapore share many similarities with respect to psychiatric services because of their geographical proximity, shared history and close cultural ties, but development has occurred at varying levels, initially asylum-based and custodial, and subsequently with growth in general hospital psychiatric units and development of community services. Inevitably, the shift has been both patchy and problematic. Like experiences in Western countries, often community services are seen as money-saving exercises. Changes in mental health laws and policy have brought additional strain on resources, with attitudes become more liberal, more cognizant of the rights of patients and promoting more humane treatment of the mentally ill. Like in the rest of the world, stigma and discrimination against mental illness, the mentally ill and mental health professionals (including psychiatrists) have affected resource allocation and acceptance of services by the population. Although change is slow, it has been a result of active leadership which has led to removing hurdles. More is needed, especially through encouraging patient advocacy and formation of patient support organizations.

In many countries in Asia a common model for training psychiatrists follows the traditional Western way, often using Western textbooks with exposure to local knowledge and practices. However, trainees are expected and indeed encouraged to spend some time overseas gaining exposure to international standards and practices. The downside is that sometimes trainees do not return after finishing their period of training.

Challenges

Another major challenge to clinicians and policymakers alike is the increased frequency of disasters faced by the region. These include both natural and man-made disasters, and mental health professionals including psychiatrists have had to attend to the mental health needs of those affected by various tragedies, building on local knowledge and expertise. Cultural values and models continue to play a major role in health care and delivery. Often patients and their families see the problems as being caused by external loci of control (e.g. 'possession' or the 'evil eye') and seek help from shamans and traditional healers. Multiple-source help-seeking is extremely common. Inevitably, there are similarities and differences. There is no doubt that culturally influenced syndromes and symptoms still exist, but the traditional way of looking at culture-bound syndromes is beginning to change. Exposure to international and globalized media and stories suggest that in many countries previously unknown psychiatric syndromes are beginning to appear.

In the section on the Far East, North and South Korea and Japan are covered. These three countries are geographically and culturally close to each other. There are obvious differences in political systems, reflecting historical development of structures which undoubtedly affect psychiatric practice and services. Epidemiological data from North Korea is limited, and the information provided relies on secondary sources. However, the major aim of sharing such information is to learn from each other, as psychiatric patients deserve the best treatments available. Local resources and policies will determine how services are planned, delivered and evaluated, but it is useful to have international standards. It is interesting to note that in Japan and South Korea emphasis on inpatient treatment and biological therapies continues irrespective of somewhat different influences. There was a strong German influence on Japanese psychiatry with an emphasis on psychopathology, whereas in South Korea the emphasis has been on psychodynamic/psychoanalytic psychiatry as a result of American influence. Both countries place a strong emphasis on psychiatric inpatient services, and indeed Japan is the only country in the world where the number of inpatient psychiatric beds is rising. With increasing longevity and the potential difficult impact of the economic downturn, services need to be reviewed and changed accordingly. Culturally acceptable and culturally developed therapies such as yoga are available but not much used. Similarly, *Tao psychotherapy* in South Korea and Morita therapy in Japan indicate that there is a clear need to explore local traditions in engaging psychiatric patients and their carers. It may be that local religious practices and values offer an acceptable format as influenced by Buddhism. People may also find using religious practices more acceptable, as they may see medicalizing their experiences as problematic. Prejudice, stigma and discrimination are all universal issues and when policymakers see mental illness as social weakness, public education becomes an urgent issue. Developing policies which are non-discriminatory and rely on social justice are critical aspects of mental health care delivery.

Within the former USSR – the Russian Federation and the Republics of Central Asia (Kazakhstan, Uzbekistan, Kyrgyzstan, Tajikistan and Turkmenistan) – it has been apparent that clinical approaches, research methodology in psychiatry and organization of mental health care were broadly similar. The underlying scientific conceptualization of mental diseases and diagnostic criteria used to diagnose and classify psychiatric disorders were based on the traditions of European and Russian psychiatry of the past two centuries, and have been not dissimilar to the practice of psychiatry elsewhere. Psychopharmacological approaches have been the mainstay since the 1950s. Although psychotherapy was available, the methods were mostly represented by suggestive approaches to psychotherapy such as hypnosis. However, behavioural treatments based on Pavlovian methods were also in vogue along with rational psychotherapy. Inevitably, in the twentieth century, the system of psychiatric care in Russia and the republics of Central

Asia of the former USSR has undergone substantial changes. Gradually the focus of psychiatric care has moved to community care and outpatient-based treatments. The geographically based and catchment-area-focused interventions have led to widespread coverage of most of the region. Interestingly, and perhaps uniquely, in many places psychiatric consultation offices were developed at factories and universities to provide psychiatric care. These were matched by similar approaches in rural regions, with psychiatric offices at district general hospitals. Geographical-area-based services were developed according to need. Interestingly, in the mid-twentieth century more large psychiatric hospitals were developed and constructed. Also, increased alcohol consumption and resulting complications added to the demand for psychiatric interventions. Addiction services were the key to managing some of these issues.

As in many countries, a rural–urban disparity in services remained, as most of the psychiatric beds were located in large cities, while in rural regions numerous obstacles remained to providing both consulting and care services, especially urgent care, due to the large distances between regional centres and remote settlements. Soviet psychiatry cared for the whole population without charges. However, in the recent times this has begun to change.

Following the collapse of the Soviet Union in 1991, Russia became the first country to have a mental health law passed, which took effect in 1993. The law considerably broadened patients' rights and restricted the possibility of unlawful actions in the course of psychiatric treatment. Economic and social changes along with cultural imperatives in the mid-1990s led to an increase in suicide rates, and addiction. Stigma against mental illness started to affect individual patients and their carers – a phenomenon not dissimilar to other countries. A shortage of human resources has reflected movement of psychiatrists out of the countries to overseas, and this has meant that more international support is needed.

In Greater China, which is the most populous nation in the world, specific issues have emerged along with the general observations noted above. China has thirty-one provincial-level administrative provinces and regions, excluding Taiwan, Hong Kong and Macao. In a fast-developing country with a culture in transition, mental health is a major global public health issue but also a serious social issue, as well as a legal issue. Mental health laws in Hong Kong were enacted over 50 years ago but in mainland China are a relatively recent development. Epidemiological studies indicate that the prevalence of psychiatric disorders is changing with the rapid social and economic developments in China. Changing lifestyles and social expectations and rapid urbanization highlight some of the additional factors which will influence rates of psychiatric disorders and help-seeking.

The mental health services in the region have been variable due to a number of reasons which are described in depth in the section. Chinese traditions, values, beliefs and changes over time have influenced help-seeking whether from traditional Chinese medicine healers or from allopathic providers, and this has been a useful co-existence assisting training in and management of psychiatric disorders.

The way forward

In this volume we present the state of play of psychiatry in different countries in Asia. Undoubtedly, there are similarities and differences. Many countries have up-to-date epidemiological data and have developed services taking into account local needs, whereas many others are lagging behind for a number of reasons. These factors are influenced by prevailing stigma, prejudice and discrimination. For cultures in transition demand may be increasing, but without any additional resources being made available to provide adequate training and services, thus creating a growing treatment gap.

In this era of rapid globalization, rapid exchange and access to information has caused increasing patient expectations of mental health professionals. Thus a better-educated population will demand better, appropriate and accessible services and it is up to the policymakers and service planners to deliver these. Full integration of mental health care services in primary care may be the best option available in many countries, which means that training of primary care physicians must start at undergraduate level. Curricula in medical schools must change and adapt to increasing recognition of psychiatric disorders. Continuing medical education programmes can offer an ongoing awareness of mental illness and evidence-based interventions available to all clinicians. New therapies and medications need to reach those who need them. In this volume we have focused on countries where some data are available, so that direct and indirect comparisons can be made and appropriate lessons learnt.

Accessibility of mental health services for all still remains a goal to be achieved in Asia. The traditional health systems are probably the first point of contact for many patients with mental illnesses. The ratio of mental health professionals to patients remains depressingly low and the availability of training is also limited. Shortage and disparity of services between urban and rural areas and even within the same city is something that needs further exploration and discussion. Health care systems must be more sensitive to the total needs of the population they serve. It is vital that we focus on cultural relativism and explore and understand the unique factors associated with each country, so that these are not lost in the advance of globalization.

Section 1

Russia and
Central Asia

Overview

Valery Krasnov

In the former USSR, the clinical approaches, research methodology in psychiatry and organization of mental health care were the same in the Russian Federation and the republics of Central Asia (Kazakhstan, Uzbekistan, Kyrgyzstan, Tajikistan and Turkmenistan). The scientific conceptualization of mental diseases and diagnostic criteria were based on the traditions of European and Russian psychiatry of the nineteenth to twentieth centuries.

In the middle of the twentieth century, clinical judgments and therapeutic approaches were in no way different from those in Europe and the USA.

Psychotropic medications had been used since 1957, i.e. at the same time as in Western European countries, and by the end of the 1960s psychopharmacology had become the main treatment for mental disorders. Lobotomy and other forms of psychosurgery were prohibited at the beginning of the 1950s. Psychotherapy was mostly represented by suggestive methods, including hypnosis; autogenic training and progressive muscular relaxation were also widely used, as well as the so-called rational psychotherapy.

The system of psychiatric care in Russia and the republics of Central Asia of the former USSR underwent substantial change during the twentieth century. Until the late 1920s, the whole of psychiatric care had been centered around psychiatric clinics, and in the 1920s and 1930s, the ideology of the so-called psychohygienic concept of psychiatric care was developed. The focus of psychiatric care shifted to outpatient units, e.g. psycho-neurological dispensaries, or special outpatient units quickly created throughout the country. The territorially focused network of such units was successful in covering most of the country. Psychiatric consulting offices were created at factories and universities, matched, in rural regions, with district outpatient units and psychiatric offices at district general hospitals.

However, psychiatric care units were generally undervalued, and to some extent, this sort of practice was similar to the concept of 'community psychiatry' developed in most countries in the late twentieth century, with some elements of sectoral psychiatric services.

However, by the mid twentieth century, the situation had started to change in some aspects, when huge hospitals (up to 2,000 beds) started to be constructed in large cities, and in general these dominated the structure of psychiatric care, although the network of district outpatient units still survived. The concentration of psychiatric care in large cities made providing aid to inhabitants of remote settlements in Siberia, the northern territories and the mountain regions

3

of Central Asia more difficult. By the early 1990s, the number of beds per 1,000 population had approached 1.5. In addition, in the early 1980s, due to widespread alcoholism (especially in the Russian Federation), the special narcological (addictological) service was detached from the general psychiatric service, with its own network of local offices, outpatient units and several special narcological clinics. Most of the psychiatric beds were located in large cities, while many difficulties remained in rural regions in providing both consulting and care services, especially urgent care, due to the large distances between regional centers and remote settlements.

Forensic psychiatric clinics and wards used to exist independently of general psychiatry. One of the definite advantages of the Soviet psychiatric care structure was its chargeless character for the whole population (as for all other types of health care). There used to be no private or commercial clinics. However, in the 1970–1980s, the drawbacks of the existing system started to come to light; first of all was the hypercentralization of the service, with all professional and technical capacities concentrated in large hospitals. Another drawback was the closed character of psychiatric facilities and their separation from general medical ones with lack of regular professional contacts. Unlike most of countries, at this period, in the USSR, there was no public control over the conditions and the quality of psychiatric care provision. With the relatively high level of psychopathological and general clinical education of the practitioners in the country, the dominant paternalism of the psychiatrists' and medical institutions' practices prevented even the slightest autonomy for patients.

It should be also mentioned that there was no special law concerning the provision of psychiatric care in the USSR at all. The regulation thereof had been prescribed by instructions from the Health Ministry. This had formed the grounds for the intervention of political pretexts into the professional psychiatric sphere and particularly was the basis for cases of abuse of psychiatric care for political reasons. Of worldwide notoriety was the practice of prejudiced psychiatric assessment and forced hospitalization to forensic psychiatric wards of so-called 'dissidents', critics of the Soviet system. These episodes were the subject of acute and mainly well-grounded criticism by human rights organizations and the World Psychiatric Association. Without recognizing and accepting this concern of several international committees, the Soviet administration, however, agreed to stop interfering in the regular professional activities of psychiatric services, allowing the professional psychiatric community to exercise reforms and democratization therein. This process was mainly executed in the already autonomous post-USSR states and was characterized by more or less common principles and solutions, matched by some locally motivated special features and directions.

In 1991 the Soviet Union fell apart and several other countries were formed (the former Union republics). Russia was the first country where a law on psychiatric care was passed. In 1992 this law was confirmed by the Parliament and it took effect in January 1993. The Russian law on psychiatric care, and guarantees of citizens' rights in its provisions, was accepted and commended by international experts. The law considerably widened patients' rights and restricted the possibility of unlawful actions in the course of psychiatric treatment.

In the 1990s Russia and most of the new countries (former Soviet republics) suffered severe crises, not only economic but also social and psychological, because of the loss of social identity and stratification of society without cohesion and psychological support in any communities. The consequences were an increase in suicide rates, migration, family problems and addiction among adolescents (which was rare in Soviet times). Until now Russia and the countries of Central Asia have been more or less in a transitional period of development.

The situation was especially painful for persons with severe mental disorders. They suffered not only from mental illness, but also from misunderstanding of their problems by society. Apart from the negative consequences mentioned above, a common burden in each country that still remains is stigmatization of the mental health sphere as a whole.

Another consequence was a shortage of qualified specialists. As is written in Chapter 2 on Kyrgyzstan:

> The emigration of high-level professionals is relevant for all ethnic groups in the country. There was an imbalance between emigration and immigration from 1990 to 2010. The majority of psychiatrists who left the country permanently were ethnic Jews, Russians, Germans and Ukrainians. Moreover, many Kyrgyz psychiatrists had already left the country to work in other countries of the region, mostly Russia, as primary care physicians. After the political instability in Kyrgyzstan in 2010, the migration flow to Russia increased.

At the same time the psychiatrists in all these countries did try to develop psychiatric care despite difficult conditions, limited budgets and other problems. New forms of mental health care are developing taking into account local conditions. Many projects have been implemented with the support of international agencies, especially in Kyrgyzstan and Uzbekistan, rather less so in Kazakhstan and Russia. Not only technical support should be mentioned, but also the provision of ethical and legislative norms in psychiatry.

Central Asia is a major part of the Asian continent. It includes five republics of the former Soviet Union: Kazakhstan, Kyrgyzstan, Tajikistan, Turkmenistan and Uzbekistan. In this section we consider the situation only in the three Asian countries and the Asian part of Russia. It has not been possible to obtain information about mental health services in Tajikistan and Turkmenistan.

1

State of mental health care in the Republic of Kazakhstan

Saya Nurmagambetova and Marat Assimov

Geographical location of the Republic of Kazakhstan

The Republic of Kazakhstan is the ninth largest country in the world, at 2,774,000 square kilometres. It is located across the junction of two continents – Europe and Asia. To the east, north and northwest Kazakhstan has borders with Russia; in the south with the Central Asian states – Uzbekistan, Kyrgyzstan and Turkmenistan; in the southeast with China. The total length of the borders is over 12,200 km, including 600 km along the Caspian Sea (in the west). Over a quarter of the territory of Kazakhstan is covered by steppes, half by deserts and semi-deserts, and the remaining quarter by mountains, lakes and rivers, and coastal areas. The water resources of Kazakhstan depend to a large extent on the rivers and lakes. The rivers are largely fed by glaciers. Kazakhstan's climate is strongly continental. Average temperatures in January range from −19°C to −4°C, in July from +19°C to +26°C. The lowest recorded temperature is −45°C, the highest +30°C.[1]

The Republic of Kazakhstan consists of 14 provinces and two cities of republican status – Astana (the capital since 1997) and Almaty (the former capital). The country's population at the beginning of 2013 was 16,967,500, of whom 9,314,100 (54.9 per cent) could be classified as urban and 7,653,400 (45.1 per cent) as rural. The population consists of 131 ethnic groups, including Kazakhs (63 per cent), Russians, Ukrainians, Germans, Uzbeks, Tatars and Uyghurs.[2] According to World Bank data, in 2012 the GNP per capita in Kazakhstan was US$12,007 and about 4.5 per cent of GDP was allocated to health care.[3]

Available data on psychiatric epidemiology

The number of registered patients with newly diagnosed mental and behavioural disorders decreased from 18,936 in 2011 to 17,079 in 2012; the incidence of such disorders per 100,000 population in those two years was, respectively, 114.4 and 101.7.

Mental and behavioural disorders in children have also slightly decreased, from 170.1 per 100,000 children in 2011 to 148.7 in 2012. Higher incidence rates are recorded in the Pavlodar (425.3) and Karaganda (339.1) regions. Mental and behavioural disorders in the adolescent population also decreased in incidence, from 166.9 per 100,000 in 2012 to 131.5 in 2011; the regions with a high incidence were Kostanai (497.0), North Kazakhstan (363.6) and Almaty (362.0).

The apparent decreases in both the incidence and the prevalence of mental and behavioural disorders may in fact result from a combination of an increase in the population of Kazakhstan and a shortage of specialists in mental health services.

At the beginning of 2013 the total number of patients with mental and behavioural disorders (excluding the use of psychoactive substances) had slightly decreased from 287,832 in 2011 to 277,133, and prevalence of mental disorders was 1,633.3 per 100,000 population (vs 1,726.1 in 2011). Notably, only 78,724 people had consulted the psychiatric services. Higher than average prevalence rates were seen in the Karaganda (1,801.2) and Kyzyl-Orda (1,801.3) regions.

In accordance with the Mental Health Ordinance Order Number 663 of the Ministry of Health of the Republic of Kazakhstan, dated September 28, 2012, since 2012 dispensary (outpatient clinic) patients with mental and behavioural disorders have been divided into two groups:

1. patients under medical supervision (dispensary);
2. patients under consultant observation (after 12 months of observation these patients can be 'removed' from this observation or transferred to dispensary supervision).

The number of children under observation decreased from 40,724 in 2011 to 37,836 in 2012 (among them, 22,853 were under dispensary supervision, and 14,983 were under consultant observation). In 2011, the prevalence of mental and behavioural disorders in children was 980 per 100,000. This indicator was high in the Karaganda (1,796.5) and East Kazakhstan (951.9) regions.

The total number of mental and behavioural disorders in adolescents in 2011 was 14,892 per 100,000. In 2012 this figure was 9,204, but counting only patients under dispensary observation.

The number of patients removed from dispensary observation due to recovery or health improvement was 1.8 per 100 patients in 2012 (3.3 in 2011).

The number of new cases with psychiatry disability was 1.3 per 100 patients in 2012 (1.0 in 2011). This figure was higher than average in the Aktobe (2.1) region and Astana (2.1).

The number of patients with disabilities under medical supervision increased from 28.9 per 100 patients in 2011 to 41.6 in 2012.

Mental health services, mental health care models, and funding

On 1 January 2013 there were 33 psychiatric clinical settings in the Republic of Kazakhstan.[4] There were 14 hospitals with 5,040 beds (5,055 beds in 2011), and also 19 dispensaries with 4,315 beds (4,385 beds in 2011). The hospitals include two national (as opposed to regional) institutions: the Republican Scientific and Practical Centre for Psychiatry, Psychotherapy and Narcology; and the Republican Psychiatric Hospital. Both offer intensive specialist supervision. The psychiatric service also includes psychiatric units within general health care services. In 2012 the number of psychiatric units was, though, only seven, with 227 beds.

In the Akmola region (only) there are beds for patients suffering from tuberculosis comorbid with mental disorders (in psychiatric institutions). In 2011 the total increased by five, to 130 beds. There are, nationally, 25 beds in forensic (guarded) psychiatric units, but these are all in one institution, the Republican Scientific and Practical Centre for Psychiatry, Psychotherapy and Narcology. The number of settings with paediatric departments is 17.

In summary, there are 9,355 beds for patients with mental and behavioural disorders: including 8,430 beds for adults, 645 for children, 150 for people with substance misuse disorders, and 130 for tuberculosis patients with mental disorders.

Considerable changes have been made in the sphere of psychiatric care since Kazakhstan gained independence in 1991, and some new problems have emerged. The total number of psychiatric beds has been reduced, especially beds in psychiatric hospitals, from 9,605 in 1991 to 5,040 in 2012, although the number of beds in dispensaries has not dropped so much, in proportion. Additionally, the number of hospital settings for rehabilitation and long-term psychosocial work has been reduced: for example, the number of workshops decreased from 23 in 1991 to two in 2011. Similarly, the number of settings for day-care patients has decreased (the number of places fell from 1,440 in 1991 to 835 in 2011). Furthermore, the number of psychiatrists decreased from 995 (0.7 per 10,000) in 1991 to 699 (0.4) in 2011. The number of psychotherapists, though, remained more or less constant (0.04 per 10,000 in 1999 and 0.05 per 10,000 in 2011).

At the same time, the number of persons registered disabled due to psychiatric disease has dramatically increased, from 16.3 in 1991 to 28.9 in 2011 (per 100 patients registered disabled). The length of hospitalisation decreased from 69.4 days in 1991 to 56.0 days in 2011, but the frequency of rehospitalisation increased (32.3 per cent in 1991 to 58.2 per cent in 2011). This suggests inefficiency within the mental health care services. Such inefficiency is associated with a dramatic worsening of the quality of life of patients with severe mental disorders, and represents a huge burden for the community. Moreover, the decrease in the number of hospital beds has not been accompanied by the development of alternative forms of care, such as social and psychological support for patients. There is thus a clear need to reconsider the government's approach to mental health care.[5]

In this light, advances have been made in recent years. Some organisational restructuring has been undertaken. For instance, as of 2012 there were 183 psychiatric offices in Kazakhstan and 35 psychotherapeutic offices, and these have provided the basis for the development of the country's system of community care. Furthermore, new forms of psychiatric care are developing, such as specialised psychiatric ambulance teams. In January 2013 there were 65 specialised mental health ambulance teams providing emergency care to patients with mental disorders in Kazakhstan; the number of patients attended in 2012 was 61,919 (56,260 in 2011). Another step has been the development of day-care and occupational therapy and rehabilitation. In 2012 there were 62 places in two occupational therapy workshops (60 places in 2011). In 2012 there were 18 day-care centres operated by 886 people (835 in 2011) and 6,540 patients were treated (5,884 in 2011).[5]

Training of professionals in mental health care

There are three universities offering undergraduate and postgraduate medical education. In addition three academic centres provide postgraduate training in the sphere of mental health.

In 2012 the number of psychiatrists increased compared with 2011, from 699 to 732, but, due to population growth, this was still the equivalent of 0.4 psychiatrists per 10,000 population, as previously. Today, 72 psychotherapists are working in Kazakhstan, or 0.04 per 10,000 population. In 2012 there were 30 medical psychologists, representing 0.02 per 10,000 population. Psychiatrists and psychotherapists have higher (university) medical education. Mental health nurses have secondary medical education, with special training in psychiatry. Medical psychologists have higher university education.

Vacant positions in psychiatry numbered 873.5 (818.25 in 2011), psychotherapists 111 (133.25 in 2011); child psychiatrists 123.0 (120.5 in 2011); and psychiatric forensic experts 58.75 (59.5 in 2011).

Mental health promotion and education for the general public

Health promotion and education are undertaken nationally, rather than at the regional level. One programme has involved training paramedics in the rescue services in mental health in order to improve their handling of disturbed people in emergency situations and thereby minimise the risk of injury.

Programmes to reduce stigma and discrimination against people at risk of developing mental disorder and those suffering from mental disorders have included the following activities:

- through the Centre for a Healthy Lifestyle, the media and other bodies, action to combat stigma and discrimination, emphasising the prevalence of mental health problems, and their generally favourable course and prognosis;
- allocation of social grants at national and local levels to implement (and analyse the results of) legislation regarding the rights of people with disabilities, so that it covers mental health, while ensuring respect for the principles of equality and justice;
- a programme of activities to combat stigma and discrimination in the employment of persons with mental health problems;
- allocation of social grants for the participation of nongovernmental organisations, individuals and groups in the provision of alternative care;
- television programmes and newspaper articles on discrimination and stigma;
- an action plan for the social inclusion (within education and training) of children and young people with mental health problems and disabilities;
- professional training;
- the adaptation of workplaces in order to ensure employment opportunities on a competitive basis for people with mental disorders.[6]

References

1. http://en.wikipedia.org/wiki/kazakhstan.
2. http://oldkazakh-tv.softdeco.net/rus/geography.
3 http://www.schizophrenianet.eu/guest/AbstractView?ABSID=7971.
4. Press-services of the Agency of Republic of Kazakhstan on statistics. May 2013.
5. Draft of the Programme 'Development and reformation of the service of mental health. Interagency cooperation'. Almaty: Republican Scientific and Practical Centre for Psychiatry, 2013
6 Katsaga A., Kuldzanov M., Karanikolos M. and Reichel B. Kazakhstan. *Health Systems in Transition*. 14(4). Geneva: WHO, 2012

2

Psychiatry in the Kyrgyz Republic

In between the Soviet past and a vague future

Elena Molchanova, Elena Kim and Tatiana Galako

Geography

Kyrgyzstan, or, officially, the Kyrgyz Republic, is one of the smallest countries in post-Soviet Central Asia, with a population of approximately five million people and a territory of 200,000 square kilometres. It is bordered by Kazakhstan to the north, Uzbekistan to the west, Tajikistan to the southwest and China to the east. Its capital and largest city is Bishkek.

Kyrgyzstan is also one of the poorest countries in the region, with 35 per cent of the population living below the poverty level, while as many as one million Kyrgyz nationals live and work abroad (Manjoo, 2010). World Bank data for 2011 show that the GNP per capita was US$1,160. The ethnic composition of the country is very complex; the major groups are ethnic Kyrgyz (67 per cent), Uzbeks (14 per cent) and Russians (10 per cent), but there are more than 80 other ethnic minorities. There is competition for fertile agricultural areas with access to water, especially in the overpopulated Fergana Valley, which is consequently predisposed to social unrest.

During a period of political instability and under a fragile interim government, ethnic violence broke out in June 2010; 400 people were killed, 375,000 were displaced, and more than a million suffered loss of property, physical injuries, or sexual or psychological violence.

Today, the geostrategic location of Kyrgyzstan – contradictorily described as 'a crossroads', 'strategic' and 'isolated' – coupled with its Soviet past, makes Kyrgyzstan of special importance in international relations. The region is believed to exemplify the contemporary geopolitics of the global superpowers, through the lens of the historic great empires (Schetter and Kuzmits, 2006; Kleveman, 2003; Rashid, 2001). It has been regarded as part of the global 'East' and 'Orient', subject to conflict and instability, Islamic and renegade groups, traditional families and silenced women (Simpson, 2009). Recent discussions about the region draw from broad frames like 'the East' and 'the West', or from ideas about 'development' and 'transition' (Simpson, 2009).

After the September 11, 2001 attacks of the Islamist militant group Al-Qaeda on New York City and Washington, DC, in the United States, the concomitant geopolitical manoeuvring and the subsequent US-led campaign in Afghanistan took the region into the 'frontline' of the global 'war on terror' (Olcott, 2005).

Psychiatric epidemiology

The multidimensional consequences of interethnic tensions, violence, and mass panic included not only political, economic and health costs, but also mental health repercussions: increased rates of reported depression, anxiety, somatoform and posttraumatic stress disorders (Molchanova *et al.*, 2011). High suicide rates among the most vulnerable of citizens, including children and teenagers, were also among the social consequences.

The official statistics underestimate the true rates of psychiatric disorder in the Kyrgyz Republic, and the data reported below reflect the iceberg phenomenon in the incidence of mental disorders. In rural areas the majority of cases of mild mental retardation remain undiagnosed and, due to culturally shaped attitudes towards elderly people, which emphasize respect, a person with dementia rarely sees a mental health care specialist. People with neurotic, somatoform and stress-related disorders prefer to address their complaints to traditional healers. Moreover, a first psychotic episode in the framework of the traditional cultural context might indicate to the client and his or her relatives the existence of supernatural abilities and is considered to be a sign of the person's future spiritual mission (*Kyrgyzchylyk*). Therefore, even when *Kyrgyzchylyk* in fact indicates the onset of what would be considered schizophrenia in a psychiatric context, it is very unlikely that the person and his or her relatives will seek professional help.

According to official data from the Statistical Committee of the Republic Centre of Mental Health (RCMH), the annual incidence of mental disorders among Kyrgyz citizens is 49.2 per 100,000 population. The prevalence of mental disorders was 916 per 100,000 population in 2012. The 'nosographic' distribution of disorders is presented in Table 2.1. Only registered cases are counted in the official statistics. Those urban citizens who are willing to receive professional help but prefer not to use official mental health institutes represent the majority of clients for specialists in Bishkek working in a non-official capacity, and they are not obliged to report new cases to the Statistical Committee of the RCMH. Therefore, the majority of reported new cases of mental disorders are patients with conditions associated with special needs, such as illness or incapacity; these patients are primarily in Bishkek and areas close to the city.

Bed numbers have decreased in recent years (Table 2.2), partly due to the development of outpatient services.

The suicide rate is 9.3 per 100,000; among teenagers it is 4.6 per 100,000. Twelve per cent of all successful suicides are committed by people with officially registered mental disorders.

Table 2.1 The prevalence of mental and behavioural disorders in the Kyrgyz Republic in 2012

Mental disorders	%
Organic, including symptomatic, mental disorders	2.6
Schizophrenia, schizotypal and delusional disorders	18.1
Mood (affective) disorders	2.7
Neurotic, stress-related and somatoform disorders, cases of mild depression	7.3
Mental retardation	45

Table 2.2 Psychiatric bed number dynamics in the Kyrgyz Republic since 2008

Year	Total number of psychiatric beds in the Kyrgyz Republic	Bed numbers per 100,000 population
2008	2,283	43.70
2009	1,943	36.82
2010	1,761	32.72
2011	1,762	32.16
2012	1,762	31.74
2013	1,665	29.40

Mental health systems and services, patterns of referral, funding and the indigenous service delivery model

The huge gap between the high number of people who need treatment and the lower number of those who actually receive professional help is partly explained by the common barriers to psychiatric treatment: the social stigmatization of mental disorder, the limited number of specialists who are primarily located only in urban areas, costs for transportation to treatment for rural individuals, underfunding and underestimation of mental health problems by local governments. The majority of psychiatric services in the Kyrgyz Republic remain concentrated within the general area of Bishkek, and particularly beneath the umbrella of the Republic Centre of Mental Health (RCMH), which provides inpatient mental health care and some outpatient care as well. In 2000, the government launched its national programme 'Mental Health of the Population of the Kyrgyz Republic in 2001–2010'. The programme anticipated a shift from institutionally based mental health care to more localized community-based services. Due to the lack of funding, however, implementation of the programme was suspended. The proposed next national programme, which will hopefully be supported by the World Bank, is in the process of development.

The current mental health care system is overly centralized (Figure 2.1) and still resembles the mental health care system in the Soviet Union. A variety of efforts have been made to improve the structure of the service but there is chronic underfunding. These efforts have included increasing the number of outpatient departments, involving psychiatrists in centres of family medicine, educating primary care physicians, advancement of the professional association of psychiatrists (Kyrgyz Psychiatric Association), and introducing a new profession – social pedagogues – who work in connection with mental health care specialists. Figure 2.1 shows the structure of the mental health care system in the Kyrgyz Republic.

Kyrgyzstan's much-needed deinstitutionalization programmes have been enthusiastically supported by numerous international donors, including the Open Society Foundation, but have produced two opposing mental health development strategies – radical and constructive approaches. The 'radical' one proposes the abolition of all mental health institutions. The followers of this model consider official psychiatry an 'evil' and psychiatric hospitals 'illegal prisons' for patients with mental disorders. Their arguments, in spite of their weakness, seem to attract aggressive representatives of human rights organizations, who understand the term 'de-stigmatization' as a synonym for 'de-psychiatrization'.

The second strategy, which seems to be much more constructive, is oriented towards the development of multidisciplinary mobile teams and strengthening community support for rural

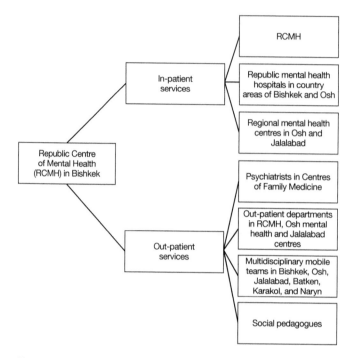

Figure 2.1 Structure of the mental health care system in the Kyrgyz Republic

regions of Kyrgyzstan under the supervision of mental health professionals. For example, the newly developed specialty of social pedagogy is intended to provide a counselling role in schools. On February 2, 2010, the Minister of Science and Education of the Kyrgyz Republic (MSEKR) signed a decree placing social pedagogues on the staff of schools countrywide. The social pedagogue is expected to contribute to the development of a healthy, safe and caring environment by advancing understanding of the emotional and social development of children and of the influences of family, community and cultural differences on student success. In response to the complex interethnic situation, and following the order of the MSEKR, 2,000 teachers from the southern region of the Kyrgyz Republic received social pedagogical training from July to November 2011. Three continuing education centres and four methodological centres have been established, and they organize and provide courses in continuing education for teachers who wish to be trained as social pedagogues. Included in the training are basic counselling skills and basic mental health screening. Every social pedagogue is connected to a specialist in the mental health sphere and can refer students to him/her when necessary.

The limited funding that the government allocates for mental health care primarily goes to the RCMH rather than community-based mental health care. Central facilities such as the RCMH, the Osh Centre of Mental Health, the Jalalabad Mental Health Centre and outpatient departments are funded, owned and operated by the national government of the Kyrgyz Republic. A variety of private psychological centres and crisis centres are mainly supported by international donors. Primary care physicians receive some basic education about affective and anxiety disorders through educational programmes run by the World Health Organization (WHO).

In theory, the pattern of referral should include several consecutive steps: (1) social worker or social pedagogue, then (2) general practitioner, then (3) psychiatrist in an outpatient ambulance and only then, if necessary, (4) a Mental Health Centre in Osh, Jalalabad or Bishkek.

In practice, this sequence is shortened, and sometimes includes only the last step, the Mental Health Centre. The rehabilitation outpatient services are in the process of development and are supported by a number of international donors.

Social/explanatory model(s) of mental illness

Explanatory models, like languages, reflect cognitive structures in the human mind: what people consider to be mental illness is closely related to what they are capable of understanding (Sapir, 1929). According to the Sapir–Whorf hypothesis, language structures are a way of thinking and perceiving the world, so explanatory models are dependent on the available lexicon (Sapir, 1929). The Kyrgyz language reflects the history and the complexity of the Kyrgyz people. For instance, Kyrgyz people have more than 130 words to describe the ages of horses (e.g. *kuluuk, tai, baitai, bishti, aigir, bae, argamak*), cattle and sheep, many terms for weather (e.g. *salkyn, jiluu, issyk, saratan, childe, muzdak*), and a rich lexicon for defining family relationships and the qualities of family members. Perhaps due to a long history of manual labour and nomadism, Kyrgyz people find it difficult to express emotional states in their own language.

Several cognitive models inform different views on mental illness in Kyrgyzstan. Two of them – distress and biological explanatory models – are more commonly subscribed to by urban citizens. According to the 'distress model', psychopathological symptoms are the results of traumatic or stressful events in everyday life. People who believe in this particular model often use psychological terminology to describe their conditions (e.g. stressful event, depression, anxiety). The idea of biological causes of mental disorders has only recently become a part of Kyrgyz contemporary usage, mainly due to the influence of the mass media. The biological model of mental illness explains the development of psychopathology in terms of biological changes – brain injury, lack of serotonin or overproduction of dopamine, etc. It is apparent, though, that in many cases this socially accepted model is not truly accepted but is presented in preference to a 'spiritual' model of mental illness that is more genuinely believed. This 'spiritual model' tends to be more explicitly used by the rural population. It includes belief in the interconnectedness of human beings with nature and the spirits of their ancestors (*Arbaktar*). This model includes a strong belief in the close connection between the health of the Kyrgyz people and their spiritual practices. According to these beliefs, psychopathology is the 'result of a misunderstanding of the spirits' demands' (Molchanova *et al.*, 2009). For example, hypochondriac disorder is often interpreted as the spirit's desire to help a person in the process of self-actualization and the spirit's task is to bring the person round to the right way. An initial psychotic episode might be considered a 'spiritual emergence' and a patient generally has to visit a number of traditional healers before a psychiatrist takes care of him or her.

Mental health workforce training

The Department of Psychiatry at Kyrgyz State Medical Academy (KSMA), established in 1942, remains the leading educational organization in mental health. Heads of the department have been Mark Goldberg, Nikolay Kantorovich, Alexandra Durandina and Valery Solozhenkin. Now the department is led by Tatiana Galako. The usual training of mental health practitioners comprises six years of education at the KSMA as a general physician and two years of residency at the RCMH or Osh Centre of Mental Health. The curriculum covers psychiatry, basic medical psychology and principles of 'doctor–patient' communication. The Department of Medical Psychology, Psychiatry and Psychotherapy of the Slavonic University in the Kyrgyz Republic was established in 1990. The curriculum there covers an introduction to 'personology', medical psychology, the basic principles of health psychology, psychopathology, psychiatry and an introduction to psychotherapy.

Training in mental health care is also provided in the education programmes for primary care physicians supported by the WHO. Around 660 primary care specialists have now received basic information on the signs and treatment of anxiety and somatoform disorders, stress-related disorders and affective disorders. Multidisciplinary mobile teams have existed in the Kyrgyz Republic since 2006; the project named 'Multidisciplinary mobile team in community treatment' was successfully developed by the NGO *Family and Society* and supported by the Soros Foundation. Since 2012 multidisciplinary mobile teams have been a useful part of the community outreach service in several cities.

Major challenges and innovations

The number of challenges for mental health professionals in the Kyrgyz Republic, in addition to those mentioned already, seems to be enormous. The most pressing ones are: the influx of international experts; the use of old treatment schemas in local mental health facilities; and the emigration of highly qualified specialists.

The influx of international experts has proved a problem because of their effect on mental health practice in Kyrgyzstan. Since the collapse of the Soviet Union in 1991, the country has become host to a multitude of international mental health activities and education programmes. But recent research (Kim, 2013) into the practices of the country's crisis centres, for instance, highlights the potential problems with such interventions. Because these crisis centres for the victims of gender/family/partner or domestic violence lack state support, they are dependent upon international agencies for funding. This, though, comes at the cost of the freedom with which specialists work with their clients. Ethnographic observations and in-depth interviews conducted with both the specialists and their clients have shown the discursive coordination of these therapeutic interactions by the global development paradigms (Kim, 2013). To illustrate, Kim found that the victims of domestic violence received legal help rather than psychological assistance. That is, psychiatrists were inclined to help the patients by referring them to law enforcement representatives and by informing them about their rights. But, considering the poorly functioning system of police protection from domestic violence, despite the existence of relevant legislation, this approach is counterproductive. The drastic inconsistency between what the professionally trained specialists know about how to do their work and what is required of them politically leads to professional frustration and a decrease in their motivation.

A difficult economic situation seems to be a common challenge for post-Soviet countries, which, in addition to the absence of mental health insurance coverage, results in prescribing medication selected on the basis of low cost rather than clinical indication. The persistent unwillingness of the Ministry of Health to include psychiatry within the single-payer system supports the old-fashioned treatment schemas, including haloperidol and other typical antipsychotics, which are available in mental health hospitals and can be used for free. At the same time, clinical protocols in psychiatry, which have been developed in recent years by specialists at the Departments of Psychiatry at both KSMA and the Slavic University, recommend innovative models of treatment.

The emigration of high-level professionals is relevant for all ethnic groups in the country. There was an imbalance between emigration and immigration from 1990 to 2010. The majority of psychiatrists who left the country permanently were ethnic Jews, Russians, Germans and Ukrainians. Moreover, many Kyrgyz psychiatrists had already left the country to work in other countries of the region, mostly Russia, as primary care physicians. After the political instability in Kyrgyzstan in 2010, the migration flow to Russia increased. Nevertheless, as a positive change, it is worth mentioning the strengthening of community support for people with mental disorders.

The Kyrgyz professional community has only recently started making efforts to establish an ethical framework for teaching, practice and research. Drawing on existing and developing ethical codes in Canada, the United Kingdom, the United States, Russia and Turkey, a group of Kyrgyz psychologists from the American University in Central Asia together with the Ethics Committee of Kyrgyz Psychiatric Association developed a draft version of the Kyrgyz Code of Ethics. The Kyrgyz Code of Ethics is based on five general principles: Respect for Human Rights, Privacy, Professionalism and Competency, Responsibility, and Integrity. The draft Code of Ethics has been recently accepted by the Kyrgyz Psychiatric Association.

Culturally sensitive community mental health care services, such as mobile teams, seem to be a way out of the cul-de-sac created by economic difficulties, social instability and the influx of culturally insensitive experts. The 'ideal' mobile team consists of four local specialists (psychiatrist, psychologist, social worker and nurse). They are familiar with their own regions and are able to reach a patient and provide help when immediate hospitalization is not required; they serve as a culturally sensitive bridge between the family and service providers in mental health centres. Mobile teams gained their good reputation during a period of interethnic conflict in Osh in 1990 and have become a service trusted both by patients and their relatives.

References

Kim, E. (2013). International Development and Research in Central Asia, Exploring the Knowledge-based Social Organization of Gender (Doctoral dissertation, University of Bonn). University of Bonn database.

Kleveman, L. (2003). *The New Great Game: Blood and Oil in Central Asia*. New York: Grove Press.

Manjoo, R. (2010). *Report of the Special Rapporteur on Violence against Women, Its Causes and Consequences*. United Nations Human Rights Council. A/HRC/14/22/Add.2.

Molchanova, E., Kim, E., Horne, S.G., Aitpaeva, G., Ashiraliev, N. and Pokhilko, D. (2009). Status of counseling and psychology in Kyrgyzstan. In L. Gerstein, P.P. Heppner, S.A. Leung and K. Norsworthy (Eds), *Handbook of Counseling and Psychology Around the Globe*. Thousand Oaks, CA: Sage Publications, pp. 265–77.

Molchanova, E., Panteleeva, L., Popkov, M. and Nelubova, T. (2011). Dinamika urovnya mezhetnicheskoi napryajennosti, obrazov 'sebja' i 'drugogo' u naselenja goroda Osh Kyrgyzskoi Respubliki v period s oktyabrja 2010 po fevral 2011 goda [Comparison of levels of interethnic tension and semantic images of the 'self' and the 'other' in periods of October 2010 and February 2011 among Osh citizens]. *Electronic Journal of Medical Psychology in Russia*, N 5: www.medpsy.ru/mprj/archiv_global/2011_5_10/nomer/nomer08.php

OECD (2012). *Kyrgyz Republic. Evolving Transition to a Market Economy. Country Assistance Programme Evaluation*. Retrieved from www.oecd.org/countries/kyrgyzstan/adb.pdf

Olcott, M.B. (2005). *Central Asia's Second Chance*. Washington DC: Carnegie Endowment for International Peace.

Rashid, A. (2001). *Taliban: Militant Islam, Oil and Fundamentalism in Central Asia*. London: IB Tauris & Co Ltd.

Sapir, E. (1929) The status of linguistics as a science. In E. Sapir *Culture, Language and Personality* (ed. D.G. Mandelbaum). Berkeley, CA: University of California Press, 1958.

Schetter, C. and Kuzmits, B. (2006). The revival of geopolitics: US policy in Afghanistan and Central Asia. In J. Rüland, T. Hanf and E. Manske (eds), *US Foreign Policy Toward the Third World: A Post-Cold War Assessment*. New York: Harpe Armonk, pp. 161–90.

Simpson, M. (2009). Local strategies in globalizing gender politics: a study of women's organizing and aid in contemporary Kyrgyzstan (Doctoral dissertation, Central European University, Budapest, 2009). Central European University database.

3

Russian Federation

Valery Krasnov and Nikolay Bokhan

Geographic and general information

The Russian Federation (Russia) is a country with a huge territory, of 17,075,000 km², spanning the eastern part of Europe and the northern part of Asia to the Pacific Ocean. Its population as of 2013 was 143.4 million, and country's GDP in 2012 reached US$3,380 billion, i.e. US$23,570 per capita.

Russia has more than 150 ethnic groups, which vary greatly in size, from the 115 million ethnic Russians to minorities numbering only several hundred persons. Between these two extremes come Tatars (5.6 million), Ukrainians (2.9 million), Bashkirs (1.7 million), Chuvashs (1.6 million), Chechens (1.4 million) and Armenians (1.1 million). The indigenous peoples of Siberia, the far east and the far north of the Asian part of Russia constitute about 0.3 per cent of the total population (500,000 persons). Most Russians, Ukrainians and Armenians can formally be described as Christian; Tatars, Bashkirs and most of the people from north Caucasus are Muslims. There are also Buddhist minorities (Kalmyks in the European part of Russia, and Buryats and Tuvinians in Siberia) and a small number of people belonging to the Judaic religion. In addition there are very small groups of pagans in remote parts of Siberia, practising shamanism. Inside Russia, however, people rarely make reference to ethnicity. People abroad use the name 'Russian' for any person speaking Russian, which is the state language in Russia, and the means of communication among the people irrespective of ethnic origin.

The north of Russia includes Siberia, Chukotka and Kamchatka (the last also being the most easterly region of the country). These areas have distinctive small indigenous populations. The far east of Russia includes the Republic of Yakutia, which is the largest administrative unit in the world, in terms of territorial size. Kamchatka is rightly regarded as a place uniquely suited to the ethnocultural investigation of the influence of the environment on the mental health of the native population. At these very high latitudes, even in modern times, with the availability of a wide range of supportive technology, socioeconomic development remains uneasy and even dangerous (Bokhan, 2009)

Siberia and the far east of Russia are home to 65 smaller indigenous groups, including Buryats (about 400,000 persons), Tuvinians and Tofalars (250,000 persons), Khakas (75,000 persons), Altaits and Shorts (92,000 persons). Buryats speak a language in the Mongolian family – whereas the other groups speak languages in the Turk, Tungustic and Samodian groups. Buryats, Tuvinians (Dashieva and Kupriyanova, 2009; Rakhmazova *et al.*, 2012), Khakas (Taliyanova and Korobitsina, 2011) and southern Altaits are representatives of a central-

Asian type of 'Mongoloid' ethnicity. Shorts, northern Altaits and some groups of Khakas belong to a south-Siberian type formed as a mixture of central-Asian Mongoloids and the ancient Caucasian population of Siberia.

Despite differences in culture and anthropomorphological traits, these groups are all experiencing a similar process of acculturation that affects the physiological as well as the social sphere. They have lived together for many years in the same territory and there is no overt discrimination or prejudice among them; indeed, there are many mixed families. However, there is in these regions a trend towards depopulation, which is sometimes viewed as being inevitable (Gumilev, 1993), but medicine and psychology assume measurement of certain parameters that may testify to these objective processes. They have high rates of alcohol and drug abuse.

Mental health policy

According to WHO, total health expenditure in Russia represents 5.2 per cent of GDP (Popovich *et al.*, 2011); this is lower than in other European countries. Care is provided free of charge for people with mental disorders but many people nonetheless make out-of-pocket payments within private and commercial services, partly because of a strong popular prejudice against official psychiatry, as well as a fear of stigmatization.

After the disaggregation of the Soviet Union in 1991, Russia was the first of the former Soviet republics to pass a law on psychiatric care, in 1992 (it came into operation in January 1993). The Russian law guarantees citizens' rights and was commended by international experts. It considerably widened patients' rights and restricted the possibility of unlawful actions in the course of psychiatric treatment. It has been successfully implemented at both federal and regional levels, but the provision of social care is inadequate.

A specific feature and principal defect of inpatient psychiatric care in Russia is its over-centralization. The majority of psychiatric hospitals have more than 500 beds and several large hospitals have more than 1,500 beds. In the past 20 years the total number of beds has decreased by 25 per cent: from 200,192 beds in 1991 to 146,427 in 2012 (see Table 3.1). Now in Russia the number of psychiatric beds per 1,000 population is 1.02 and is still continuing to fall. However, the decrease in the number of psychiatric beds has not always been combined with an increase in extramural forms of psychiatric care.

The task of rebuilding the large hospitals remains, but economic difficulties hinder this. The public health system struggles to provide mentally ill people with suitable employment and adaptation in the setting of a market economy. The number of people registered disabled due to a mental disorder was 1,033,308 in 2011 (Gurovich, 2012); and there are few sheltered jobs for them (only 3.3 per cent). While many appear to live on the streets, most of them are in fact either inpatients of specialized institutions ('internats') for the chronically mentally ill (without active therapy) or live at home under the informal care of their relatives and the formal care of a visiting specialist from a local dispensary. 'Dispensary' is the traditional name for an outpatient clinic.

The unfavourable living conditions in many psychiatric clinics (rooms with many beds, lack of space and equipment) raise serious ethical and legal issues. Moreover, many effective remedies are costly and so remain unavailable to many patients, especially outpatients. Economic difficulties of this transitional period in Russia's social development make it unlikely that these problems will be overcome in the short term. Until recently, psychiatry was not a priority in the state's health care strategy, unlike paediatrics and cardiosurgery.

Table 3.1 Resources available for administration of psychiatric care in Russia[a]

Institutions	1999	2008	2012
Psychiatric dispensaries	164	145	102
Dispensary departments in psychiatric hospitals	122	123	170
Narcological dispensaries (for alcoholics and drug addicts)	171	144	101
Psychotherapeutic units in general outpatient clinics	1,118	1,107	830
Psychiatric hospitals	278	257	224
Narcological hospitals	13	12	11
Total number of beds in psychiatric hospitals (including psychiatric beds in general hospitals)	170,440 (14,015)	155,834 (13,890)	146,427 (13,915)
Number of beds in narcological hospitals	28,700	26,550	24,250

a Current statistical data has been taken from the website of the Ministry of Public Health of the Russian Federation

Table 3.2 Specialists rendering psychiatric care in Russia

Specialists	1999	2008	2012
Psychiatrists (including psychotherapists)	15,860 3,248	16,184 3,438	13,287 1,717
Narcologists (specialists rendering care for people suffering from alcohol and other substance abuse)	4,470	5,012	5,457
Specialists in social work (with higher education)	70	772	911
Social workers	840	1,857	1,606
Clinical psychologists (working in psychiatric and narcological institutions)	1,407	3,050	3,568

The whole system of psychiatric care has shown contradictory tendencies in its development (Table 3.1). On the one hand, taking into account the shortages in state budget allocations, the provision of psychiatric care through local psychiatric dispensaries that are open to the general public and connected to local psychiatric hospitals is a practical expedient. On the other hand, stigma and societal prejudices against psychiatry and psychiatric institutions hinder the development of psychiatric dispensaries. Many psychiatrists, especially psychotherapists, have left the public sector to work in private practice (Table 3.2). Only about 30–35 per cent of all mentally ill patients apply for psychiatric assistance in a dispensary. The prevalence of mental disorders registered in psychiatric institutions reached 2,951.1 per 100,000 population in 2011. In addition, approximately 25–30 per cent of primary-care patients need psychiatric consultations (Krasnov, 2008). The need has arisen to reform outpatient psychiatric care, and the development of alternative forms of care is also required.

Suicide and substance abuse

Suicide statistics vary widely by region within Russia. Siberia has the highest rate. In the Altay Republic the rate is 67.3 per 100,000, in Nenets Autonomous District it is 64.1 and in Buryatia it is 64.0.

The lowest rates of suicide are seen in the north Caucasus. In the Chechen Republic the rate is 0.8 per 100,000 and in Dagestan it is 2.8. This is due to the traditional culture of the predominantly rural Muslim population, as Islam prohibits suicide. The Russian national average rate was 20.1 per 100,000 in 2012. This is one of the highest national rates in the world (Table 3.3). Over the last two decades, though, it has decreased substantially, from 38.7 in 1999. The rate among men is six times higher than among women, probably because of the higher rate of alcohol consumption among men. Across the whole population, alcohol consumption in Russia is the equivalent of approximately 14–15 litres of spirit (primarily vodka) per capita (Nemtsov, 2011).

The prevalence of alcoholism has been more or less stable over last decade, at around 1,792.5 per 100,000 population. The male/female ratio is 5:1. Other addictions appear to have increased in prevalence over recent years, from a total of 252.2 per 100,000 population in 2008 to 382 per 100,000 of population in 2012; among these, opioid dependence is the dominant form of addiction.

Reforms in psychiatric care

Several important changes have been made in the last decade in the development of psychiatric care. First of all, a significant number of psychologists and social workers have been added to the staff of psychiatric institutions, to support a transition from a largely medical to a biopsychosocial model of mental health care and a team approach to its provision (see also Table 3.1).

Table 3.3 Suicide rates per 100,000 by country, year and sex per year (WHO, 2012, data)

Rank	Country	Male	Female	Average	Year
1	Greenland	116.9	45.0	83.0	2011
2	Lithuania	54.7	10.8	31.0	2012
3	South Korea	38.2	18.0	28.0	2013
4	Guyana	39.0	13.4	26.4	2006
5	Kazakhstan	43.0	9.4	25.6	2008
6	China			22.23	2011
7	Belarus			20.5	2012
8.	Slovenia	34.6	9.4	21.8	2011
9	Hungary	37.4	8.5	21.7	2009
10	Japan			21.7	2012
11	Sri Lanka	34.8	9.24	21.7	2012
12	Latvia			20.8	2010
13	Russia			20.1	2012
13	Ukraine			19.8	2012
14	Croatia			19.7	2002
...					
51	Kyrgyzstan	14.1	3.6	8.8	2009
73	Uzbekistan	7.0	1.7	4.3	2005

Second, the structure of the mental health service has changed, with a greater emphasis on the development of care in the community, where a system of psychosocial rehabilitation is organized. In addition, special clinics for people in a first episode of psychosis, hostels and other types of protected housing have been established, and interaction with social services has been facilitated. Assertive treatment teams have been set up and 'hospital at home' – psychoeducation and psychosocial work with families – is now provided. NGOs are not yet sufficiently involved but are now increasingly engaged in mental health provision (Gurovich, 2005, 2012; Krasnov and Gurovich, 2012).

The problem of mental health care for indigenous populations in Siberia and the north requires the development of cross-cultural psychiatry, with an integrated understanding of the role of psychological issues, culture, religion, mythology, traditions and customs. Addiction psychiatry, psychology and psychotherapy are required. In particular, alcohol addiction is a problem. Alcohol use among the indigenous inhabitants of southern Siberia exceeds alcohol use by Caucasians living in the same region, as shown by long-term epidemiological investigations (Nikitin, 2007)

Geographic and ethnic patterns of mental health

The extreme climate, and long dark winters, combined with the low density of population and isolation and remoteness of villages, nevertheless accompanied by the development of large industrial complexes within the high-tempo socioeconomic development of the far northern territories, represent risk factors for the development of mental disorders. This is combined with limited local labour resources and the large-scale immigration of workers from elsewhere in Russia.

Despite their historical and enduring contact with Slavs, most of the indigenous inhabitants of southern Siberia have maintained their traditional culture and have administrative territorial autonomy.

The quality of life and mental health of the smaller ethnic groups of Russia (and especially the circumpolar populations) have been greatly influenced by acculturation, or the 'stress of modernization'.

Ethnocultural factors can influence the clinical manifestation and management of various types of disorder. For instance, Tuvinians and Buryats are highly tolerant of persons with senile psychoses, which is culturally conditioned by their respectful attitude towards the elderly. Among Buryats (continental Mongoloids), explosiveness in a state of alcohol intoxication is common. Arctic Mongoloids are characterized by an absence of vegetative signs of abstinence from alcohol, low rates of alcohol psychoses and a low prevalence of female alcoholism. Interestingly, the frequency of mental pathology in the Buryat Mongol population differs widely across family/tribal groups. Currently more than 270,000 Buryats could be classified as continental Mongoloids and about 660,000 ethnic Russians live in Buryatiya (other groups are much smaller). In a clinical/epidemiological investigation (Dashiyeva and Kupriyanova, 2009) of the population of remote districts of Buryatiya, high rates of alcohol dependence were found in male Buryats (up to 60.8 per cent of those examined) and of neurotic disorders in women (21.1 per cent) (Rakhmazova et al., 2012). In Primorsky Krai, among Udegeans and Nanaits rates of addiction in men were as high as 36.9 per cent, and in women 20.3 per cent. Quickness of formation of a withdrawal syndrome, acts of brutality while intoxicated, acceptance of therapy and a family history of alcoholism are typical (Bokhan et al., 2006; Badyrgy et al., 2012; Artemyev, 2012). Dependence on more than one substance was a trigger for the formation of child/adolescent pathology.

High rates of neuropsychiatric disorders and alcoholism among north-Asian and Arctic Mongoloids (Republics of Sakha/Yakutia, Buryatiya, Tyva), as well as among Mongoloids of Baykal and south-Siberian types, have been described repeatedly but they remain insufficiently studied; nevertheless, these groups do appear to be vulnerable to social stress and the formation of a number of affective and addictive states (Semke and Bokhan, 2008; Semke and Chukhrova, 2009).

Among the more mixed populations typical of the east-Asian part of Russia, the multifactorial concept of mental disorders appears to be more generally applicable. This concept supposes an important role of three basic factors in the aetiology of these diseases: social, psychological and individual/biological (biochemical, genetic, constitutional, morphological). The particular weight and significance of this triad is associated with the peculiarities of populations living under specific conditions and needs distinct ethnocultural investigation. The specific contributions of each of this triad of factors to mental disorders varies.

There are some differences in the symptoms of mental disorders among Caucasian people living in Siberia and some of the small indigenous minorities. For instance, the presentation of schizophrenia and the content of mental disturbances – delusions and hallucinations – in Buryats can reflect religious beliefs: shamanism, Lamaism, Buddhism. Thus, the most frequent delusions concern ideas of supernatural abilities of clairvoyance and healing powers, and patients imagining themselves to be a lama or shaman (Shaman [шаман] – a mediator communicating with spirits, who does aid recovery from mental disorders in some local areas in east Russia). Depressive spectrum disorders in Buryats are characterized by the presence of complaints of a somatic character often themselves attributed to the violation of a taboo.

Psychopharmacological therapy in cases of culture-bound delusion is usually insufficient, and the basic delusional story persists, perhaps because of patients' beliefs in its correctness within their religious frameworks.

In Russia, an area of urgent research interest is the choice of substances of abuse among specific groups, especially Mongoloid peoples. Low tolerance, early loss of situational control, early development of amnesic forms of intoxication and alcohol-related personality changes, notably with brutal behaviour, have been noted. The greatest rates of progression to alcoholism and the greatest rates of resistance to treatment have been observed in the native Arctic population (Semke and Bokhan, 2008). The key may be to understand the problem of their heightened rates of alcoholism.

Thus, for modern Russia a priority is the development of cross-cultural psychiatry and addiction psychiatry services. New forms of psychiatric, psychological and psychotherapeutic help are needed by the indigenous populations of the eastern region of Russia. On the threshold of acceptance of ICD-11, the theoretical significance and practical value of distinguishing different 'risk groups', pre-morbid states, and, for instance, prognostic criteria for borderline personality and addictive disorders have become all the more evident (Bokhan and Ovchinnikov, 2014). In the development of preventive activities by healthcare agencies, a complex of medico-social and sociocultural interventions are required, ones which have a flexible structure and which strive not to violate human rights. The elaboration of cross-cultural aspects of personality disorder represents an important theoretical stimulus connected with the crystallization of a biopsychosocial paradigm and sociotherapeutic preventive measures.

Research activity in the mental health sphere

As there is an urgent need for reforms in mental health care, Russian psychiatrists regard applied clinical–organizational studies as the main scientific task in their work. Epidemiology, the testing of new models of treatment, especially multidisciplinary teamwork approaches to treatment and rehabilitation, and involvement of NGOs are priorities for most researchers and research groups (Gurovich, 2005, 2012). The recognition and treatment of depressive and anxiety disorders within primary care are also an important focus of scientific and practical effort, as are optimal forms of working relationships and joint research with general practitioners, cardiologists, neurologists and other specialists (Krasnov, 2008, 2011). Socially oriented studies have in recent years been supported by a special federal programme (2007–2011). In particular regions, study of the mental health of populations living for a long time under the strain of a state of emergency, and even during periods of reconstruction and reconciliation, as in the Chechen Republic, has led to the development of appropriate mental health care interventions (Idrissov and Krasnov, 2009).

Russia's multi-ethnic population presents specific problems in relation to psychiatric care in some regions. Recently, new branches of research and clinical psychiatry have emerged in Russia, such as ecological and ethnocultural psychiatry (Semke et al., 1999; Semke and Bokhan, 2008; Bokhan et al., 2013).

Further development of the scientific basis of mental health care in Russia is likely to have a multidisciplinary focus on the ethnic or territorial parameters of the mental health of the population: the epidemiology, pathogenesis, phenomenology, clinical assessment, diagnosis and prevention of mental disorders (including addictions and psychosomatic disorders) across different age and social groups; the ethnocultural assessment of suicidal and aggressive behaviour; gender differences; problems of comorbidity; therapeutic resistance in addictive, borderline, affective and schizophreniform disorders; the contribution of migration, acculturation stress, anthropogenic and extreme geographic factors (principally long winter nights in the far north); medico-social indices and substance abuse; the predictors of the formation, clinical dynamics and prevention of addictive states among indigenous and smaller ethnic groups in Siberia, the far east and far north; the biological, molecular-genetic, neurophysiological and experimental-psychological investigations of mental disorders in different ethnic populations; ethnocultural aspects of the prevention of mental and behavioural disorders in different social groups; and the mental health consequences for ethnic groups of the industrialization of some remote regions of Russia. Indeed, all these issues are being studied at the school of cross-cultural psychiatry in Tomsk (Semke et al.,1999; Semke and Bokhan, 2008; Bokhan and Ovchinnikov, 2014).

Education in psychiatry

Postgraduate education for clinical practice (after six years of formal medical education) comprises an additional two-year course termed 'ordinature' and then 500 hours of specialization in forensic psychiatry, narcology or psychotherapy (psychotherapy is possible only after at least three years of practical work in psychiatry). There are also courses on psychogeriatrics, child psychiatry, psychosomatics and the organization of psychiatric services. All doctors have to validate their professional status in certificate confirmation courses, once every five years. There are also a variety of training schemes for clinical psychologists and social workers.

But, taking into consideration the wide differences in socioeconomic and sociocultural conditions across Russia's huge territory, the system of psychiatric education is lacking in certain key regards. For instance, there is no special training course in cross-cultural psychiatry and addiction, where an acquaintance at least, on the part of psychiatrists and psychologists, with the religious notions typical of Buddhism and shamanism, say, and the development of other aspects of professional ethnocultural competence, would help in the elaboration of strategies for prevention, and treatment and rehabilitation within mental health care. In this respect, psychological training in Buddhism might serve as a basis for the elaboration of new psychotherapeutic methods of treatment for the indigenous population of Siberia, especially for patients with culture-bound disorders.

Conclusion

In 2007–2012 the Federal Programme of Emergency Measures in Socially Important Diseases did help to develop some projects in psychiatry, and to improve conditions in many psychiatric institutions. Several attempts to establish such a programme in previous years failed because of financial difficulties and a conflict of priorities (areas such as cardiology, oncology and paediatrics are generally given primacy). Some mental health problems are being solved with the help of regional programmes for the improvement of psychiatric care, especially the development of psychosocial approaches in mental health care and the transition from the medical model to a more comprehensive biopsychosocial model of care with multidisciplinary working.

In programmes for the prevention of dependence in indigenous populations in Siberia, along with modern psychopharmacological approaches, considerable emphasis is given to traditional methods of treatment, necessary for the treatment of culture-bound mental disorders among Buryats. The development of personalized medicine within a cross-cultural psychiatric approach will help to meet the ethical norms of psychiatry, psychology and prevention. Awareness on the part of psychiatrists and psychologists of the religious notions typical of Buddhism and shamanism will help in the elaboration of preventive and treatment programmes.

Modern Russia is characterized by dynamism and instability. Social psychiatry and the assessment of the psychogenic factors underlying the most common psychopathological disorders of personality, neurotic and addictive disorders, have particular relevance in Russia, especially its eastern regions, with their multiethnic populations and multicultural lifestyles, combined with immigrant labour. Under these conditions the mental health of the population depends on the structure and content of the microsocial and macrosocial environment: each societal stratum has its own social and ethnic characteristics, which determine, for example, responses to stress, and thereby indirectly determine individual and societal well-being. The effective organization of psychiatric help in Russia needs a systemic analysis of the 'inner' and 'outer' space of the individual through the prism of national traditions and customs, but incorporating universal values.

Bibliography

Artemyev, I. A. (2012) 'Alcoholism in polyethnic subpopulations of the circumpolar zone of north-eastern regions of Russia'. *Siberian Herald of Psychiatry and Addiction Psychiatry*. 72: 32–5 (in Russian).

Badyrgy, I. O., Bokhan, N. A., Mandel, A. I., Mongush, Ch. K. and Peshkovskaya, A. G. (2012) 'Medico-social indices of the drug situation among the population of Republic of Tyva'. *Siberian Herald of Psychiatry and Addiction Psychiatry*. 72: 29–32 (in Russian).

Bokhan, N. (2009) 'Clinical-ethnocultural peculiarities of alcoholism among the aboriginal population of Kamchatka'. *World Cultural Psychiatry Review*. Supplement S1: 119–22.

Bokhan, N. A. and Ovchinnikov, A. A. (2014) *Dissociative model of addiction formation*. Saint-Louis, MO, USA: Publishing House Science and Innovation Center.

Bokhan, N. A., Mandel, A. I. and Gusamov, R. R. (2006) 'Mental and behavioral disorders in substance use among adolescents under conditions of the far north'. *Alaska Medicine*. 49: 251–4.

Bokhan, N. A., Mandel, A. I., Aslanbekova, N. V. and Peshkovskaya, A. G. (2013) 'Ethnoterritorial heterogeneity of formation of alcohol dependence in the native population of Siberia'. *Zhurnal Nevrologii and Psikhiatrii Imeni SS Korsakova*. 113: 9–14 (in Russian).

Dashiyeva, B. and Kupriyanova, I. (2009) 'Factors influencing on mental health state of schoolchildren from Buryat rural population'. *World Cultural Psychiatry Research Review*. 1: 139–41.

Gumilev, L. N. (1993) *Ethnosphere: History of people and history of nature.* Moscow: Ekopros.

Gurovich, I. Y. (2005) 'Reform of psychiatric care in the Russian Federation. Current status and problems'. *Social and Clinical Psychiatry.* 4: 12–18 (in Russian).

Gurovich, I. (2012) 'The state of the psychiatric care system in Russia: Current challenges against background shrinking of the inpatient care'. *Social and Clinical Psychiatry.* 4: 5–10 (in Russian).

Idrissov, K. and Krasnov, V. (2009) 'Mental health of the population of the Chechen Republic: A dynamic population 2002–2008 study'. *Zhurnal nevrologii I psikhiatrii imeni SS Korsakova.* 7: 76–81 (in Russian).

Krasnov, V. (2002) 'Ethical problems of contemporary Russian psychiatry'. *Independent Psychiatric Journal.* 3: 12–17 (in Russian).

Krasnov, V. (ed.) (2008). *Improvement of early diagnostics of mental disorders (on the basis of interrelationship with primary care specialists).* Moscow: Medpractica-M (in Russian).

Krasnov, V. (2011) *Affective spectrum disorders.* Moscow: Practicheskya meditsina.

Krasnov, V. and Gurovich, I. (2012) 'History and current conditions of Russian psychiatry'. *International Review of Psychiatry.* 24(4): 328–33.

Nemtsov, A. (2011) *Contemporary history of alcohol in Russia. Newest period.* Stockholm: Sodertorns hogskola.

Nikitin, Yu. (2007) 'Health of Chukotka population: Results and prospects'. In : *Current problems of medicine.* Abakan: Khakassic State University (in Russian).

Popovich, L., Potapchik, E., Shishkin, S., Richardson, E., Vacroux, A. and Mathivet, B. (2011) 'Russian Federation'. *Health systems in transition.* 13(7). Geneva: World Health Organization.

Rakhmazova, L. D., Semke, A. V. and Ochirova, I. B. (2012) 'Prevalence of schizophrenia in Buryatiya'. *Siberian Herald of Psychiatry and Addiction Psychiatry.* 72: 18–20.

Semke, V. and Bokhan, N. (2008) *Cross-cultural addictology.* Tomsk: Publishing TSU (in Russian).

Semke, V. and Chukhrova, M. G. (2009) *Mental health of the indigenous population of the east of Russia.* Tomsk, Novosibirsk: Publishing House Nauka (in Russian).

Semke, V., Bokhan, N. and Galaktionov, O. (1999) *Essays of ethnology and ethnopsychotherapy.* Tomsk: Publishing TSU (in Russian).

Sokolova, Z. (2000) *People of West Siberia. Ethnographic survey.* Moscow: Nauka.

Taliyanova, T. I. and Korobitsina, T. V. (2011) 'Peculiarities of alcohol use in patients – natives of Republic of Khakasia suffering from alcohol dependence'. *Siberian Herald of Psychiatry and Addiction Psychiatry.* 66: 85–8.

WHO (2012) *Suicide rates per 100,000 people per year, country, and sex.* Geneva: World Health Organization.

4

State of mental health care in the Republic of Uzbekistan

Grigoriy Kharabara and Nargiza Khodjaeva

The geography of the Republic

The Republic of Uzbekistan is located in the middle of Central Asia. Its capital is Tashkent. Its territory runs 925 km north–south and 1,400 km east–west, totalling 448,971 km². Its neighbouring states are Kyrgyzstan to the northeast, Kazakhstan to the northwest, Turkmenistan to the southwest, Tajikistan to the southeast and Afghanistan to the south. The total length of the country's borders is 6,621 km.

Among the member states of the Commonwealth of Independent States (CIS, the organization of former Soviet republics), Uzbekistan has the fifth largest area and the third largest population (about 30 million people). Uzbekistan is a multi-ethnic state with more than 120 nationalities and ethnic groups, including Uzbeks (80 per cent), Russians (5.5 per cent), Tadjiks (5 per cent), Kazakhs (3 per cent), Karakalpaks (2.5 per cent) and others (1.5 per cent). According to the World Bank, GNP per capita was US$1,717 in 2011.

Following the declaration of Uzbekistan as a sovereign state on 31 August 1991, the Republic acceded to the Universal Declaration of Human Rights by a resolution of Parliament, and in 1992 the Convention on the Rights of the Child was ratified. In 1997 Uzbekistan acceded to the Universal Declaration of Human Rights and the Human Genome. Uzbekistan also signed other international treaties of the United Nations: the International Covenant on Civil and Political Rights; the International Covenant on Economic, Social and Cultural Rights; the Convention on the Elimination of All Forms of Discrimination against Women; the Convention on the Elimination of All Forms of Racial Discrimination; and the Convention against Torture and Other Cruel, Inhuman or Degrading Treatment or Punishment, among others.

The law 'On Psychiatric Care' governing the activities of psychiatric services and the legal status of persons with mental disorders was implemented in the Republic in 2000. This legislation enshrined orders of the Ministry of Health in order to prevent human rights violations and discrimination and to empower people with mental disorders. In addition, 'On Psychiatric Care' guarantees the delivery of psychiatric care.

Other legislation regulates the rights of persons who have committed criminal offenses, or who are on trial or who are being investigated on felony charges, and who have been found to suffer from mental illness, or are believed may suffer from such disease. The Legislative Chamber of the Republic on 12 July 2012 passed the law 'On amendments and additions to some legislative acts of the Republic of Uzbekistan in connection with the further reform of the judicial system', under which such persons can be placed in medical facilities at the pre-trial stage for forensic psychiatric examination by order of an investigator, prosecutor or the court; amendments and additions to existing legislation provide for similar judicial procedures during the course of a trial.

Organizational aspects of mental health care and psychiatric epidemiology

Mental health services (preventive and curative care and maternal and child health) are the responsibility of the Central Organization Department of the Ministry of Health. The Ministry has a chief freelance psychiatrist, one child psychiatrist, and chief freelance consultants in forensic psychiatry, psychotherapy and self-harm. In the 14 regional health authorities, Head Specialists are responsible for specialized mental health services in the regions; in each region there is a Chief Psychiatrist and senior specialists in paediatric and forensic psychiatry, psychotherapy and self-harm services.

Within each region, the leading psychiatric institution has organizational and methodological advisory departments; they annually submit reports to the national organizational and methodological advisory department. The mental health of the population is annually reported at the medical boards or at boards of the Ministry of Health.

According to dispensary (outpatient clinic) statistics, in 2012, the overall incidence of mental and behavioural disorders was 120 per 100,000. The highest rate was observed in Tashkent city (253.6) and the lowest in the Tashkent region (70) and the Republic of Karakalpakstan (70.8) (a 3.6-fold difference). Tashkent city is the capital of the country, and has a well-developed infrastructure, including the mental health care system. In contrast, the rest of the Tashkent region is a rural area without a well-developed care system, and with few qualified specialists. Residents of the villages often keep mental disorders secret within the family. Among a cohort of people registered at a dispensary and under clinical supervision in all 14 regions in Uzbekistan (365,849), 10.9 per cent were in receipt of mental health care; villagers accounted for 58.3 per cent of this group. The overall prevalence of mental disorders per 100,000 of the rural population was 1,464. Analysis of prevalence by regions shows fluctuations – from 1,544.9 (Andijan) to 917.4 (Navoi) (a 1.7-fold difference).

In 2012, again according to dispensary statistics, the prevalence of mental disorders was 1,229 per 100,000 of population (men 57.8 per cent, women 42.2 per cent):

- Persons suffering from mental retardation – 38.8 per cent (including those with autism and other developmental disorders);
- Persons with non-psychotic mental disorders – 34.6 per cent;
- Persons with psychosis or a dementia – 26.6 per cent, including schizophrenia – 64.6 per cent of the group with a psychosis.

Among patients attending the dispensaries in 2012, 24.4 per cent were disabled by mental illness; 1.3 per cent of all patients had previously committed socially dangerous acts and were consequently registered in a special file.

In children, mental and behavioural disorders (22.6 per cent) are the leading cause of mental health problems but most of them are transient. According to medical examinations of children aged 0 to 14 years who were involved in school-based survey, 1.3 per 100 examined were retarded in neuropsychological development.

Mental health services: multidisciplinary approach to treatment and rehabilitation

Outpatient mental health care is mainly provided by what are termed psychoneurologic dispensaries which consist of multidisciplinary teams, with members such as psychiatrists, psychotherapists and nurses providing medical advice or clinical supervision. Community-based care is provided in day hospitals, in specialized psychiatric and psychotherapeutic offices established on the basis of district outpatient health care facilities. To provide community-based mental health care in 2012, Uzbekistan's 22 psychoneurologic dispensaries and three dispensary departments in psychiatric hospitals arranged 2,598 visits per day. The actual number of visits (including preventive examinations) amounted to 5,220,343.

Nationally, there are 275 outpatient clinics with psychiatric (neuropsychiatric) offices (including the 22 dispensaries and three hospital dispensary departments mentioned above) and 444 psychotherapy offices.

To provide medical assistance to the rural population in 2012 the Republic had 3,191 rural medical centres and 456 branches. A decree from the Ministry of Health stipulates a list of qualifying diseases and the medical services to be provided in rural medical stations by a general practitioner. The chapter 'Mental disorders and diseases in adults, adolescents and children' sets out the criteria for diagnosis, treatment, emergency care, referral to specialists in regional medical organizations, rehabilitation and clinical examination.

Outpatient forensic psychiatric examination is provided by 15 commissions, and all outpatient forensic expert committees operate within the psychiatric institutions.

Nine psychiatric institutions have psychiatric 'hospitals at home' and 'infant psychiatry' services, which monitor the health of infants (0 to 4 years) at risk. Day-care centres operate in 11 regions; they have a total of 678 places for day-care patients, but this is a substantial decrease from the total in 1991, when there were 1,222 places. The number of working placements (similar to sheltered workshops in the West) in the workshops of psychiatric institutions decreased 10.5 times and reached 120 compared with 1,263 in 1991.

A national model for emergency medical assistance has been put in place in the Republic. It had previously been decentralized but is now coordinated by an integrated Republican Scientific Centre of Emergency Medicine (RSCEM), which has branches in all regional centres. The RSCEM has a national organization to tackle self-harm, which has its own regional offices. These offer psychosocial assistance ('hotlines' or 'crisis hospitals') for people with suicidal behaviour and suicidal dangerous states who are not registered in the psychiatric dispensary and not in need of psychiatric registration.

Inpatient psychiatric care in the country is delivered through 12 psychiatric hospitals with a total of 4,515 psychiatric beds, 17 psychiatric dispensaries with a 24-hour psychiatric capacity of 2,941 beds, and 185 beds in seven psychosomatic departments of the general hospitals. Again, the number of psychosomatic beds has decreased since 1991, from 13,095 to 7,641, including 330 for children, 245 for adolescents, 310 for people with psychoactive substance abuse problems and 237 for patients with concomitant tuberculosis.

In addition, the Republic has 880 inpatient forensic beds: 505 at the Republican Psychiatric Hospital of the Ministry of Health, which can provide intensive supervision; 275 in forensic departments in psychiatric hospitals (100 beds in forensic psychiatric hospitals, and 175 in specialist psychiatric rehabilitation wards in psychiatric hospitals); and 100 at the Republican Hospital of the Ministry of Internal Affairs. The number of psychiatric beds for the period 1991–2012 decreased 2.4-fold, from 6.2 (1991) to 2.6 (2012) per 10,000 population.

According to data on social support and rehabilitation from the Ministry of National Education, in all regions of the country there are schools for children with speech and IQ disturbances, and boarding schools for children with conduct disorders. Within the Ministry of Labour and Social Protection there are homes for people with severe and disabling mental disorders.

There are 42,302 children with special educational needs being educated in 85 specialist boarding schools, 26 boarding schools with sanatorium facilities and 183 specialist preschools. These educational institutions are an integral and equal part of the education system. In line with the national model of inclusive education, in 5,900 educational institutions the educational process is organized for the 28,890 children with disabilities and various educational needs.

Among the ten most prevalent chronic health problems and disabilities for men and women of the Republic, ranked according to their weight in the total number of disability-adjusted life years, neuropsychiatric disorders accounted for 16.6 per cent of men and 21.9 per cent of women ('Highlights on health in Uzbekistan', 2005). The mental health service is financed solely by the government; in this respect it is in a less privileged position than other services, which additionally receive payments for private health care.

Expenditure on mental health services amounted to 2.1 per cent of total health care spending in 2012. Due to insufficient funding, the physical infrastructure remains inadequate, and many psychiatric institutions do not meet the requirements for technical equipment (heating, ventilation, sanitary equipment, artificial lighting, etc.). Most psychiatric institutions do not meet the requirements for planning, design and operation. In only six districts has the diagnostic equipment been updated in the last two decades. All other psychiatric institutions have outdated electroencephalography, X-ray equipment and other medical equipment.

Training in mental health

Medical education proceeds in three stages:

1. Undergraduate courses in medicine last seven years, and successful students can qualify as general practitioners;
2. Postgraduate training (e.g. for psychiatrists), covers a further two (clinical residency in clinical settings) to three years (MSc programme and its clinical bases);
3. A doctorate, taking another three years, qualifies specialists in medical science and education.

The training of mental health specialists is provided by the Department of Psychiatry at the country's six medical universities. Medical schools also provide training in 'medical psychology'.

In Uzbekistan three levels of training are recognized for doctors: first, second and higher. These are assigned through examination and there are various postgraduate training schemes for psychiatrists for these higher qualifications. The training and retraining of doctors is carried out in specialist training courses: psychiatry, child and adolescent psychiatry, psychotherapy, forensic psychiatry, self-harm, medical psychology and narcology. Professional time is specifically allocated for attendance at these courses, though this differs for general practitioners, family physicians and specialists.

The number of specialists within mental health care (together with experts in the departments of psychiatry and in administrative positions) at the beginning of 2013 amounted to 936: 662 specialists for the adult population; 157 child psychiatrists; 56 adolescent psychiatrists;

20 psychotherapists; 12 forensic psychiatrists; four specialists in dealing with self-harm behaviour; 11 specialists in sexual pathology; and 14 medical psychologists. Among these working professionals, five had the degree of Doctor of Medical Sciences and 19 were Doctoral Candidates of Medical Sciences.

Nationally, there are 0.28 psychiatrists per 10,000 people, which is 1.8 times less than in 1991. The decline is likely to be due to the stigmatization of psychiatry and the low salaries despite hard work.

There are 2,578 nurses in psychiatric institutions (0.9 per 10,000 population). According to WHO recommendations, an adequate ratio is about four certified nurses per psychiatrist, while in the Republic this ratio is 3.1:1.

Given the shortage of personnel, steps have been taken to integrate mental health services with primary care by reconsidering the education of general practitioners, family physicians and nurses in mental health care.

With the technical and financial support of the WHO Country Office, 'Guidelines for health professionals on mental health legislation' and a textbook entitled *Mental health in the primary health care system of the Republic of Uzbekistan* have been published. Annually for the past five years training courses and seminars on integrating mental health services with primary care have been conducted for the directors of pre- and postgraduate training programmes for general practitioners.

In 2009 a cross-sectional 'Strategy for suicide prevention in the Republic of Uzbekistan for 2010–2020' was developed and approved and in 2010 the textbook *Implementing strategies to prevent suicides in the Republic of Uzbekistan for 2010–2020* was published.

Prevention and rehabilitation programmes: perspectives for improving mental health services

It is well known that the primary prevention of mental disorders largely depends on activities outside the formal provision of psychiatric services (they relate instead to family planning, maternal health, environmental health, specific activities in the field of obstetrics and paediatrics, and in many other sectors). Such actions have been successfully implemented in Uzbekistan. They have included maternal immunization against rubella; a decrease in the incidence of Down's syndrome using cytodiagnosis and selective abortion; identification of congenital hypothyroidism; screening for phenylketonuria and supply of dietary products that do not contain phenylalanine; detection of human immunodeficiency virus; measures specific to infant and early childhood; immunization against measles and pertussis; the management of meningococcal meningitis in children; and the identification and treatment of chronic bacteriuria and pyelonephritis.

In order to develop healthy families and reduce the incidence of hereditary diseases, a system of compulsory pre-marital medical examination of couples planning marriage was introduced for a variety of diseases, such as HIV, tuberculosis, mental disorders, substance abuse and venereo-logic diseases. Additional measures to improve the reproductive health of mothers in order to prevent the birth of children with congenital malformations have been introduced: an annual survey of more than 420,000 women in early pregnancy, and the provision of dietary supplements containing micronutrients such as folic acid. An issue with regard to diseases related to iodine deficiency has been successfully resolved.

Taking into consideration that some hereditary diseases and chromosomal syndromes are accompanied by disturbances of mental development, modern technologies for the early detection of a wide range of metabolic disorders are included in this programme. According to the State Statistics Committee, the incidence of children born with congenital anomalies decreased by 14 per cent in comparison with 2000. Activities for the early detection of congenital and genetic diseases averted in 2012 the birth of 3,408 children with severe debilitating hereditary diseases. In 2012 the method of tandem mass spectrometry was for the first time introduced in screening centres for the early diagnosis of inherited metabolic disorders that lead to mental retardation.

Given the existing resources and staff shortages, the governmental order of the Republic of 25 July 2013 'On measures for further improvement of the psychiatric service of the Republic of Uzbekistan' approved a programme of further development of the material–technical base of psychiatric services for the period 2013–2017. The programme includes basic parameters for the reconstruction and overhaul of mental health facilities and psychiatric institutions, including the replacement of medical equipment. The programme extends to the improvement of the legal framework; prevention, early diagnosis and effective treatment of mental disorders; provision of psychiatric services with highly qualified personnel; research within the field of psychiatry; and the facilitation of international cooperation in this field. In order to implement the programme, 30 specialized working groups were created, one of which is responsible for the development and implementation of regional education programmes for different segments of the population about the prevalence and primary manifestations of mental illnesses and their treatment. The Press Service of the Ministry was charged with the development and approval of meetings, interviews, lectures, 'round tables', television and radio programmes, and articles that could help to counter stigma.

The General Directorate of Science and Educational Institutions of the Ministry of Health identifies the short-term and long-term priorities for psychiatry; it also evaluates innovative ideas for the development of mental health care across the population.

The Ministry of Finance has provided an extra-budgetary fund for reconstruction, refurbishment and equipment of educational and medical institutions within an annual appropriation provided by the state budget, as well as soft loans and grants from foreign states, international financial institutions and other sources not prohibited by law. The budget for the programme is estimated to be more than US$83 million.

References

Guidelines for health professionals on mental health legislation' (2005) Ministry of Public Health, Tashkent.

'Highlights on health in Uzbekistan' (2005) Geneva: WHO European Office.

Implementation of suicide prevention strategy in the Republic of Uzbekistan for 2010–2020 (2010) Ministry of Public Health, Tashkent.

Mental health in the primary health care system of the Republic of Uzbekistan (2007) Ministry of Public Health, Tashkent.

Situation analysis of mental health service in Uzbekistan and the ways of reforms in 1991–2012 (2013) Ministry of Public Health, Tashkent.

WHO–AIMS report on the mental health system in Uzbekistan (2007) Geneva: WHO.

Section 2

Indian subcontinent

Overview

Diversity in unity and adversity

Santosh K. Chaturvedi and Geetha Desai

The Indian subcontinent includes Bangladesh, Bhutan, India, Nepal, Pakistan and Sri Lanka. The chapters in this section present an overview of epidemiological aspects of mental health problems, mental health services and mental health legislation in these countries. The focus is also on the indigenous and traditional aspects of mental health services which are very much an integral part of the health system.

Few common themes emerge while glancing over the descriptions of mental health services in these six countries of the Indian subcontinent. All the countries are thickly populated (and naturally have large numbers of persons with mental health problems); have very few mental health professionals, especially psychiatrists, for their burden of mental health problems; have political instability and internal conflicts to a lesser or greater extent; suffer from periodic natural disasters and socioeconomic adversity; have numerous unique traditional methods of mental health and medical care; and continue to survive and thrive. By way of development, these nations are becoming urbanized in haphazard ways leading to many societal changes, and erosion of the traditional values and lifestyles. This has thrown challenges at the mental health systems as these transitional societies bring new concerns.

Mental health is a neglected field in all the countries in the subcontinent. The focus in healthcare is more on infectious diseases, nutritional deficiencies, and, among the non-communicable diseases, on cancer, cardiovascular disease and diabetes. Major mental disorders in the subcontinent are depression, schizophrenia, and somatoform and dissociative disorders. There are no recent large-scale, national epidemiological data on mental illness in some of the countries in the subcontinent. However, many epidemiological studies have been conducted in India since the 1960s and there are systematic reviews which give a fair idea of the prevalence of psychiatric disorders. In the Indian subcontinent, the mental health burden is predominantly from common mental disorders, followed by substance abuse and then severe mental disorders.

The mental health services have been gradually evolving over the years, however, growth in these countries is at different levels. Despite mental health problems being recognized as a major health concern, the development of services has not kept pace with other specialties. Mental asylums have been gradually replaced by mental hospitals or institutions. There has also been significant growth in the number of general hospital psychiatry units. Community psychiatry mainly focuses on epilepsy, mental retardation and psychoses.

The specialist mental health infrastructure is limited in the subcontinent. In Pakistan, for a population of 190 million, there are 520 psychiatrists and less than 3,000 psychiatric inpatient beds. There are 18 NGOs in Pakistan involved in individual assistance activities such as counseling, housing or support groups. In Bangladesh, a mental health service is only available in tertiary care provided by about 220 qualified psychiatrists and other support service personnel. At the tertiary care level, there is only one National Institute of Mental Health with 200 beds, and one mental hospital with 500 beds. In Nepal there are 65 psychiatrists, one child psychiatrist, 14 clinical psychologists and more than 48 mental health nurses, but no psychiatric social workers. There are very few psychiatrists and mental health professionals in Bhutan. There are 63 mental health outpatient clinics, all integrated with inpatient facilities and one day-care facility in the country. There are 63 community-based community psychiatry inpatient units with an approximate total of 100 beds. India has more than 5,000 psychiatrists, a number which is inadequate for the vast population. About 450 postgraduates qualify as psychiatrists every year in India, but there are hardly any jobs for them. Most cities and towns have private psychiatrists providing services, and usually very busy clinics. There is a discrepancy between the mental health services provided in the urban and rural areas, with hardly any psychiatrists in the rural areas.

The mental health policies and legislation are ancient in some of the countries of the subcontinent, and are being reviewed in some of them. In Pakistan, a Mental Health Ordinance was passed in 2001; mental health policy was last revised in 2003. In Nepal, the National Mental Health Policy and Plan was developed by the Ministry of Health in 1997 but still exists only theoretically. In Bhutan, the National Mental Health Programme (NMHP) was initiated in 1997 under the Eighth Five Year Plan, with the primary focus on community mental health care. A mental health policy drafted by a committee under the leadership of the Sri Lanka College of Psychiatrists was approved by the Government of Sri Lanka for the first time in 2005 (Mental Health Policy 2005). The Indian Lunacy Act 1912 was replaced by the Mental Health Act 1987, which is in the process of being amended. The Mental Health Care Bill 2011, is awaiting approval by the Indian parliament. There have been concerns about human rights violations against patients with mental illness in the subcontinent. Legislation related to mental health has not evolved at a uniform pace.

Psychiatric training in the subcontinent has gradually evolved over the last few decades. Many of the trained mental health professionals have been practising outside the subcontinent leading to a shortage of mental health professionals in their own countries. The training has predominantly been influenced by Western mental health frameworks, which has its own advantages and disadvantages. The biggest disadvantage would be lack of understanding of the cultural aspects of mental illness presentations, help-seeking behaviours and indigenous practices. There has been significant growth in the subspecialties of psychiatry, like addiction medicine, child psychiatry, consultation liaison psychiatry and community psychiatry, through fellowship programmes. In Bangladesh, the course curriculum for postgraduate qualification in psychiatry is standardized in both a fellowship and residency programme. Besides formal courses regular short-term training is going on for general practitioners and other health professionals. Postgraduate courses are also available in all countries, except Bhutan.

A notable observation is the use of local idioms for distress and folk illnesses, which reflect abnormal illness behaviour among persons with mental health problems. Factors that impede diagnosis and treatment of mental disorders include stigma, discrimination and misconceptions about mental disorders. Traditional medicine is popular in most countries of the subcontinent, including Bhutan, and is usually the first point of contact in the health care system, for patients. In the all the countries, traditional, alternative and complementary systems of health care are popular, easily accessible and relatively low cost. People also have faith in religious healers and religious places for care of the mentally ill.

Accessibility of mental health services to all still remains a goal to be achieved in the Indian subcontinent. The traditional health systems are probably the first point of contact for patients with mental illnesses as well. The ratio of mental health professionals to patients is still low. However, the large number of persons with untreated mental health problems to be expected with this acute shortage of services, are neither reported nor seen wandering! What is interesting is that despite the drawbacks the outcome of schizophrenia seems to be better in these countries. It is important to understand the unique factors associated with this outcome so that we do not lose them in the advance of globalization.

In the Indian subcontinent mental health problems and services have more in common with each other, than with the rest of the world, including common psychosocial problems and common solutions. However, diversity exists, despite the similarity of problems and adversities. It is time the countries in the Indian subcontinent collaborated with each other, not only in research and academically, but also in services.

5

The Bangladesh perspective

*Golam Rabbani, Helal Uddin Ahmed,
Geetha Desai and Dinesh Bhugra*

Country overview

History

Bangladesh is a comparatively young country, having become a separate entity only relatively recently. After having been part of the British Raj and then pre-Independence India, Bengal province was divided into what became known as East Pakistan in 1947. Following the Indo-Pakistani war in 1971, the country became independent and was renamed Bangladesh. The history of the country is strongly influenced by a number of external factors, and this is reflected in its growth and development, both in general as well as in medicine and psychiatry. The nation's history is also reflected in its agricultural, industrial and socio-economic development.

Physical geography

Bangladesh forms a part of the structure of the Indian subcontinent and is considered a South East Asian country. It geographical spread covers an area of 147,570 square kilometers with geographical borders with India and Myanmar and the Bay of Bengal to its south.

Population

The population of Bangladesh is roughly around 152 million. The country has one of the highest population densities in the world at a population of 1,015/square kilometer. A significant proportion of the population is young; however, only about half of the population is literate, with literacy rate of about 51.8 percent.

The main language of Bangladesh is 'Bangla' (Figure 5.1). The vast majority of the population (about 83 percent) is Muslim, with 16 percent Hindu and 1 percent reported as other religions including Buddhist and Christian, or other. The annual population growth rate is about 2 percent.

Health care structure

The doctor/patient ratio in Bangladesh is 1:3,800. This includes only doctors working in the national health system, and does not include those offering other approaches such as traditional

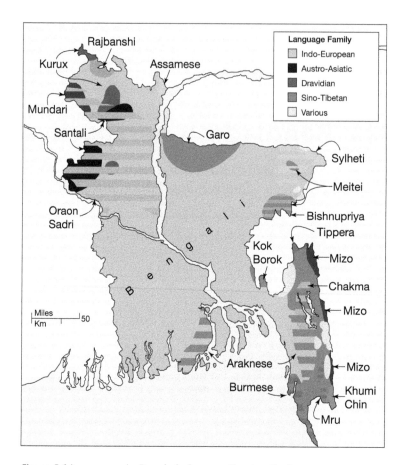

Figure 5.1 Languages in Bangladesh according to ethnic group

Source: http://en.wikipedia.org/wiki/Languages_of_Bangladesh#mediaviewer/File:Languages_of_Bangladesh_map.svg

medicine. In 2012, the average life expectancy of the population was 70.06 years with male life expectancy being somewhat lower than that of women at 68.21 years and 71.98 years, respectively. The infant mortality rate is 49/1,000 and the maternal mortality rate 240/100,000 live births.

Like most of the world and surrounding countries, the entire professional (allopathic) health care system is organized in three tiers. These three levels are primary care at district or sub-district levels, secondary care and supra-regional care. Primary care includes 18,000 community health clinics, 1,500 union sub centers and 460 Upazila (sub district) health complexes. The secondary level includes district hospitals in 64 districts. The medical colleges, super-specialized tertiary hospitals, include teaching hospitals and one medical university (see below).

Mental health care structure

Manpower

As is the case in neighboring countries, modern psychiatric care in Bangladesh remains inadequate with limited human and financial resources allocated to mental health care. Only

220 psychiatrists serve the whole nation. Psychiatric nurses, psychiatric social workers, occupational therapists, speech therapists and physiotherapists are even scarcer, and this has led to increasing stress and expectations being placed on those who continue to work in Bangladesh, sometimes in very difficult circumstances. There are only 50 trained clinical psychologists in the whole country. Most mental health professionals including psychiatrists work in tertiary care and are concentrated in the urban areas, leaving large parts of rural Bangladesh totally without cover. Furthermore, most psychiatrists are either in private practice or in a mixture of teaching and private practice in cities.

The budget allocation for mental health is only 0.44 percent of the total health budget in the public sector.

Hospitals

There is one national Institute of Mental Health in Bangladesh situated in Dhaka, with postgraduate training capacity, 200 inpatient beds and an outpatient service. Another mental hospital with 500 beds situated in Pabna district in the northern part of Bangladesh has been in service since 1957. There are psychiatric departments in Bangabandhu Sheikh Mujib Medical University (BSMMU), and government and private medical colleges with inpatient and outpatient services and also training facilities. In all there are in total roughly 817 beds for mentally ill people in Bangladesh in the whole of public sector.

Prevalence of mental disorders

In line with many countries, the prevalence rates of psychiatric disorders are remarkably high in Bangladesh. A national survey on mental disorders among adults (2003–2005) showed that 16.1 percent had psychiatric morbidity and among them 8.4 percent had anxiety disorders, 4.6 percent major depressive disorders, 1.1 percent psychosis, 0.6 percent bipolar mood disorders and 0.1 percent schizophrenia. Another WHO-supported community-based survey of children (2009) found an 18.4 percent prevalence of mental disorders among children aged 5–18 years. This study revealed that other than the mental disorders, 3.8 percent of children had mental retardation (MR) (a term still used in Bangladesh), 2 percent had epilepsy and 0.8 percent had substance abuse problems. Research on treatment gaps in Bangladesh (2012) found the treatment gap for epilepsy was more than 77 percent. The treatment gap for psychiatric disorders is likely to be higher.

Psychiatric services, referral and service delivery model

The history of modern mental health services in Bangladesh is relatively recent, going back less than 60 years. In 1957, a 60-bed temporary mental hospital in the Pabna district was established in an abandoned building called Sitlai House. Construction of a permanent mental hospital building was started at the same time in that area in an abandoned 'Asram' (prayer center) named Sat Sangha which is located near the river Padma, in Pabna. Initially this Pabna mental hospital had 200 beds, which was gradually increased to 500 beds in stages.

During this period the government of Pakistan (Bangladesh was East Pakistan at that time) allocated funds to each medical college to establish mental health clinics. Unfortunately, however, little funding was utilized in East Pakistan (Bangladesh) for that purpose. After independence and separation from West Pakistan, a small scheme named 'Organization of training on mental health' was introduced in medical colleges to develop mental health services. In only

1972 a department of psychiatry was established in the Institute of Post Graduate Medicine and Research (IPGM&R) (now known as Bangabandhu Sheik Mujib Medical University). Postgraduate courses in psychiatric training started in 1975 at the University of Dhaka and Bangladesh College of Physicians and Surgeons (BCPS). In 1981 the National Institute of Mental Health was established in order to develop and provide mental health services along with training to foster skilled manpower in mental health. This institute started offering inpatient services in 2001 and now is functioning as a research institute with postgraduate facilities, and providing supra-regional mental health services to the nation.

The health services and mental health system are integrated into the overall strategy for the national health care system. At present, there is no separate formal health system for mental health although mental health services in the community are being provided by making proper use of the current general health facilities with the development of links and referrals between villages and nearby mental health facilities. Primary care facilities in the country generally include union health centers, Upazila (sub district) health complexes and community clinics. Different levels of primary care workers provide services. Essential mental health services that are available at the Upazila level include early identification of mental disorders, such as schizophrenia, depressive disorder, anxiety disorders, bipolar mood disorder, mental retardation and obsessive compulsive disorder as well as treatment for these conditions. As in neighboring countries, managing epilepsy is often part of psychiatrists' remit. The ongoing management of stable psychiatric patients and appropriate referral to other levels of care when required is part of the service. In addition some recognition of and attention to the mental health needs of people with physical health problems are becoming part of the mental health services, especially at district general hospitals, along with increasing recognition of mental health promotion and prevention.

In Bangladesh, there are 22 government medical colleges and 57 private medical colleges, and more are in development, again in line with neighboring countries. Most of these medical colleges do have departments of psychiatry but are not well equipped in terms of manpower so the teaching of psychiatry is confined to a short period with limited clinical exposure. Tertiary psychiatric services are delivered through the 500-bed Mental Hospital, Pabna, 250 kilometers away from the capital city, Dhaka. The National Institute of Mental Health has been based in Dhaka, serving as the overall research, training, education and service development, planning and delivery coordinator at the national and international level. It has 200 inpatient beds with outpatient and emergency services. The institute also provides tertiary services at the national level and conducts academic activities with a postgraduate course in psychiatry. As in many countries, including others in South East Asia, private psychiatric services are common and people have to pay for these services either out of their own pocket or via limited insurance claims. Psychiatric services are also provided by qualified psychiatrists in private consultation centers, private mental hospitals and clinics.

For a developing country like Bangladesh, community mental health services are essential, but unfortunately the country does not have a policy or the resources to develop and deliver community mental health programs; all the major services are largely confined to big urban centers. The approach of providing mental health services through integration with existing primary health care has been accepted as a matter of principle and a possible way to provide mental health services to people in the community but there is a long way to go.

In the whole country there are only 50 outpatient centers of which very few (only 4 percent) cater exclusively for children and adolescents. The most common condition treated in outpatients is schizophrenia (30 percent), followed by mood disorders (20 percent), and common mental disorders such as anxiety, depression and phobias (20 percent). The availability of medications depends upon the cost and local availability. Over half (58 percent) of psychiatric outpatient facilities have at least one psychotropic medicine of each therapeutic class (anti-psychotic, antidepressant, mood stabilizer, anti-anxiety and antiepileptic) freely available in the facility or at a pharmacy near the facility.

Inevitably some patients with severe mental disorders will need hospital treatment. This is available at district general hospitals or psychiatry units of nearby medical colleges which are able to provide accessible 24-hour psychiatric care. There is no doubt that for such a large population with high prevalence rates the overall services and facilities are not adequate, with a limited number of inpatient beds in the public sector (Figure 5.2). Inpatient beds are not entirely free: 60 percent are completely free of charge but patients and their relatives have to pay limited amount for the use of the remaining 40 percent.

The National Institute of Mental Health has inpatient facilities for adult psychiatry; child, adolescent and family psychiatry; geriatric and organic psychiatry; psychotherapy; and forensic (prison) psychiatry. In Bangabandhu Sheikh Mujib Medical University 25 percent of beds in the department of psychiatry are allocated to children and adolescents. The National Institute of Mental Health has a child guidance clinic and a geriatric clinic.

Mental Health Act

Bangladesh's has no mental health act yet; however, a draft has been completed and hopefully the Mental Health Act: Bangladesh will be enacted very soon.

Patterns of referral

In Bangladesh, as in most countries around the world, basic health care is provided through primary health care clinics. The government policy is to train all physicians in mental health care using the primary care system but this has not worked in practice. The district hospitals with a capacity of 110–200 beds provide secondary care; however, these hospitals do not always have psychiatrists available largely owing to a lack of human resources. Regarding tertiary care, Bangladesh has one mental hospital with 500 beds, one national institute with 200 beds, one department with 40 beds in the medical university, and beds in medical colleges, to cater to patients referred from other services (Figure 5.2).

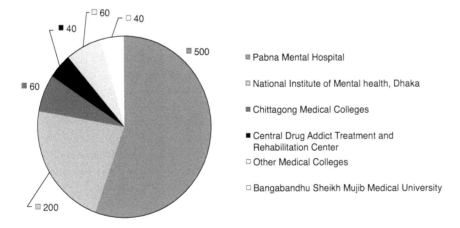

Figure 5.2 Distribution of psychiatric beds in public hospitals in Bangladesh

Expenditure in mental
health 0.44%

Other health expenditure
99.56%

Figure 5.3 Expenditure on mental health as a percentage of the total health budget in
Bangladesh.

Source: Based on W World Health Organization and Ministry of Health and Family Welfare Bangladesh. *WHO–AIMS
report on mental health system in Bangladesh: A report of the assessment of the mental health system in Bangladesh using
the World Health Organization – Assessment Instrument for Mental Health Systems (WHO–AIMS)*. Dhaka: World Health
Organization, 2007. http://www.who.int/mental_health/bangladesh_who_aims_report.pdf.

Funding

The budget for health care including mental health in Bangladesh is very inadequate. According
to the WHO-AIMS report on mental health system in Bangladesh (2007), only 0.44 percent
of the total health budget was allocated to mental health (Figure 5.3). Most patients have to
pay out of their own pocket. The cheapest antipsychotic drug is Taka 5.00 (US$0.07) per day
and the cheapest antidepressant is Taka 3.00 (US$0.04) per day. No formal health insurance is
offered by the government.

Lack of awareness

In common with many low and middle income countries, social inequalities play a role in mental
health and knowledge of psychiatric disorders in Bangladesh, and the resulting stigma attached
to such disorders is extremely high. Though the level of mass education is improving and rising
day by day, awareness about mental health remains very poor indeed with stereotypical images
and attitudes which have to be challenged. Myths about mental disorders, such as mental illness
being caused by black magic, the evil eye or evil spirits, continue to persist along with old-
fashioned views like: masturbation can cause mental illness and generalized weakness, marriage
can cure mental illness, and mental illness can be cured by taking holy water and wearing a
sacred locket (*Tabij*). It is important that professional and government initiatives be developed
to educate both the policy makers and the population in general.

Liaison psychiatry: a novel approach

As mentioned above, in common with rest of the world the first port of call in the professional sector for patients in Bangladesh is the primary care physician or other medical specialist, rather than psychiatrists either in the public or private sectors. Some patients will have seen religious healers as the first point of help. Owing to poor sanitation and infections, organic causes of psychiatric disorders are common, as is epilepsy. More importantly, however, patients may present with physical symptoms such as headache, general bodily aches and pains, feelings of tiredness, weakness, and functional symptoms affecting several organs or systems which are vague in nature for which they may be investigated excessively and often unnecessarily. Often depression and/or anxiety are at the root of these complaints, sometimes combined with substance abuse. Inevitably patients will be seen repeatedly by medical specialists and their underlying psychological disorder will be ignored with the focus remaining on somatic manifestations in the specialist's field of expertise.

It is also highly likely that many patients with physical illness will have psychiatric morbidity which gets ignored in medical clinics. For example, patients with chronic physical conditions such as diabetes, hypertension or chronic arthritis may also suffer from anxiety or depression which will need to be treated in its own right.

As mentioned above, the treatment gap for psychiatric conditions is huge. As long ago as 1978 a cross-sectional study conducted in an urban area (Dhaka city) showed that 29 percent of patients had existing psychiatric morbidity but they sought treatment from medical specialists. Between 30 and 40 percent of patients attending general practitioners, specialists and primary health centers have mental illness but they present with physical complaints. Their treatment may be inadequate and incomplete as far as psychiatric conditions are concerned, thus highlighting perhaps an inadequate level of training in the mental health aspects of medical diagnoses at both undergraduate and postgraduate levels.

Consultation–liaison psychiatry can prove to be helpful in these circumstances but inadequate training and low numbers of clinicians in the field make this extremely difficult. Training and educational packages teaching diagnostic and management strategies and appropriate skills may prove to be extremely helpful in primary care as well as non-psychiatric secondary care. Such an approach will improve therapeutic engagement and outcomes.

Training in mental health: multidisciplinary issues

Undergraduate training

Four percent of the training of medical doctors at the undergraduate level is devoted to mental health, whereas it is even less for nurses at 2 percent and primary health care workers receive none. This is obviously inadequate; mental health training needs to be increased and included for all health care professionals. This situation is beginning to change slowly, as within the last seven years primary health care workers, paramedics and opinion leaders have been trained by the National Institute of Mental Health in common mental health problems, psychosocial care after disasters and autism.

Postgraduate training

Postgraduate training facilities are limited to tertiary care hospitals. Three types of postgraduate course are offered to graduate doctors: Fellowship in Psychiatry (FCPS) by the Bangladesh College of Physicians and Surgeons; a Residency Program in Psychiatry (Doctor of Medicine, MD) by Bangabandhu Sheikh Mujib Medical University, Dhaka; and a Master of Philosophy (MPhil) in Psychiatry by medical colleges. The Fellowship and Residency require five years' intensive training, and the MPhil requires two years of training.

Training for general physicians and other health professionals

Although within the last few years about 7,000 general physicians and about 4,000 nurses and other health professionals have been trained in basic identification, diagnosis and management of mental disorders, this is not yet universal. Over a dozen training manuals have been published and made available, and these are also being used by other South East Asian countries. After a short training course general physicians are expected to be able to:

- Set standards of clinical care based on modern psychiatric principles.
- Carry out specialized treatment of patients referred by other specialist colleagues as well as from other referral sources.
- Provide clinical support and supervision to staff.
- Actively participate in teaching, training and curriculum development in mental health.
- Encourage and actively participate in mental health education of the community.
- Carry out research in mental health.

Mental health – development and future prospects

The development of mental health in Bangladesh can be summarized as follows (see also Figure 5.4):

- 1957: Establishment of country's first mental hospital in Pabna district.
- 1979: Postgraduate courses (MPhil, FCPS) in psychiatry started.
- 1981: Establishment of National Institute of Mental Health which took over 20 years to function fully.
- 2001: Postgraduate qualification in psychiatry (MD in Psychiatry) introduced.
- 2003–2012: Baseline data on mental health generated by national survey on mental disorders; community survey on child mental health; estimation and recognition of treatment gap in epilepsy; and other research.
- 2014: Finalization of the draft Mental Health Act, Bangladesh.
- 2021: Integration of mental health service in primary health care.

Folk therapies

Folk therapies for mental disorders are popular in Bangladesh. This may reflect the explanatory models used by patients and their families but a lack of access to professional services also makes such an option attractive. There are several indigenous treatment models for mental health in Bangladesh like the spiritual method, and Kabiraj, Unani, Ayurvedic, Djinn (evil spirits) treatments, etc. A large number of people, especially from rural backgrounds, seek these methods and many use modern medical treatments and indigenous treatments simultaneously. But awareness about mental health is increasing rapidly and these folk therapies are becoming less popular. Legislation has been put into place against malpractice and harmful practices, and general education is playing a role in eradicating harmful folk therapies. A special training and

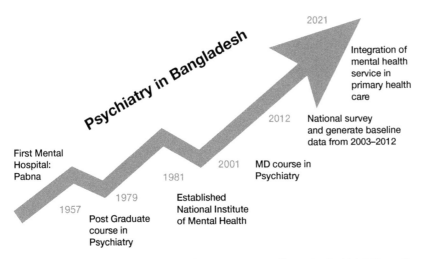

Figure 5.4 Psychiatry in Bangladesh: future prospects (figure by Dr Helal Ahmed)

awareness program is also being provided by the National Institute of Mental Health for folk healers.

e-health program

Bangladesh has entered a new era of technology in the past five years. Greater use and acceptance of technology has led to increasing technological support for the health care delivery system. The e-health program is ongoing for maternal and child health. Plans are being developed to incorporate an e-health program for mental health as part of which it is proposed that the community clinics or Upazila health complexes will act as satellite centers equipped with web cameras, internet and cell phones, while the tertiary care hospitals like the National Institute of Mental Health or Bangabandhu Sheikh Mujib Medical University will act as supporting centers with round-the-clock psychiatric services. This e-mental health system will have major advantages in increasing access to services while supervising staff from a distance, cutting travel costs and ensuring that quality services are available. As Bangladesh has a very limited number of psychiatrists and most of them work in tertiary care hospitals, people in remote areas have no easy direct access to them, and for this reason a suitable e-mental health program will be very effective and justified.

Conclusions

There is little doubt that Bangladesh has numerous challenges to overcome in ensuring universal delivery of mental health services with limited resources; however, some of these challenges can be easily overcome by a number of initiatives to reduce the mental health treatment gap. This may be achieved by increasing the number of trained mental health professionals, creating awareness about mental health among the public to reduce stigma, and utilizing e-mental health options. The involvement of government and nongovernmental agencies can bring about this desired change.

Bibliography

Alam MN. Psychiatric morbidity in general practice. *Bangladesh Medical Research Council Bulletin*, 1978; 4:38–42.

Ali, AMM Shawkat. *Politics and land system in Bangladesh*, Dhaka: National Institute of Local Government, 1986.

Bhugra D. The colonized psyche: British influence on Indian psychiatry, in D Bhugra and R Littlewood (eds) *Colonialism and psychiatry*, New Delhi: Oxford University Press, 2001, pp. 46–76.

Chowdhury, Subrata Roy. *The genesis of Bangladesh: A study in international legal norms and permissive conscience*, Asia Publishing House, 1972.

Curriculum for Fellowship in Psychiatry (FCPS), Bangladesh College of Physicians and Surgeons, 2008.

Curriculum for Residency Program in Psychiatry (Doctor of Medicine – MD), Bangabandhu Sheikh Mujib Medical University, 2010.

Curriculum for the Medical Graduation (MBBS-Curriculum), Directorate of Health Services, Bangladesh.

Daily ProthomAlo, 12 April 2010.

Fact Sheet: Published by the National Institute of Mental Health, Dhaka, Bangladesh.

Firoz AHM, Karim ME, Alam MF, Rahman AHMM, Zaman MM. Prevalence, medical care, awareness and attitude towards mental illness in Bangladesh. *Bangladesh Journal of Psychiatry*, June 2006; 20(1):9–36.

http://en.wikipedia.org/wiki/Economy_of_Bangladesh#cite_note-CIAFactbook-2012-02-05-1.

http://www.who.int/gho/countries/bgd.pdf.

Islam MM, Ali M, Ferroni P, Underwood P, Alam MF. Prevalence of psychiatric disorders in an urban community in Bangladesh. *General Hospital Psychiatry*, September–October 2003; 353–7.

Mechanic D. Barriers to help-seeking, detection, and adequate treatment for anxiety and mood disorders: implications for health care policy. *Journal of Clinical Psychiatry*, 2007; 68(Suppl. 2):20–6.

Ministry of Health and Family Welfare – Bangladesh, National Institute of Mental Health, World Health Organization – Bangladesh, *Integration of mental health services with primary health care in Bangladesh*, 2011.

National Institute of Mental Health, Bangladesh. *Integration of mental health services with primary health care in Bangladesh*, October 2011.

Rabbani MG, Alam MF, Ahmed HU et al. Prevalence of mental disorders, mental retardation, epilepsy and substance abuse in children, *Bangladesh Journal of Psychiatry*, June 2009; 23(1):11–53.

Saraceno B, van Ommeren M, Batniji R et al. Barriers to improvement of mental health services in low-income and middle-income countries. *The Lancet*, 2007; 370(9593):1164–74.

Bangladesh Bureau of Statistics (BBS). *Statistical yearbook of Bangladesh – 2012*. http://www.bbs.gov.bd/home.aspx.

World Health Organization. *Mental health atlas 2011*. Geneva: World Health Organization, 2011.

World Health Organization, Regional Office for South-East Asia. *Report of the informal consultation on strengthening mental health systems through community-based approaches*. Bali, 19–22 December 2010. New Delhi: WHOSEARO, 2011.

World Health Organization. *The world health report 2001 – Mental health: New understanding, new hope*. Geneva: World Health Organization, 2001.

World Health Organization and Ministry of Health and Family Welfare Bangladesh. *WHO-AIMS report on mental health system in Bangladesh: A report of the assessment of the mental health system in Bangladesh using the World Health Organization – Assessment Instrument for Mental Health Systems (WHO-AIMS)*. Dhaka: World Health Organization, 2007. http://www.who.int/mental_health/bangladesh_who_aims_report.pdf.

6

Mental health report for Bhutan

Arun Kandasamy and Pooja H. Shetty

Demographics

Bhutan is located in South Central Asia. The capital city is Thimphu and the currency is the Ngultrum. The main language used in the country is Dzongkha, and the main ethnic group are the 'Drukpa', of mixed Tibetan and Bhutanese origin. Religious groups include Buddhists and Hindus.

Bhutan consists of 20 administrative districts called Dzongkhags (Pelzang, 2012). Bhutan covers an area of 47,000 square kilometres and has a population of 708,484. According to World Bank 2010 criteria, Bhutan is a lower-middle-income country. The Health budget is 5.5 per cent of total Gross Domestic Product (WHO, 2011).

Gross National Happiness (GNH), as a philosophy and concept was first articulated in Bhutan by the Fourth King, His Majesty Jigme Singye Wangchuck in 1972 and proposed a unique objective measure of Quality of Life. The concept was operationalized in the form of the GNH Index. This has nine dimensions and 33 indicators. The 33 indicators are grouped under the following dimensions (Ura *et al.*, 2012a):

1.	Psychological well-being,	4
2.	Health,	4
3.	Time use,	2
4.	Education,	4
5.	Cultural diversity and resilience,	4
6.	Good governance,	4
7.	Community vitality,	4
8.	Ecological diversity and resilience,	4
9.	Living standards	3
Total		33

In a 2010 survey developed by the Centre for Bhutan Studies, the GNH Index value is 0.743 and shows that overall, 40.9 per cent of Bhutanese are identified as happy (meaning they are extensively or deeply happy), and the remaining 59.1 per cent enjoy sufficiency in 56.6 per cent of the domains on average (Ura *et al.*, 2012b).

Mental health and mental illness in Bhutan

Between 1999 and 2001 records from the tertiary care Jigme Dorji Wangchuck National Referral Hospital in Thimphu, showed that over 1,500 patients with psychiatric disorders were treated. Forty per cent had depression and 31 per cent had anxiety and stress-related disorders, with epilepsy at 8 per cent and alcohol disorders at 7 per cent. Psychosis is relatively rare compared to depression and anxiety.

In 2002, the first pilot survey was carried out in three regions of Bhutan. The study, covering a population of 45,000, showed the prevalence of mental illness as less than 1 per cent, broken down as 25 per cent epilepsy, 18 per cent depression, 14 per cent mental retardation, 6 per cent psychosis, 6 per cent suicide and a high comorbidity of alcohol dependence (30 per cent) (Dorji, 2004). The number of new cases of mental disorders recorded as being treated at the National Referral Hospital (NRH) was 2,846 in the year 2008.

Neuropsychiatric-condition-related DALYs (Disability Adjusted Life Years) were 19 per cent, coming second only to cardiovascular diseases (22 per cent) in the overall contribution of non-communicable diseases (62 per cent) to DALYs (Engelgau et al., 2011).

Table 6.1 Data on prevalence of mental illness in Bhutan

Common diagnoses	Outpatient facilities (%)	Community-based inpatient units (%)
Substance abuse		27
Mood disorders	22	32
Neurotic disorders	17	12
Schizophrenia	5	19
Others	54	10

(courtesy: WHO–AIMS, 2007)

Alcohol and drug use in Bhutan

Being socially acceptable, alcohol use is high in Bhutanese society. Local alcohol includes homemade wines such as *bangchang, sinchang* and *tongba*, and *Ara* which is a home-distilled spirit (Dorji, 2007). With development, Bhutan has thrown open its borders to the import and export of alcohol and is home to over 3,000 licensed bars. According to leading psychiatrist Chencho Dorji, prevalence studies show a high rate of alcohol use in Bhutanese society, and 20 per cent drink regularly with an average of five bottles of alcohol per week. He has suggested population-based approaches to curtail alcohol supply and demand, which would go a long way in preventing the adverse effect that alcohol is beginning to have on Gross National Happiness (Dorji, 2007).

According to traffic police reports, the most common cause of deaths due to road traffic accidents is alcohol use. Evaluation of deaths in medical wards (between the years 2001 and 2003) found that 30 per cent were alcohol-related (Dorji, 2004, 2007).

Bhutan banned tobacco products in 2004. A mental health survey in 2002 showed that 20 per cent of respondents were using nicotine. Following the ban, smoking significantly reduced (Dorji, 2004). For other drugs, there are informal reports of abuse, predominantly prescription drugs and inhalation of solvents.

Health system in Bhutan

Health services are provided completely through the public sector in Bhutan. The total number of hospital beds is 1,078 and there are 145 medical doctors in service (Dorji, 2008). To provide primary care, there are 35 physician-based primary health care units (29 district hospitals and six Basic Health Units, Grade 1) and 170 non-physician-based primary health care clinics or Basic Health Units. All these units are associated with traditional medicine practices provided by the government.

The majority of physician-based primary health care units, unlike non-physician-based units, have assessment and treatment protocols for key mental illnesses. These units have interactions with mental health professionals and send referrals to tertiary care. Health workers at these units are allowed to prescribe, though only the psychotropics that the government has made available freely at these clinics.

There are 63 mental health outpatient clinics, all integrated with inpatient facilities, and one day-care facility in the country. There are 63 community-based community psychiatry inpatient units with an approximate total of 100 beds. These beds are in general hospitals and made available for patients with psychiatric illnesses. The majority of patients are treated in outpatient settings and admissions are significantly lower.

There is no separate psychiatric facility for children and adolescents. Forensic patients do not have a separate facility and are treated in police custody. There are no mental hospitals or community-based residential facilities for psychiatric patients in Bhutan.

As of 2006 there were two psychiatrists (0.29 per 100,000 population) and 100 doctors and 370 nurses, not specialized in psychiatry. Per bed, in community-based psychiatric inpatient units, there are 0.01 psychiatrists, 0.33 medical doctors, 3.7 nurses and 1.70 support staff. There are no psychologists, psychosocial workers or occupational therapists (WHO–AIMS, 2007).

Table 6.2 Mental health care service delivery in Bhutan (adapted from WHO–AIMS, 2007)

Facilities	Personnel
35 Physician-based PHUs	1 Psychiatrist
170 Non-physician-based PHUs	3 Psychiatric nurses
63 Mental health OP clinics and Community IP units	No psychologists, psychiatric social workers or occupational therapists
1 Day-care facility at tertiary care general hospital	PHU doctors, nurses and health workers receive refresher training in mental health
No psychiatric facility	
All PHUs are integrated with traditional medicine/indigenous units	
No medical college	145 doctors in Bhutan, including specialists

PHU: Primary health care unit; OP: Outpatient; IP: Inpatient

Plans and policies for mental health

A National Mental Health Programme (NMHP) was initiated in 1997 under the Eighth Five Year Plan, with the primary focus on community mental health care. Currently, most patients are receiving treatment for mental illnesses at a tertiary centre due to lack of trained personnel in primary health care centres. A comprehensive mental health plan was framed in 1997 that includes specific goals, a time frame and budget plan for the delivery of mental health care services (WHO, 2007). The components are community mental health services, integration into primary care, resources, consumer participation, advocacy, financing, quality improvement and a monitoring system. There is no separate law/act for mental health or any human rights policies for the mentally ill.

From the essential drug list, at the least one drug from each of the classes of psychotropics has been made available at treatment facilities, making them free of cost to patients. All mental disorders are covered by social insurance schemes.

The National Mental Health Authority is the regulatory and supervisory body for instituting the mental health plan. The Information and Communication Bureau of the Ministry of Health is in charge of public education and awareness programmes.

School-based counsellors and health educators conduct activities to promote mental health in schools. Funds have been allotted to the mental health programme in the Tenth Five Year Plan (2008–2013). The important points on the agenda are:

- Increasing the manpower: training psychiatrists, psychologists, psychiatric social workers, occupational therapists, psychiatric nurses, and drug and alcohol counsellors.
- To open electroconvulsive therapy units and a drug and alcohol treatment detoxification and rehabilitation centre.
- Development of training programmes and frequent refresher training in mental health.
- Increasing the number of psychiatric beds.
- Improving information, education and communication activities.

Training

There are no medical colleges in Bhutan, so Bhutan must send candidates to neighbouring countries such as Bangladesh, India, Myanmar and Sri Lanka for their MBBS courses.

The degree of training that a medical doctor receives in mental health during their undergraduate course is unclear and varies widely. All primary health care doctors receive two-day refresher training in mental health. Nine per cent of medical training for nurses and 10 per cent for non-doctor/non-nurse primary health care workers is devoted to mental illnesses. They also receive refresher training. Health workers receive more refresher training as they work independently to provide services in the community.

Traditional medicine and mental health

Traditional medicine is popular in Bhutan and is usually the first point of contact in the health care system for patients. A study that looked at the extent of religious practice associated with illness and hospitalization found that 92.5 per cent of inpatients at a referral hospital ($n=106$) felt that religious care facilities should be available at hospitals (Pelzang, 2010). Though it is not possible to generalize, this section gives an overview of the role of religion and tradition in health care. The Buddhist system of medicine known as *gSo-BA Rig-PA* that is currently practised in Bhutan, Tibet and Mongolia is 2,500 years old and it entails the use of over 2,200 traditional prescription drugs. This system follows the principle that imbalance of one of the three elements of *rLung* (Air), *mKhris-pa* (Bile) and *Bad-kan* (Phlegm) causes illness, and it also follows the Buddhist philosophy that all suffering is caused by ignorance. Hence, treatment interventions involve not only herbal medicines, physiotherapy and minor surgery but also spiritual healing (Wangchuk *et al.*, 2007). There are also local healing practices that are not formalized. Recognizing the need for integration of traditional medicine into so-called modern medical practice, Traditional Medicine Units are now associated with hospitals and Basic Health Units to provide care. These units function under the supervision of the Institute of Traditional Medicine Services (ITMS) (Wangchuk, 2008). This has been recognized by the World Health Organization as an important way of providing primary health care services.

The way forward

From review of the existing literature, it is clear that Bhutan has well-integrated traditional and modern medicine systems that are acceptable and accessible to its people. With increasing awareness about mental illness, and studies showing the prevalence of mental illness in Bhutanese society, this system of health care services may cater well to patients with mental illness in the community. There is a need for increased training, increased manpower and increased funding for mental health care services. The funds allocated to the mental health programme in the Tenth Five Year Plan (2008–2013) take all this into account, and if successfully implemented will go a long way towards overcoming the deficits in resources.

There is a need also for more research on mental illness – its prevalence, phenomenology, cultural presentations, explanatory models, comorbidities, disability and treatment interventions. The method of combining traditional practices with so-called modern medicine, and with treatment interventions in line with Buddhist spiritual philosophies is another unique area for research. The effect of mental illness on the concept of Gross National Happiness would be another interesting area of research and might throw light on the burden of mental illness in Bhutanese society. The world as a whole is moving towards de-centralization, and while this country nestled in the Himalayas woke to the need for mental health care services just over a decade ago, this service was born with a community-based approach. Slowly though steadily, Bhutan has risen to the challenge of caring for the mentally ill.

Acknowledgment

We thank Dr Chencho Dorji for sending three weblinks to articles that he wrote on mental health in Bhutan, and allowing us to use and quote them in this chapter.

References

Dorji C (2004) Achieving Gross National happiness through community-based mental health services in Bhutan, *Gross National Happiness and Development*, Proceedings of the First International Conference on Operationalization of Gross National Happiness, pp. 599–627. Available from: http://archiv.ub.uni-heidelberg.de/savifadok/volltexte/2010/1358.

Dorji C (2007) The myth behind alcohol happiness, *Rethinking Development*, Proceedings of Second International Conference on Gross National Happiness, Centre for Bhutan Studies, Thimphu, pp. 64–77. Available from: www.bhutanstudies.org.bt/rethinking-development/.

Dorji C (2008) Bhutanese health care reform: a paradigm shift in health care to increase Gross National Happiness, *Gross National Happiness: Practice and Measurement*, Proceedings of the Fourth International Conference on Gross National Happiness, Centre for Bhutan Studies, Thimphu, pp. 413–36. Available from: http://archiv.ub.uni-heidelberg.de/savifadok/volltexte/2013/2642.

Engelgau MM, El-Saharty S, Kudesia P, Rajan V and Rosenhouse PS (2011) Capitalizing on the demographic transition: tackling non communicable diseases in South Asia, World Bank. Available from: http://go.worldbank.org/92XR19LUC0.

Pelzang R (2010) Religious practice of the patients and families during illness and hospitalization in Bhutan, *Journal of Bhutan Studies*, 22: 77–97.

Pelzang R (2012) Mental health care in Bhutan: policy and issues, *WHO South-East Asia Journal of Public Health*, 1(3): 339–46.

Tenth Five Year Plan (2008–2013) Volume 2: *Programme profile, 2009*, Royal Government of Bhutan, Gross National Happiness Commission.

Ura Karma, Alkire Sabina, ZangmoTshoki and Wangdi Karma (2012a) *A short guide to Gross National Happiness Index*, Centre for Bhutan Studies, Thimphu. Available from: www.grossnationalhappiness.com/wp-content/uploads/2012/04/Short-GNH-Index-edited.pdf (accessed 28 February 2014).

Ura Karma, Alkire Sabina, ZangmoTshoki and Wangdi Karma (2012b) An extensive analysis of GNH Index, Centre for Bhutan Studies, Thimphu. Available from: www.grossnationalhappiness.com/wp-content/uploads/2012/10/An%20Extensive%20Analysis%20of%20GNH%20Index.pdf (accessed 28 February 2014).

Wangchuk P (2008) Health impacts of traditional medicines and bio-prospecting: a world scenario accentuating Bhutan's perspective, *Journal of Bhutan Studies*, 18: 116–34.

Wangchuk P, Wangchuk D and Aagaard-Hansen J (2007) Traditional Bhutanese medicine (*gSo-BA Rig-PA*): an integrated part of the formal health care services, *Southeast Asian Journal of Tropical Medicine and Public Health*, 38(1): 161–7.

WHO–AIMS (2007) Report on Mental Health System in Bhutan, WHO and Ministry of Health, Thimphu, Bhutan. Available from: www.healthinternetwork.com/mental_health/who_aims_country_reports/en/.

World Health Organization (2011) *Mental Health Atlas 2011*. Available from: www.who.int/mental_health/publications/mental_health_atlas_2011/en/.

Additional resource

Tobgyay T, Dorji T, Pelzom D and Gibbons RV (2011) Progress and delivery of health care in Bhutan, the Land of the Thunder Dragon and Gross National Happiness, *Tropical Medicine & International Health*, 16: 731–6.

7

Mental health in India I

Epidemiology, services and health systems

Santosh K. Chaturvedi and T. Sivakumar

Introduction

India is the seventh largest country in the world with an approximate area of 3.3 million square kilometers. With a population of more than 1.2 billion, India is the second most populous country in the world. Every sixth person in the world is an Indian. Based on 2010 World Bank criteria, India belongs to the lower-middle-income group. It is a Himalayan task to organize mental health services for the diverse predominantly rural population. Economic constraints, scarcity of trained mental health professionals, 'brain drain', stigma and bureaucracy compound the problem (Thara *et al.*, 2004).

Country geography

India has immense diversity in geography, languages, and social and cultural practices. The Indian peninsula is separated from mainland Asia by the Himalayas. The country is surrounded by the Bay of Bengal to the east, the Arabian Sea to the west, and the Indian Ocean to the south. The mainland comprises four regions, namely the great mountain zone, the plains of the Ganga and the Indus, the desert region and the southern peninsula.

India's history and culture span back to the beginning of human civilization. Harappan civilization along the Indus River has been documented dating back to 2,500 BC. India has integrated people who have migrated from the diverse cultures surrounding it. All the five major racial types (Australoid, Mongoloid, Europoid, Caucasian and Negroid) are represented in the Indian population (National Portal of India, 2014).

Hinduism (80 percent) is the most commonly practiced religion followed by Islam (13 percent), Christianity, Sikhism, Buddhist, Jainism and others (National Portal of India, 2014). The Indian constitution recognizes 22 different languages out of which Hindi is an Official Language (National Portal of India, 2014). English continues to be used for official purposes.

India has a federal system of governance consisting of Central Government, 28 states and seven union territories (National Portal of India, 2014). India has a predominantly young population with 37 percent being under the age of 18 years (WHO, 2011). The proportion above 60 is 5 percent. The literacy rate is 82 percent for men and 66 percent for women (National Portal of India, 2014). The life expectancy at birth is 65.8 years for males and 68.1 years for females (National Portal of India, 2014).

Psychiatric epidemiology

According to the National Commission on Macroeconomics and Health, about 80 million people will need care for various mental disorders in all age groups by 2015 (Ministry of Health and Family Welfare, Government of India, 2005). The treatment gap is as high as 70–80 percent (Ministry of Health and Family Welfare, Government of India., 2005). The suicide rate for males is 12.2 per 100,000 population and for females is 9.1 per 100,000 population (WHO, 2011).

Community-based epidemiological studies on mental and behavioral disorders show prevalence rates ranging from 9.5 to 102/1,000 population (Math and Srinivasaraju, 2010). This has been attributed to several factors like underreporting and differing 'case' definitions, diagnostic methods and sampling procedures (Math and Srinivasaraju, 2010).

A meta-analysis covering 33,572 persons in 6,550 families over 13 studies showed a prevalence of 58.2 per 1,000 population (Reddy and Chandrashekar, 1998).

Ganguli reviewed 15 regional representative psychiatric epidemiological studies and reported a national prevalence rate for 'all mental disorders' of 70.5 (rural), 73 (urban) and 73 (rural + urban) per 1,000 population (Ganguli, 2000; Gururaj et al., 2005). A conservative median estimate value of persons with mental and behavioral disorders of 65 per 1,000 population has been derived from the above mentioned studies (see Table 7.1).

Both studies report that prevalence of mental disorders in urban areas is higher: 2 times according to Reddy and Chandrashekar (1998); 1.6 times according to Ganguli (2000) than in rural areas.

Reddy and Chandrashekar (1998) reported that mental retardation and alcohol/drug addiction had higher prevalence among males, while affective disorders and neuroses had higher prevalence among females.

Table 7.1 Prevalence of psychiatric disorders in India

	Reddy and Chandrashekar (1998)	Ganguli (2000)
Prevalence of psychiatric disorders (per 1,000 population)	58.2	73.0
Rural prevalence of psychiatric disorders (per 1,000 population)	48.9	70.5
Urban prevalence of psychiatric disorders (per 1,000 population)	80.6	73.0
Prevalence of schizophrenia (per 1,000 population)	2.7	2.5
Prevalence of affective disorders (per 1,000 population)	12.3*	34.0
Prevalence of mental retardation (per 1,000 population)	6.9	5.3
Prevalence of hysteria (per 1,000 population)	4.5	3.3

* (excluding neurotic depression)

In an ICMR (Indian Council for Medical Research) multisite study on schizophrenia, prevalence rates ranged from 1.8/1,000 in Bangalore to 3.1/1,000 in Patiala (Gururaj *et al.*, 2005). The incidence rate for schizophrenia has been calculated to be 4/1,000 population (Gururaj *et al.*, 2005).

A world mental health survey initiative collected data using multistage household probability samples from 11 sites across India: Bangalore, Bhavnagar, Chandigarh, Dibrugarh, Faridabad, Imphal, Lucknow, Pondicherry, Pune, Ranchi and Tirupati. All interviews were carried out face-to-face by trained lay interviewers using WMH–CIDI. Disorders were assessed using ICD-10 and DSM-IV criteria. The results from the Indian sites are awaited.

A large-scale survey of psychiatric disorders is to be conducted by NIMHANS (National Institute for Mental Health and Neurosciences), Bangalore, throughout the country shortly.

Child psychiatry epidemiology

An ICMR-funded community epidemiological study on psychiatric disorders among the 0–16 years age group in Bangalore and Lucknow showed a lower prevalence of psychiatric disorders (about 12 percent) than similar studies conducted in the West. Other studies conducted in school children revealed a lower prevalence (Table 7.2). In school children, teachers' rating of psychiatric disorders was higher than parents' rating (Malhotra *et al.*, 2002). The most common diagnosis was enuresis in all studies.

Substance abuse epidemiology

The epidemiology of substance abuse in India has been studied by national household surveys (NHS), drug abuse monitoring systems (DAMS) and rapid assessment surveys (RAS) (Ray and Chopra, 2012).

Table 7.2 Prevalence of child psychiatric disorders in India

Study	Site	Sample size	Age group	Results
Hackett *et al.*, 1999	Calicut	1,403	8–12 years Community	9.4% prevalence
PGIMER (Malhotra and Pradhan, 2013; Malhotra *et al.*, 2002, 2009; Shah *et al.*, 2005)	Chandigarh	963	4–11 years School children	At baseline, 6.33% prevalence Annual incidence rate of disorders 18/1,000/year
NIMHANS (Srinath *et al.*, 2005)	Bangalore	2,064	0–16 years Community (rural + urban)	12.5% prevalence among 0–16 years age group 13.8% prevalence among 0–3 years age group 12% among 4–16 years age group
KGMC (Shah *et al.*, 2005)	Lucknow	2,325	0–16 years Community (rural + urban)	12.1% prevalence in 0–16 years age group

Table 7.3 Prevalence of substance use in India

Drug type	Current prevalence (%)	Prevalence (in millions)	Dependence (ICD-10) (%)
Alcohol	21.4	62.5	16.8
Cannabis	3.0	8.7	25.7
Heroin	0.2	2.0	22.3
Opium	0.4		
Other opiates	0.1		

A national household survey, the first nationwide survey to determine the prevalence of licit and illicit drug use was conducted on a sample of 40,697 males aged 12–60 years drawn from 25 states (Ray, 2004). Data were collected by trained interviewers from March 2000 to November 2001 and the diagnosis of dependence was established using ICD-10 criteria (Ray, 2004). The results are shown in Table 7.3. Among drug users, 22.3 percent were poly drug users (Ray, 2004).

Over the last few decades, there has been an increase in pharmaceutical drug abuse (including prescription opioids and inhalants) (Ray and Chopra, 2012; Basu *et al.*, 2012). An increasing number of patients have sought treatment for opiate dependence in recent years (Ray and Chopra, 2012). Experts have emphasized the need for a national drug abuse monitoring system (Ray and Chopra, 2012).

Geriatric age group/mental illness among the elderly

With increased life expectancy, the proportion of older adults is projected to increase from 7.5 percent (in 2006) to 12.4 percent (in 2026) (Tiwari and Pandey, 2012). The prevalence of DSM-IV dementia in rural India has been found to be 0.3 percent (Llibre Rodriguez *et al.*, 2008). The 10/66 dementia research group studied prevalence of DSM-IV dementia in urban Chennai (0.9 percent) and rural Vellore (0.8 percent) in Tamil Nadu (Prince, 2009). An ICMR epidemiological study conducted in rural and urban Lucknow found that 17.3 percent of urban and 23.6 percent of rural older adults aged 60 years and above suffer from syndromal mental health problems and 4.2 percent of urban and 2.5 percent of rural older adults suffer from sub-syndromal mental health problems (Tiwari and Pandey, 2012).

Services available, mental health systems, patterns of referral, funding and the indigenous service delivery model

Services available

Traditionally, mental health services were provided by faith healers and religious bodies. Ayurvedic literature speaks about mental illness and remedies.

Allopathic mental health services are provided by the government, NGOs and a booming private sector. They provide outpatient and inpatient services. Mental hospitals with closed and open wards have existed from pre-independence days. General hospital psychiatry units have played an important role in expanding the reach of mental health services to the population. Private psychiatry has surged over the last few decades in private hospitals, clinics and corporate hospitals.

Table 7.4 Data on availability of mental health facilities in India (WHO, 2011)

	Total number of facilities/beds	Rate per 100,000 population
Mental health outpatient facilities	4,000	0.329
Psychiatric beds in general hospitals	10,000	0.823
Mental hospitals	43	0.004
Beds in mental hospitals	17,835	1.469

Mental hospitals

Most psychiatric beds are confined to large custodial mental health hospitals which cater to a limited population (Table 7.4). There are 43 state-run mental hospitals in the country (Sinha and Kaur, 2011). Deficits in staffing and infrastructure have been a major issue. In its 1998 review, the National Human Rights Commission found mental hospitals to be highly unsatisfactory. They were criticized for their jail-like structures without basic amenities in many instances.

Following an initial review, funds were provided to mental hospitals. A subsequent review showed positive changes (Nagaraja and Murthy, 2008). However, many posts have remained vacant despite creation of new positions. Recently, the National Human Rights Commission moved the supreme court to ensure that the government allocates adequate resources for mental hospitals (Venkatesan, 2013).

According to the WHO India Mental Health Profile 2011 (WHO, 2011), the admission rate to mental hospitals is 14.52 per 100,000 population. The majority of patients (62 percent) in mental hospitals stay for less than a year (WHO, 2011). About 14 percent of patients stay for more than 5 years (WHO, 2011). Data pertaining to outpatient treatment in mental hospitals are not available.

General hospital psychiatric units

The first general hospital psychiatric unit (GHPU) was established at R. G. Kar Medical college in 1933 (Agarwal, 2004). There has been a dramatic increase in GHPUs since the 1960s, which also paved the way for consultation liaison psychiatry. The GHPU units attached to the medical colleges throughout the country provide services closer to the community with less stigma. GHPUs provide both outpatient and inpatient services. They mainly provide open ward facilities where patients are admitted in the company of family members.

As per norms set up by the Medical Council of India, all medical colleges have a department of psychiatry. With the proliferation of private medical colleges across the country, their faculty and infrastructure can potentially offer accessible and affordable psychiatric services to the masses (Thirunavukarasu, 2011).

Private clinics

Private sector psychiatrist services are mainly concentrated in urban areas. Mostly they are run by a psychiatrist who provides outpatient services. Some of them also offer inpatient services in hospitals which are tightly regulated. They offer diagnostic services and pharmacologically oriented management. Though expensive, they have helped in taking mental health services closer to the population. Some corporate hospitals also have outpatient and inpatient psychiatry services.

Indigenous medicine

Besides psychiatric practice according to modern medical practice, many other systems of health care are prevalent. These are based on scientific and systematic methods like ayurveda, siddha, unani, homeopathy and naturopathy.

Ancient Indian texts by Charaka and Vagbhatta describe the phenomenology of mental illnesses and their classification (Neki, 1973). Some mental disorders are considered as disease processes while others are attributed to supernatural powers or unfavorable stellar positions (Neki, 1973).

Ayurvedic practitioners have used *Rauwolfia serpentina* for hundreds of years to treat insanity (*oonmad* in sanskrit). Its tranquilizing effects were reported by Sen and Bose in 1931 (Bhatara *et al.*, 1997). Reserpine was isolated from *Rauwolfia serpentine* in 1952 and used subsequently in psychotic patients (Kline, 1954). There is increasing interest in investigating these treatments according to rigorous scientific methods (Patwardhan and Mashelkar, 2009).

Community-based programs

The National Mental Health Programme (NMHP) was implemented in 1982. Under the NMHP, community mental health services are provided through the District Mental Health Programme (DMHP) which integrates mental health care in primary care with supervision and support from a mental health team at the district level. DMHP performance has been unsatisfactory for various reasons, including a top-down prescriptive model, fragmentation of the mental health sector among different departments, lack of coordination, inadequate support from professionals, lack of monitoring and lack of awareness in the community (Murthy, 2011; Patel and Copeland, 2011). Innovations like Primary Health Centre-based rural mental health programs, general practitioner-based urban mental health programs, school-based mental health programs and home-based follow-up of psychiatric patients have not been consistently pursued (Agarwal, 2004). As of 2011, 127 districts were covered under the DMHP (Murthy, 2011).

Non-governmental organizations

Several non-governmental organizations (NGOs) play an important role in delivering psychiatric services (Patel and Thara, 2003). The Schizophrenia Research Foundation (Chennai), Richmond Fellowship Society (Bangalore, Delhi and Lucknow), Family Fellowship (Bangalore) and Medico-Pastoral Association (Bangalore) offer care to patients with chronic mental illness in different settings like outpatient care, daycare, halfway homes and long-stay homes. Sneha (Chennai) is involved in suicide intervention and runs a 24/7 suicide helpline (Vijaykumar, 2007). The Alzheimer's and Related Disorders Society of India (ARDSI) in Kerala, offers help to elderly people with mental health issues. Sangath (Goa) works on community-based rehabilitation, child mental health and treatment of common mental disorders (Chatterjee *et al.*, 2009; Patel *et al.*, 2010). Banyan (Chennai) and the Bapu Trust (Pune) work for homeless mentally ill women and provide community mental health services. T. T. Ranganathan Research Foundation (Chennai) works in the area of substance abuse/dependence. Self-help and support groups consisting largely of the families of people with mental illness (AMEND, Bangalore) have taken up advocacy at national and international level.

Traditional healers

The traditional healer is a multipurpose community leader who deals with all aspects of maladaptation in society. Different motivating factors have been described for seeking faith healing including cultural beliefs, inadequate level of recovery using modern psychiatric treatment and financial difficulties in obtaining medical treatment (Sethi *et al.*, 1977). People from lower socioeconomic strata, usually females, are a major part of the healers' clientele (Sethi *et al.*, 1977).

They are easily accessible and accepted by people who believe that they are gifted with magical powers. As they belong to the same community/socioeconomic background, this helps them comprehend patients' dialect/gestures when communicating symptoms (Trivedi and Sethi, 1979). They contribute a sizeable share of the private health sector.

Studies have revealed that a quarter of their clientele present with psychiatric problems. No consistent method has been reported in their approach to assessment and suggesting a remedy (Trivedi and Sethi, 1979). They utilize various indigenous precepts prevalent in the society. They may offer a variety of magical, religious and ritual suggestions (including witchcraft, sorcery, exorcism, prayer, penance, casting of spells, flogging), and dietary, herbal and biomedical interventions. They support clients' beliefs that their problem is due to external factors, which aids in recovery (Trivedi and Sethi, 1979).

Religious treatments

Some temples, mosques and churches are culturally inclined to offer cures to the mentally ill. Patients are engaged in rituals (bathing in the temple tank and circumambulating the temple) and prayers. The religious settings also offer shelter to patients left alone by their family. Some places have a better track record than others.

A study on temple healing showed that an affectionate and caring atmosphere lowered Brief Psychiatric Rating scale (BPRS) count without medication (Raguram et al., 2002). Religious settings have been reported to show benefits by mechanisms of role playing, imitation, identification, spontaneity, catharsis, therapeutic community, psychodrama and social modelling (Satija et al., 1981).

In an accidental fire in one such shelter in Erwadi (Tamil Nadu), 26 mentally ill patients who were chained were burned to death in August 2011 (Thara et al., 2004). There were calls to shut down all such institutions in the aftermath. It has been pointed out that such places exist because of a lack of feasible and effective alternatives, which need to be provided (Tharyan, 2008).

Mental health systems

Policy and plan

As of now, India has a mental health plan but does not have an officially approved mental health policy. However, mental health is specifically mentioned in the general health policy (WHO, 2011). The Ministry of Health and Family Welfare has appointed a policy group to prepare a mental health policy and plan (Mental Health Policy Group, 2011).

The mental health plan was revised in 2009 which included guidelines for the implementation of the mental health plan, funding, shifting services to the community and integrating mental health services into primary care.

In the Twelfth Five Year Plan, the Indian government is likely to include mental illnesses as non-communicable disorders and set national targets to reduce their incidence.

Legislation

The Mental Health Act (1987) and Persons with Disability Act (1995) have been revised. The Mental Health Care Bill (2013) and Right to Persons with Disability Act (2013) have been tabled in parliament. Both bills are in line with the United Nations Convention on the Rights of Persons with Disabilities. Both bills were prepared after consulting multiple stakeholders in an inclusive and transparent manner.

For the first time, Indian mental health legislation has defined mental illness as 'Mental illness means a disorder of mood, thought, perception, orientation, and memory which causes significant distress to a person or impairs a person's behaviour, judgment, and ability to recognize reality or impairs a person's ability to meet the demands of daily life and includes mental conditions associated with the abuse of alcohol and drugs, but does not include mental retardation' (Ministry of Health and Family Welfare, Government of India, 2013). The inclusion of alcohol and drug abuse is a welcome change.

There are several positive aspects to the revised Mental Health Care Bill (2013). The bill provides the right to access mental health care and treatment from mental health services run or funded by the appropriate government. If a particular district has no public mental health services, the individual has a right to access private services and get refunded. The bill mandates the government to provide essential psychotropic medications free of cost. The insurance companies cannot exclude mental illness and have to consider it on a par with physical illnesses.

A longstanding demand to decriminalize suicide has been incorporated in the bill (Sachan, 2013).

Though the bill has incorporated progressive principles like a 'mental health review commission' and 'advance directives', concerns have been raised whether Indian society and the mental health system is ready for them (Kala, 2013). Critics have pointed out that they are likely to create administrative bottlenecks which will be detrimental to patient treatment (Kala, 2013; Sachan, 2013).

The 2013 bill bans unmodified electroconvulsive therapy (ECT) (Ministry of Health and Family Welfare, Government of India, 2013). A position statement on unmodified ECT by the Indian Psychiatric Society recommends that unmodified ECT should not be used as a routine form of treatment but can be considered on a case-by-case basis when expected benefits outweigh the risks (Andrade et al., 2012). Examples of circumstances where unmodified ECT may be considered include emergency situations where anaesthesia facilities are not available or when there are medical contraindications to anesthesia (Andrade et al., 2012). The position statement clarifies that it is unacceptable to use unmodified ECT for convenience (Andrade et al., 2012).

According to the 2013 bill, ECT can be administered to minors only on a case-by-case basis after permission from a mental health review commission (Ministry of Health and Family Welfare, Government of India, 2013).

Human resources

There are more than 5,000 psychiatrists in the country though the exact number is difficult to ascertain. The average national deficit in psychiatrists is 77 percent. Psychiatrists are mainly concentrated in urban areas. Currently, India has the training infrastructure to produce approximately 320 psychiatrists, 50 clinical psychologists, 25 psychiatric social workers and 185 psychiatric nurses per year (Sinha and Kaur, 2011) (Table 7.5).

To address the shortage of mental health professionals, 11 centers of excellence in mental health, 120 postgraduate departments in mental health specialties (MD/DPM/DNB in psychiatry, MPhil/PhD in clinical psychology, MPhil/PhD in psychiatric social work, Diploma/MSc in psychiatric nursing), upgrading of medical college psychiatric wings and modernization of state-run mental hospitals will be supported under the Eleventh Five Year Plan (Sinha and Kaur, 2011).

Patterns of referral

In India, substantial numbers of patients suffering from mental disorders seek non-professional care (Chadda et al., 2001). Several studies in different parts of India have shown that faith healers

Table 7.5 Workforce and training in India (WHO, 2011)

	Health professionals working in the mental health sector (rate per 100,000)	Training of health professions in educational institutions (rate per 100,000)
Psychiatrists	0.301	0.0364
Nurses	0.166	0.016
Psychologists	0.047	0.010
Social workers	0.033	0.003

are the first care providers for many psychiatric patients (Jain *et al.*, 2012; Lahariya *et al.*, 2010; Trivedi and Jilani, 2011).

In India, various factors have been implicated in delaying initiation of treatment, including cultural myths, magico-religious models of psychiatric illness, availability/accessibility of mental health services, stigma of mental illness and accommodation of untreated mentally ill patients in extended family groups (Trivedi and Jilani, 2011). Early engagement with psychiatric services can improve prognosis by shortening the duration of untreated illness.

In contrast to pathways to care in mental illness, more than 90 percent of patients attending a de-addiction center were self-referred (Kattimani *et al.*, 2013).

Further research is needed to delineate psychiatric pathways of care and their determinants in India. This will help policy makers plan and provide cost effective pathways of care for psychiatric patients according to community needs. In addition, there is a need to increase awareness about psychiatric disorders and services among the public.

Funding

India spends 4.16 percent of the gross domestic product on health (WHO, 2011). However, only 0.06 percent of the total health budget is spent on mental health by the central government (WHO, 2011). Kerala had ring-fenced 2 percent of the health budget for mental health for 2007–8 (Raja *et al.*, 2010). Data on ring-fencing of budgets by the central and other state governments are not available.

A positive aspect is that there has been increased funding for mental health over a period of time. Mental health in the Eleventh Five Year Plan had three-fold increased funding as compared with the Tenth Five Year Plan (WHO, 2003).

As government-sponsored mental health services are inadequate, many people have to access services by out-of-pocket spending, which is likely to have an adverse impact on the income and savings of patients' families (WHO, 2013). Insurance coverage is rare among the general population. As of now, medical insurance does not cover mental illness treatment. The new Mental Health Care Bill (2013) (introduced in the Rajya Sabha – the Council of States) states that all insurers should make provisions for medical insurance for treatment of mental illness as for physical illness.

Data about expenditure on medicines for mental and behavioral disorders at country level are not available (WHO, 2011). It is estimated that nearly 50 percent of out-of-pocket mental health expenditure in Indian households is met by loans and another 40 percent is met from household income or savings (WHO, 2013). In a study conducted in a catchment area of primary health centers in Goa, 15 percent of women with depressive disorder reported having spent more than 10 percent of their household income on health-related expenses (Patel *et al.*, 2007).

Indigenous service model

Despite the lack of a robust system to take care of the homeless mentally ill, and contrary to expectations, they are given food, shelter and in some cases a haircut and shave by the community (Tharyan, 2008). Instances of volunteers helping patients, of village women forming self-help groups to liaise with psychiatrists to supervise treatment of the mentally ill, and of a symbiotic relationship between an untreated mentally ill person and the public have been described (Tharyan, 2008). Existing community resources need to be optimally utilized to care for the mentally ill.

Conclusion

Being a lower-middle-income country, India faces multiple challenges in providing affordable and accessible mental health care services to its public. As the population ages, geriatric mental health issues are likely to increase over the next few decades. With urbanization and disintegration of the extended family system, issues related to substance use are on the increase.

Though we still have a long way to go, there have been several positive developments for mental health over the last decade in legislation, policy and political will. More financial resources are being allotted to increase the number of trained mental health professionals and improve services. A planned and concerted effort from all stakeholders is necessary to face the challenges in improving mental health services.

References

Agarwal, S. (ed.) (2004). *Mental Health: An Indian Perspective, 1946–2003.* Published for Directorate General of Health Services Ministry of Health and Family Welfare, Elsevier, New Delhi.

Andrade, C., Shah, N., Tharyan, P., Reddy, M.S., Thirunavukarasu, M., Kallivayalil, R.A., Nagpal, R., Bohra, N.K., Sharma, A., Mohandas, E. (2012). Position statement and guidelines on unmodified electroconvulsive therapy. *Indian J. Psychiatry* 54, 119–33. doi:10.4103/0019–5545.99530

Basu, D., Aggarwal, M., Das, P.P., Mattoo, S.K., Kulhara, P., Varma, V.K. (2012). Changing pattern of substance abuse in patients attending a de-addiction centre in north India (1978–2008). *Indian J. Med. Res.* 135, 830–6.

Bhatara, V.S., Sharma, J.N., Gupta, S., Gupta, Y.K. (1997). Images in psychiatry. *Rauwolfia serpentina*: the first herbal antipsychotic. *Am. J. Psychiatry* 154, 894.

Chadda, R.K., Agarwal, V., Singh, M.C., Raheja, D. (2001). Help seeking behaviour of psychiatric patients before seeking care at a mental hospital. *Int. J. Soc. Psychiatry* 47, 71–8.

Chatterjee, S., Pillai, A., Jain, S., Cohen, A., Patel, V. (2009). Outcomes of people with psychotic disorders in a community-based rehabilitation programme in rural India. *Br. J. Psychiatry* 195, 433–9. doi:10.1192/bjp.bp.108.057596

Ganguli, H. (2000). Epidemiological findings on prevalence of mental disorders in India. *Indian J. Psychiatry* 42, 14.

Gururaj, G., Girish, N., Isaac, M. (2005). Mental, neurological and substance abuse disorders: Strategies towards a systems approach, in: *Burden of Disease in India.* National Commission on Macroeconomics and Health, Ministry of Health and Family Welfare, New Delhi, pp. 226–50.

Hackett, R., Hackett, L., Bhakta, P., Gowers, S. (1999). The prevalence and associations of psychiatric disorder in children in Kerala, South India. *J. Child Psychol. Psychiatry* 40, 801–7. doi:10.1111/1469–7610.00495

Jain, N., Gautam, S., Jain, S., Gupta, I.D., Batra, L., Sharma, R., Singh, H. (2012). Pathway to psychiatric care in a tertiary mental health facility in Jaipur, India. *Asian J. Psychiatry* 5, 303–8. doi:10.1016/j.ajp.2012.04.003

Kala, A. (2013). Time to face new realities; mental health care bill – 2013. *Indian J. Psychiatry* 55, 216. doi:10.4103/0019–5545.117129

Kattimani, S., Bharadwaj, B., Kumaran, A. (2013). Referral patterns in de-addiction services: An experience from a single centre. *Indian J. Med. Res.* 138, 360–1.

Kline, N.S. (1954). Use of *Rauwolfia serpentina* benth. in neuropsychiatric conditions. *Ann. N. Y. Acad. Sci.* 59, 107–32. doi:10.1111/j.1749–6632.1954.tb45922.x

Lahariya, C., Singhal, S., Gupta, S., Mishra, A. (2010). Pathway of care among psychiatric patients attending a mental health institution in central India. *Indian J. Psychiatry* 52, 333–8. doi:10.4103/0019–5545. 74308

Llibre Rodriguez, J.J., Ferri, C.P., Acosta, D., Guerra, M., Huang, Y., Jacob, K.S., Krishnamoorthy, E.S., Salas, A., Sosa, A.L., Acosta, I., Dewey, M.E., Gaona, C., Jotheeswaran, A.T., Li, S., Rodriguez, D., Rodriguez, G., Kumar, P.S., Valhuerdi, A., Prince, M., 10/66 Dementia Research Group (2008). Prevalence of dementia in Latin America, India, and China: A population-based cross-sectional survey. *The Lancet* 372, 464–74. doi:10.1016/S0140–6736(08)61002–8

Malhotra, S. K., Pradhan, B. (2013). Childhood psychiatric disorders in North-India: Prevalence, incidence and implications. *Adolesc. Psychiatry* 3, 87–9.

Malhotra, S., Kohli, A., Arun, P. (2002). Prevalence of psychiatric disorders in school children in Chandigarh, India. *Indian J. Med. Res.* 116, 21–8.

Malhotra, S., Kohli, A., Kapoor, M., Pradhan, B. (2009). Incidence of childhood psychiatric disorders in India. *Indian J. Psychiatry* 51, 101–7. doi:10.4103/0019–5545.49449

Math, S., Srinivasaraju, R. (2010). Indian psychiatric epidemiological studies: Learning from the past. *Indian J. Psychiatry* 52, 95. doi:10.4103/0019–5545.69220

Mental Health Policy Group (2011). http://mhpolicy.org/ (accessed 1.4.12).

Ministry of Health and Family Welfare, Government of India (2005). Report of the National Commission on Macroeconomics and Health.

Ministry of Health and Family Welfare, Government of India (2013). The Mental Health Care Bill, 2013, as introduced in the Rajya Sabha.

Murthy, R.S. (2011). Mental health initiatives in India (1947–2010). *Natl. Med. J. India* 24, 98–107.

Nagaraja, D., Murthy, P. (eds) (2008). *Mental Health Care and Human Rights*, First ed. National Human Rights Commission, New Delhi.

National Portal of India (2014). http://india.gov.in/india-glance/profile (accessed 1.2.14).

Neki, J.S. (1973). Psychiatry in south-east Asia. *Br. J. Psychiatry* 123, 257–69. doi:10.1192/bjp.123.3.257

Patel, V., Copeland, J. (2011). The great push for mental health: Why it matters for India. *Indian J. Med. Res.* 134, 407–9.

Patel, V., Thara, R. (2003). *Meeting the Mental Health Needs of Developing Countries: NGO Innovations in India*. SAGE, London.

Patel, V., Chisholm, D., Kirkwood, B.R., Mabey, D. (2007). Prioritizing health problems in women in developing countries: Comparing the financial burden of reproductive tract infections, anaemia and depressive disorders in a community survey in India. *Trop. Med. Int. Health* 12, 130–9. doi:10.1111/j.1365–3156.2006.01756.x

Patel, V., Weiss, H.A., Chowdhary, N., Naik, S., Pednekar, S., Chatterjee, S., De Silva, M.J., Bhat, B., Araya, R., King, M., Simon, G., Verdeli, H., Kirkwood, B.R. (2010). Effectiveness of an intervention led by lay health counsellors for depressive and anxiety disorders in primary care in Goa, India (MANAS): A cluster randomised controlled trial. *The Lancet* 376, 2086–95. doi:10.1016/S0140–6736(10) 61508–5

Patwardhan, B., Mashelkar, R.A. (2009). Traditional medicine-inspired approaches to drug discovery: Can Ayurveda show the way forward? *Drug Discov. Today* 14, 804–11. doi:10.1016/j.drudis.2009.05.009

Prince, M.J. (2009). The 10/66 dementia research group – 10 years on. *Indian J. Psychiatry* 51, 8.

Raguram, R., Venkateswaran, A., Ramakrishna, J., Weiss, M.G. (2002). Traditional community resources for mental health: A report of temple healing from India. *BMJ* 325, 38–40.

Raja, S., Wood, S.K., de Menil, V., Mannarath, S.C. (2010). Mapping mental health finances in Ghana, Uganda, Sri Lanka, India and Lao PDR. *Int. J. Ment. Health Syst.* 4, 11. doi:10.1186/1752–4458–4-11

Ray, R. (ed.) (2004). *The Extent, Pattern and Trends of Drug Abuse in India – National Survey*. Ministry of Social Justice and Empowerment and United Nations Office on Drugs and Crime.

Ray, R., Chopra, A. (2012). Monitoring of substance abuse in India – Initiatives and experiences. *Indian J. Med. Res.* 135, 806–8.

Reddy, V., Chandrashekar, C. (1998). Prevalence of mental and behavioural disorders in India: A meta-analysis. *Indian J. Psychiatry* 40, 149.

Sachan, D. (2013). Mental health bill set to revolutionise care in India. *The Lancet* 382, 296. doi:10.1016/S0140–6736(13)61620–7

Satija, D.C., Singh, D., Nathawat, S.S., Sharma, V. (1981). A psychiatric study of patients attending Mehandipur Balaji Temple. *Indian J. Psychiatry* 23, 247–50.

Sethi, B.B., Trivedi, J.K., Sitholey, P. (1977). Traditional healing practices in psychiatry. *Indian J. Psychiatry* 19, 9.

Shah, B., Parhee, R., Kumar, N., Khanna, T., Singh, R., Kumar, N. (2005). Mental Health Research in India (Technical Monograph on ICMR Mental Health Studies).

Sinha, S., Kaur, J. (2011). National mental health programme: Manpower development scheme of eleventh five-year plan. *Indian J. Psychiatry* 53, 261. doi:10.4103/0019–5545.86821

Srinath, S., Girimaji, S.C., Gururaj, G., Seshadri, S., Subbakrishna, D.K., Bhola, P., Kumar, N. (2005). Epidemiological study of child and adolescent psychiatric disorders in urban and rural areas of Bangalore, India. *Indian J. Med. Res.* 122, 67–79.

Thara, R., Padmavati, R., Srinivasan, T.N. (2004). Focus on psychiatry in India. *Br. J. Psychiatry* 184, 366–73.

Tharyan, A. (2008). Mental health services: Indigenous models of care in the community. *Indian J. Med. Ethics* 5, 75–8.

Thirunavukarasu, M. (2011). Closing the treatment gap. *Indian J. Psychiatry* 53, 199. doi:10.4103/0019–5545.86803

Tiwari, S.C., Pandey, N.M. (2012). Status and requirements of geriatric mental health services in India: An evidence-based commentary. *Indian J. Psychiatry* 54, 8–14. doi:10.4103/0019–5545.94639

Trivedi, J.K., Jilani, A.Q. (2011). Pathway of psychiatric care. *Indian J. Psychiatry* 53, 97–8. doi:10.4103/0019–5545.82530

Trivedi, J.K., Sethi, B.B. (1979). Motivational factors and diagnostic break-up of patients seeking traditional healing methods. *Indian J. Psychiatry* 21, 240.

Venkatesan, J. (2013). SC issues notice to States, centre on condition of mental hospitals. *The Hindu*, 9 July.

Vijaykumar, L. (2007). Suicide and its prevention: The urgent need in India. *Indian J. Psychiatry* 49, 81–4. doi:10.4103/0019–5545.33252

WHO (2003). Mental health financing (Mental health policy and service guidance package). World Health Organization, Geneva.

WHO (2011). India mental health profile. World Health Organization, Geneva.

WHO (2013). Investing in mental health: Evidence for action. World Health Organization, Geneva.

8

Mental health in India II

Training and explanatory models

Sydney Moirangthem, Geetha Desai and
Santosh K. Chaturvedi

Introduction: explanatory models

Very often the role of a clinician or a physician is not limited to just finding a manual-guided diagnosis of an illness, it also entails the need to see how the patient looks at his suffering and understands it.[1,2] A patient's perspective can provide a bird's eye view through which any management plan can be viewed to analyze whether the options being planned will be of any meaningful effectiveness in improving the patient's symptoms and restoring his or her functionality.[3] For chronic non-communicable illness in general and psychiatric disorders in particular, the influence of differences in culture and context of illness interpretation often affect the outcome of a treatment plan or model.[4–6]

A number of terms, including 'explanatory models', 'common sense representations', and 'implicit theories' have been used to describe the influence of culture and context on patient and physician perspectives.[7,8] More often than not, physicians and patients have different perspectives.

Explanatory models[9,10] (EMs), a term coined by Kleinman, denotes the 'notions about an episode of sickness and its treatment that are employed by all those engaged in the clinical process'.

Discordance in perspectives happens when the patient and the team engaged view the illness from each of their own perspectives. A modern physician diagnoses and treats diseases (abnormalities in the structure and function of body organs and systems) whereas patients suffer illnesses (experiences of unwanted changes in states of being and social function). Such discordance in patient and physician explanatory models can hamper the treatment process and lead to poor health outcomes.

Many methods have been proposed to identify the dimensions of the exploratory models and many studies have suggested various contexts to be explored by physicians during the information-gathering phase of the medical interview[11] including cause, treatment, severity, coping, locus of control and meaning of illness.[12,13]

Religious overview of mental illness in India

Hinduism[14]

Many consider Hinduism more a way of life than an actual religion. It is rooted in the Vedic system of beliefs handed down the generations from time immemorial both in oral and textual form. The term "Vedic" refers to the *Vedas* (knowledge) that are the oldest religious texts of Hinduism. *Rig Veda* and *Atharva Veda* are among the four major Vedas, which refer to a myriad of illnesses and their treatments. *Atharva Veda* describes illnesses that have supernatural causes but are treatable with traditional healing practices like incantations, exorcism, and the use of herbal plants and traditional medicine. Ayurveda is a part of *Atharva Veda* and deals with various physical and mental conditions and has been practiced in India for many centuries. The Ayurvedic beliefs state that mental health depends upon the *karma* (actions), *vayu* (air) and *swabhav* (personal nature) of the individual.

Accordingly, mental disorders are a reflection of abstract metaphysical entities, supernatural agents, sorcery or witchcraft. Ill health is also an outcome of an imbalance among three kinds of bodily fluids or forces called *Dosha*, and factors which contribute to these imbalances include inappropriate diet, disrespect to the gods, teachers or others, excessive fear or joy leading to mental shock and faulty bodily activity. Hence, treatments are suggested in the form of herbs and ointments, charms and prayers, moral or emotional persuasion, etc. All these beliefs still today influence causal models and help-seeking behavior.

Islam[15]

Muslim beliefs and ethnic sub-cultures are heterogeneous. They are often perceived as a monolithic group, stereotyped and subjected to significant interpersonal and structural differences.

There are contextual differences among practices and beliefs about health and illness and important commonalities across Muslim groups. A fundamental tenet of Islam is that there is one God (Allah is used universally by Muslims, regardless of ethnic group or language of origin) and Allah causes everything, including illnesses.

Although influenced by local cultures, the Islamic faith premises that human beings are made up of both body and soul; the unity of which results in a psyche (*nafs*) that reflects itself in behaviors. Human behavior is the result of the dynamic interplay between material and non-material forces and is in control of human consciousness. For a total understanding of man, a study of both these forces is necessary. While the body is in need of physical pleasure and tends to overstep its bounds, the spiritual intelligence in man intervenes to strike a balance in the human personality. Ongoing purification of thought and deeds brings a person closer to God and keeps a person mentally healthy. The neglect of religious practices enables evil forces to take control of the individual devoid of spiritual content.

An illness is also believed to be a method to get connected with God. It is not considered as something unwanted but rather it is a mechanism of the body that serves to cleanse, purify, and balance the person on the physical, emotional, mental and spiritual planes. This core belief holds true for both physical and mental illness.

Having a strong belief in this concept, many Muslims read the Qur'an to ward off evil and the influences of negative thoughts on the person. A common belief among Muslims is possession by Genies (spiritual beings), called by different names in different parts of South East Asia and India. For Muslims, the neglect of religious values and a deviation from *fitrah* (a state of inherent goodness) may also result in psychological disturbance. Among Muslims, a belief in predestination can also be a deterrent to seeking mental health care and the faithful may use various folk and traditional practices to overcome psychological distress in life. Very often a religious faith-healer, the Imam (often seen as an indirect agent of Allah's will and a facilitator of the healing process) is consulted to seek relief from a mental illness.

Explanatory models for mental illness

Schizophrenia

The explanatory model for severe mental illness, and schizophrenia in particular, has an admixture of religio-cultural underpinnings. There are few studies of the EMs for psychosis/schizophrenia (causation and help-seeking behavior) from India, and whatever is available does not always offer a uniform explanation. This could be due to the fact that the country is multi-cultural, multi-ethnic and no particular religion or culture totally dominates the rest.

What is found to be uniform in most of the studies is the widely held belief of the general public and the caregivers that some supernatural powers are responsible for most of the features of a mental pathology, either as a punishment for sins committed in the past or in past lives, or as a means to attain atonement. As an outcome of such a belief, many patients and their caregivers seek the help of faith healers to get rid of patients' symptoms. It has been shown that indigenous healing methods are considered complementary to the medical management of mental illness.[16]

Some studies carried out to evaluate the causal models and help-seeking behavior in patients with schizophrenia suggest that although some patients do have biomedical models, many patients have non-biomedical causal models of schizophrenia.[17] A study from Tamil Nadu, which evaluated the causal models as understood by patients with schizophrenia, reported that 70 percent of patients with schizophrenia had many non-biomedical causal models.[18]

Another study[19] showed that a minority of the subjects identified as having psychological problems, considered psychosis as a disease, attributed it to black magic or evil spirits, and felt that help should be sought from a nurse/doctor/hospital or traditional healers and the temple. However, the majority also attributed the problems to economic difficulties. A majority of subjects in the sample held to at least one non-biomedical explanation for the psychosis (e.g. black magic, evil spirits, non-disease concept), and sought treatment from traditional healers or temples and not from a medical center.

In a study carried out in North India[20] among a set of patients suffering from schizophrenia, on being asked about the cause of their problem, about one-third of the patients attributed their illness to sorcery/witchcraft (*Jaadu Tona*). This was the most commonly attributed supernatural cause followed by planetary/celestial influences (*Grah Nakchatra*), bad deeds in a previous life (*Karma*), spirit intrusion (*Opari Kasar*), evil spirits (*Buri Atma*), ghosts (*Bhoot-Pret*) and divine wrath (*Devi Devta Prakop*). Overall, about two-thirds of the sample attributed their symptoms to one of the above causes and about 40 percent attributed their symptoms to more than one of the above causes. Additionally, 63 percent of patients also accepted that stress can lead to the development of mental illness and 70 percent also agreed that change in neuro-chemical balance can lead to symptoms of mental illness.

Across all studies, most patients and care-givers believed in magico-religious treatment and many considered it to be the only option for mental illness. A significant percentage though, will add prayers and other forms of religious treatment to the medical care. Over decades, this practice has not changed much, though people coming to health centers to seek help have actually increased in number.

Depressive disorder

Even though the biological underpinnings of depressive disorder are well known, studies from various parts of the world suggest many patients with depression and common mental disorders have non-medical causal models for their illness.

There is a paucity of studies from India which have evaluated the explanatory models of patients presenting with the common mental disorders, depression and post-partum depression. The studies available have shown that many patients have non-medical causal models of illness and they prefer to visit local faith healers before seeking help from medical professionals.[21] The popularity of native healers arises from the fact that they are easily accessible and available, and provide culturally sensitive care.[22,23]

A study[24] in a cohort of married women suffering from major depressive disorder found they gave expression to their problems primarily through somatic complaints (non-specific bodily aches and pains, autonomic symptoms, gynecological symptoms, weakness and fatigue, and sleep problems). Economic difficulties and difficulties with interpersonal relationships (particularly related to marital relationships) were the most common causal models. However, those women rarely considered biomedical concepts, for example, the notion that they might suffer from an illness or that their complaints were due to a biochemical disturbance in the brain. Despite the lack of a biomedical concept, most of the participants had sought medical help for their somatic complaints.

Depressive disorders being more common in women, many studies from India and other parts of the world are mostly limited to the female population.[25] Most of these studies are community based and have evaluated rural populations. Even when it is reported that the patients have sought psychiatric treatment or at least reported to a mental health care facility, many of them drop out of treatment and follow-up. Very often, patients are non-adherent to treatment.[25] Some studies from north India suggest that the help-seeking behavior for depressive disorders no longer shows a female predominant distribution.[26] Many of the studies carried out in India found multiple explanatory models, but common to all are attributions to past-life deeds, influence of supernatural powers, familial attributes passed down through generations, psychosocial factors and life events, and some 'unknown medical reasons'.

A study[27] to evaluate the EMs for depressive disorders in north India using open-ended questions has shown that nearly three-quarters of the sample reported at least one explanation for their depression, of which psychological factors were the most commonly reported followed by social factors. On further probing, it was found that the most frequently reported explanations were categorized to the Karma-deed-heredity group, followed by psychological weakness, nerves-related and social causes in descending order. Further, most patients had more than one explanatory model for their symptoms. According to 'the Karma theory', one's actions and deeds are automatic and mechanical, determined by a fundamental law of nature that is also automatic and mechanical. It is not something that is imposed by God or as a system of punishment or reward, nor is it something that the gods can interfere with.[21] Indian personality is understood as dependence-prone, traditional and religious.[21] Hence, there is a tendency to find explanations for a problem beyond an individual and very often the individual has no control over it. This tendency to find an 'external explanation' often becomes a hindrance to seeking medical help, and often an expectation that somebody else will take care of the individual's problem comes into play.

A study in South India[28] shows that most patients attended with a set of somatic symptoms as presenting features of depression, as a purely psychological symptom of depression was stigmatizing, and hence was not the preferred presentation. Moreover, socio-cultural values validate the use of somatic complaints as indicators of an underlying problem of a psychological nature.

Common mental disorders

Common mental disorders (CMDs) are among the most frequent causes of morbidity and disability in India and worldwide. Several studies have examined the mental health needs of patients attending primary care centers in India and have documented that 17 to 46 percent of patients attending these facilities suffer from CMDs.[22] These patients are frequent users of medical facilities and are a major burden to their families, health care services and society. A criticism of the studies on somatization has been the absence of data on culture and local beliefs concerning somatic complaints.

Many studies have shown that a significant proportion of patients with unexplained somatic symptoms held a combination of medical and non-medical views about their condition. A substantial proportion of patients thought that they had specific physical diseases, attributed their problems to a variety of causes, considered their conditions as serious, and feared death and major disability.[28]

Somatoform disorders

In somatoform disorders, the presenting symptoms suggest a physical disorder, but there are no demonstrable organic findings from conventional bio-chemical and imaging studies, and there is often strong evidence for a link to psychological factors or conflicts. Very often, the users of clinical services are women from minority communities, though many studies suggest that distribution is not specific to one community. The presenting complaints are usually aches and pains, fatigue, tiredness and vague autonomic features.[29,30] Most of the patients initially do not report any obvious psychosocial factor/s. What was a common denominator in all were that most women lived in an impoverished, restrictive, social environment, where complaining of somatic symptoms was acceptable, without any stigma. The presentation of physical complaints becomes the only means for these women to seek medical help, though the cause of their presentation is not usually a medical disorder.[31,32]

In a study[33] of patients coming to a tertiary level psychiatric service in north India for somatoform disorder, the most common subtype was persistent somatoform pain disorder irrespective of gender. The most common explanations given for their problems belonged to the category of psychological factors (68.7 percent) followed by weakness (67.7 percent), karma/deed/hereditary (53.5 percent) and social causes (51 percent).

Culture bound syndromes

Dhat syndrome

Culture-bound syndrome is a term used to describe the uniqueness of some syndromes to specific cultures. Culture-bound syndromes have been discussed under a variety of names and are defined as 'episodic and dramatic reactions specific to a particular community – locally defined as discrete patterns of behaviour'.[34] However, it has been proposed[35,36] that these form a unique and distinctive class of generic phenomena, and that such syndromes exist among and afflict only 'others' – people who by some criterion are outside the 'mainstream' population (however defined).

Dhat (semen-loss anxiety) has been considered to be an exotic 'neurosis of the Orient'. It is a culture-bound syndrome characterized by excessive concern about loss of semen, vague somatic symptoms, fatigue, weakness and loss of appetite prevalent predominantly in the natives of the Indian subcontinent.[37,38] The patient attributes the symptoms to loss of semen in urine or through masturbation or excessive sexual activity. The word 'Dhat' derives from the word 'Dhatu' which means the elixir of life in Sanskrit.[39] The traditional medicinal system of Ayurveda considered semen as the most precious among the seven 'Dhatus' in the human body. It was believed that it takes 40 drops of normal venous blood to be converted into one drop of bone marrow blood and that 40 drops of bone marrow blood convert into a drop of semen. Hence, conservation of semen by all possible means was important.[40]

There have been attempts to explain how this belief system arose in the Indian psyche. One explanation is that these people do not understand the complex anatomy and physiology of the penis and believe that the blood that is collected in the cavernous spaces during erection gets converted into semen and so they are losing blood (and, thus energy) with each sexual act.[41,42]

Sexuality is considered a taboo in India, and sexual matters are generally not discussed in Indian families. The tabooed nature of sex and discussions related to it in Indian cultural context make it difficult for individuals to have discussions with peer groups, which prevents normalization of the experience of semen loss. Extreme concern over semen loss, either spontaneously or through masturbation, leads to presentations characterized by predominantly somatic complaints, anxiety, depressive symptoms and, rarely, psychotic symptoms.

The majority of men from rural India seek help from practitioners of traditional systems of medicine for their sexual problems.[43] Both allopathic and the alternative systems have different explanatory models and approaches in managing such cases. In one community-based study, 50 percent of traditional practitioners conveyed that semen loss is a physical illness and results from western influences, including the media which encourages masturbation. The traditional belief is that such weakness can be treated properly only by traditional systems of therapy, as modern medicines are strong, have a lot of side effects and offer only short-term benefits.[44] The allopathic system of medicine however, terms it a culture-bound syndrome in which an exaggerated response to a physiological phenomenon occurs, to be dealt with by proper psycho-education, relaxation techniques and management of concurrent depressive, somatic or anxiety symptoms with appropriate medication.[45].

Female Dhat syndrome

In females, Dhat syndrome is not reported as commonly as in males. Nevertheless, female Dhat syndrome does present in clinical settings. In clinical practice, in gynecological, medical and psychiatric clinics, women frequently attribute their physical symptoms (vague aches and pains, dysuria, asthenia) to their passing of a white discharge per vagina (WDPV). Ujla (whiteness), SwetaPradara (white discharge), safedpaani (white water) and bilihoguvudu (white going) are some common terms by which the passing of WDPV is referred to by women. Most often, the reasons given were things like dietary factors, excess of heat (or cold) in the body, emotional factors/stress, activity of any nature and tubectomy.[45]

Suicide

The WHO estimates that about 170,000 deaths by suicide occur in India every year. Suicide death rates in India are among the highest in the world. A large proportion of adult suicide deaths occur between the ages of 15 and 29 years, especially in women. Public health interventions such as restrictions on access to pesticides might prevent many suicide deaths in India.[46]

Suicide is recognized as a preventable cause of death that constitutes a major global public health problem, and it is particularly important in India. A profile of relatively higher risk for young adults, compared with the elderly, is a feature of suicide in India, where it is also the leading cause of death for women of childbearing age. Active surveillance, compared with data from passive reporting in police and crime bureau records, has highlighted the extent of suicide for young adolescents in the 10–19 year-old age group, with rates from a community study by Christian Medical College, Vellore, south India, as high as 148 per 100,000 for young women and 58 per 100,000 for young men.[47]

Reasons for suicide reported by family, friends, and the popular press typically focus on the triggers and underlying problems, which may be regarded as causes of suicidal behavior. Newspaper accounts may refer to financial disaster, disturbed relationships, marital problems, and a variety of other issues and conflicts.[48]

Community studies of suicide in south India highlight the underappreciated role of ongoing stress and chronic pain as reasons for suicide, in contrast with overestimation of the role of psychiatric disorders based on uncritical use of symptom checklists that are too easy to apply. Furthermore, attention to social determinants, such as economic problems leading to farmers' suicides, suggests an alternative to the primary role of psychopathology.[48]

Substance abuse

The socio-cultural history of alcohol consumption and other substance abuse differs significantly across the world and understanding explanatory models is an important step in the clinical process. There are four broad causal attributions for alcohol abuse: psychosocial causes (financial stressors and marital discord), peer influences, availability of disposable income and drinking for pleasure. The impact of substance abuse is felt on social life, family life, health and family finances which are all adversely affected.[49]

Mental health work force training in India

The initiation of mental health services in India started at the time of independence when the general health sector itself was at a minimal level. Most of the care was provided by the families in their homes at a community level, ranging from committal to isolation, and the majority of patients could not get access to organized mental health services. In the first decade post independence, there were only 10,000 beds for the mentally ill in a country of nearly 300 million people.

The following six decades however saw some changes in the mental health care initiatives, services and delivery system. There have been continuous efforts to address the needs of mentally ill persons and their families, building on the strengths of the community. The first two decades of independent India were devoted to doubling the number of mental hospital beds and humanizing the services at hospitals. The period saw the emergence of an innovation in the mental health care delivery system – the active involvement of the family in the planning and delivery of care of the mentally ill. This initiative was started by a psychiatrist in Amritsar, Dr Vidya Sagar. It happened at a time where the rest of the world, particularly the West excluded the family from the treatment net, and the families were seen as detrimental and toxic to care.

The early 1970s witnessed the setting up of general hospital psychiatric beds. This was a slow and silent change but in many ways revolutionized the whole approach to care for the mentally ill. The birth of community psychiatry began in 1975, when a new initiative to integrate mental health with general health services, was adopted to develop the mental health services. Community psychiatry in India is almost 40 years old. It started as an isolated extension of psychiatric clinics in primary health centers, and today the integration of mental health care into general services covers over 127 districts (about 20 percent of the population) in the country.

The National Mental Health Programme (NMHP) was formulated in 1982 to develop a national-level initiative for mental health care based on the community psychiatry approach. During the past three decades, there have been a large number of other community initiatives to address a wide variety of mental health needs of the community through programs on suicide prevention, care of the elderly, substance misuse and disaster mental health care, and by setting up daycare centers, half-way homes, longstay homes and rehabilitation facilities. The rapid growth of psychiatry in the private sector is another important recent development. Though mainly confined to large urban centers, private sector psychiatry is providing valuable services to the community. The District Mental Health Programme (DMHP) is now becoming the nodal unit to implement and coordinate the NMHP at the district level, integrating with primary health care.

Formal medical education

In India most of the hospitals, medical colleges and universities are funded by both the central and state governments, though the level of care, standards and funding may vary across organizations. The health system in the government sector works in a three-tier structure. Primary care is concerned with a specific and well-defined area in a district. The secondary tier is constituted by the district hospitals. The tertiary level comprises various state-level medical colleges or universities and the centrally funded hospitals with super and sub-specialties. Every year nearly 45,000 students graduate from medical schools including government funded and privately established medical colleges and universities.

The exposure to psychiatry training for medical undergraduates in India is minimal. In the whole of the five and half years of training, an average medical undergraduate undergoes only two weeks of clinical training and attends about 30 theory classes (this may range from 25 to 50 classes depending on the medical center).

Residency training in psychiatry[50-52]

Training in psychiatry, as for any other postgraduate specialty, is a three-year residency system with an exit examination at the end of the training period leading to the degree of the Doctor of Medicine (MD). A shorter two-year diploma (Diploma in Psychological Medicine) is offered in a few training centers.

Competition for postgraduate training is intense, with limited training posts available. Currently, there are about 450 training places annually for psychiatry, which is low considering the demand for psychiatric care in such a large population.

Training posts are spread across various state medical colleges. However, there are a few central institutions that offer postgraduate training, namely: the National Institute of Mental Health and Neurosciences (NIMHANS) in Bangalore; the Post Graduate Institute of Medical Education and Research (PGIMER) in Chandigarh; the All India Institute of Medical Sciences in Delhi (AIIMS); and the Central Institute of Psychiatry in Ranchi. Training in these institutions, and some centers in Mumbai and Chennai (formerly Madras), is highly sought after. Standards of training vary across institutions but training standards in some institutions are high. In institutions like NIMHANS and PGIMER, doctors undertake a comprehensive training program covering placement in outpatient and inpatient services, addiction medicine, liaison psychiatry, psychotherapy, child psychiatry, forensic psychiatry, community psychiatry and neurology.

Very few centers offer sub/super specialty training and they are limited to child psychiatry and addiction medicine.

At the time of writing, India has approximately 5,500 psychiatrists, and there are perhaps more Indian psychiatrists working out of the country.

Other mental health professionals from the fields of clinical psychology, psychiatric social work and psychiatric nursing add to the mental health work force.

Training of primary care physicians in mental health[53]

As a part of the National Mental Health Programme (which commenced in 1982) and the District Mental Health Program, all primary care doctors posted to a district are to be trained in mental health care for three days at a designated place near their place of work which can either be a district hospital or a nodal center or the medical college of that district.

Medical officers who work in primary health care centers are the first contact for any health-related problems. In their routine clinical practice, they are unlikely to see patients with severe mental illnesses, but more often see patients with common mental disorders like depression, anxiety disorders and somatoform disorders. The prevalence of common mental disorders in general/primary health care settings has been reported to vary from 20 to 45 percent. Such illnesses, if left untreated, can cause significant functional impairment. Thus, it is important for primary care physicians to be familiar with these disorders so as to identify and manage such patients effectively in their clinical practice.

Complementary and alternative therapies for mental illness

Music therapy

In Indian culture, music has been present since the time of Vedas as a therapy for many illnesses, including mental illness. The traditional system of medicine, i.e. Ayurveda, holds that *doshas* like *vata*, *pitta* and *kapha* (wind, bile and phlegm, respectively) can be modulated through music therapy, and that the Ragas in the Indian system of music are believed to act on specific chakras or energy centers, to bring about harmony in the body and consequent healing. Music and healing were ad libitum, meaningfully ingrained group activities that were as natural to everyone as other daily rituals. The historical records of various cultures echo this, and give numerous accounts of music being used as a mode of treatment for its healing abilities.[54] Research on the impact of music therapy on psychiatric problems in India is limited and no randomized controlled trial has compared the efficacy of music therapy for mental illness, either as a primary treatment modality or as an adjunct. However, several anecdotal reports suggest the efficacy of music therapy as an adjunct to usual care.

A randomized single blind study[55] carried out on 272 patients in Mumbai with chronic schizophrenia enhanced with music therapy for a one-month period in addition to their usual care showed that it may prove an effective tool in the holistic rehabilitation of schizophrenia, as an adjunct to various pharmacological and psychosocial treatments. The sub-scores on the Positive and Negative Symptom Scale for Schizophrenia (PANSS) showed a significant difference in the group whose treatment was supplemented with music therapy.

Yoga

Yoga or *yuj* (in Sanskrit) means 'to yoke' or 'to unite'.

The attainment of self-realization or *mukti* is considered to be the highest and most ideal goal according to Hindu philosophy. Hence, many believe that the practice of yoga or its subtypes/subdivisions (Mantrayoga, Layayoga, Hathayoga and Rajayoga) is probably a precursor that acts as a way to achieve the perfect physical and mental balance.

With the growth of science and modern medicine, yoga or practices based on its principles have crept in to influence the outcome and quality of life of an individual. Most evidence has shown the principles of yoga to be beneficial in chronic non-communicable lifestyle diseases like diabetes mellitus, hypertension and pain conditions.[56-58]

The benefits of yoga in the alleviation of symptoms of mental morbidities have already been documented in the complementary and alternative systems of Indian medicine like Ayurveda and Unnani but there are not many studies of yoga from the allopathic system's perspective. However, recent evidence suggests that the practice of yoga and its principles are beneficial in modern psychiatry.[59] Yoga has been found to be useful in depressive disorders and augments the therapeutic effects of antidepressants.[60] A few studies state an efficacy that is similar to antidepressants in mild forms of depressive disorder.[61] In anxiety disorders, it reduces the autonomic symptoms of anxiety, which also helps in reducing or controlling the cognitive components.[62] In severe mental illness like schizophrenia, it has been noted that chronic patients can tolerate the positive symptoms of the illness better with the practice of yoga.[63-65] In sub-syndromal or mild stressful situations, yoga helps in improving coping in addition to increasing the endurance of the individual, both physical and psychological.[66]

References

1. Cole SA, Bird J. *The medical interview: the three function approach*. St. Louis: Mosby; 2000.
2. Barley G, Boyle D, and Johnston MA Rowing downstream and the rhythm of medical interviewing. *Medical Encounter* 2001; 16: 6–8.
3. Schouten BC, Meeuwesen L. Cultural differences in medical communication: a review of the literature. *Patient Educ. Couns.* 2006; 64: 21–34.
4. Helman CG. Communication in primary care: the role of patient and practitioner explanatory models. *Soc. Sci. Med.* 1985; 20: 923–31.
5. Haidet P, Paterniti D. 'Building' a history rather than 'taking' one: a perspective on data sharing during the medical interview. *Arch. Intern. Med.* 2003; 163: 1134–40.
6. Heijmans M, de Ridder D. Assessing illness representations of chronic illness: explorations of their disease-specific nature. *J. Behav. Med.* 1998; 21: 485–503.
7. Leventhal H. The role of theory in the study of adherence to treatment and doctor–patient interactions. *Med. Care* 1985; 23: 556–63.
8. Williams GH, Wood PH. Common-sense beliefs about illness: a mediating role for the doctor. *The Lancet* 1986; 2: 1435–7.
9. Kleinman A. *Patients and healers in the context of culture*. Berkeley, CA: University of California Press; 1980.
10. Kleinman AM, Eisenberg L, Good B. Culture, illness and care. Clinical lessons from anthropological and cross-cultural research. *Ann. Intern. Med.* 1978; 88: 251–8.
11. Helman CG. Communication in primary care: the role of patient and practitioner explanatory models. *Soc. Sci. Med.* 1985; 20: 923–31.
12. Leventhal H, Diefenbach M, Leventhal EA. Illness cognition: using common sense to understand treatment adherence and affect cognition interactions. *Cognit. Ther. Research* 1992; 16: 143–63.
13. Meyer D, Leventhal H, Gutmann M. Common-sense models of illness: the example of hypertension. *Health Psychol.* 1985; 4: 115–35.
14. Bhugra D. Psychiatry in ancient Indian texts: A review. *Hist. Psychiatry* 1992; 3: 167–86.

15. Al-Krenawi A. Mental health practice in Arab countries. *Current Opinion in Psychiatry* 2005; 18: 560–4. http://dx.doi.org/10.1097/01.yco.0000179498.46182.8b

16. Kulhara P, Avasthi A, Sharma A. Magico-religious beliefs in schizophrenia: A study from North India. *Psychopathology* 2000; 33: 62–8.

17. Saravanan B, Jacob KS, Deepak MG, Prince M, David AS, Bhugra D. Perceptions about psychosis and psychiatric services: a qualitative study from Vellore, India. *Soc. Psychiatry Psychiatr. Epidemiol.* 2008; 43: 231–8.

18. Saravanan B, Jacob KS, Johnson S, Prince M, Bhugra D, David AS. Belief models in first episode schizophrenia in South India. *Soc. Psychiatry Psychiatr. Epidemiol.* 2007; 42: 446–51.

19. Compion J, Bhugra D. Experiences of religious healing in psychiatric patients in South India. *Soc. Psychiatry Psychiatr. Epidemiol.* 1997; 32: 215–21.

20. Kate N, Grover S, Kulhara P, Nehra R. Supernatural beliefs, aetiological models and help seeking behaviour in patients with schizophrenia. *Indian J. Psychiatry* 2012; 21: 49–54.

21. Chowdhury AN, Chakraborty AK, Weiss MG. Community mental health and concepts of mental illness in the Sundarban Delta of West Bengal, India. *Anthropology & Medicine* 2001; 8: 109–29.

22. Gupta R, Khandelwal SK, Varma VK, Wig NN, Rao U, Tripathi BM. Depressive symptoms – an inter-centre comparison. *Indian J. Psychiatry* 1982; 24: 380–2.

23. Patel V, Pereira J, Mann AH. Somatic and psychological models of common mental disorder in primary care in India. *Psychol. Med.* 1998; 28: 135–43.

24. Pereira B, Andrew G, Pednekar S, Pai R, Pelto P, Patel V. The explanatory models of depression in low income countries: listening to women in India. *J. Affect. Disord.* 2007; 102: 209–18.

25. Shankar R, Saravanan, BB, Jacob KS. Explanatory models of common mental disorders among traditional healers and their patients in rural South India. *Int. J. Soc. Psychiatry* 2006; 52: 221–33.

26. Chakraborty K, Avasthi A, Grover S, Kumar S. Functional somatic complaints in depression: an overview. *Asian J. Psychiatr.* 2010; 3: 99–107.

27. Grover S, Kumar V, Chakrabarti S, Hollikatti P, Singh P, Tyagi S, Kulhara P, Avasthi A. Explanatory models in patients with first episode depression: a study from North India. *Asian J. Psychiatr.* 2012; 5: 251–7.

28. Nambi SK, Prasad J, Singh D, Abraham V, Kuruvilla A, Jacob KS. Explanatory models and common mental disorders among patients with unexplained somatic symptoms attending a primary care facility in Tamil Nadu. *Natl. Med. J. India* 2002; 15: 331–5.

29. Janakiramaiah N, Subbakrishna DK. Somatic neurosis in Muslim women in India. *Social Psychiatry* 1980; 15: 263–6.

30. Janakiramaiah N. Somatic neurosis in middle-aged Hindu women. *Int. J. Soc. Psychiatry* 1983; 29: 113–16.

31. Chaturvedi SK, Michael A, Sarmukaddam S. Somatizers in psychiatric care. *Indian J. Psychiatry* 1987; 29(4): 337–42.

32. Chaturvedi SK, Upadhyaya MP, Shivajirao S. Somatic symptoms in a community clinic. *Indian J. Psychiatry* 1988; 30(4): 369–74.

33. Grover S, Aneja J, Sharma A, Malhotra R, Varma S, Basu D, Avasthi A. Explanatory models of somatoform disorder patients attending a psychiatry outpatient clinic: a study from North India. *Int. J. Soc. Psychiatry* 2013 Sep 11. [Epub ahead of print.]

34. Littlewoods R, Lipsedge M. Culture bound syndromes. In *Recent Advances in Clinical Psychiatry* (ed. Granville-Grossman K). Edinburgh: Churchill Livingstone; 1985. pp. 105–42.

35. Hughes CC, Wintrobe RM. Culture bound syndromes and the cultural context of clinical psychiatry. In *Review of Psychiatry* (eds Oldham JM, Riba M). Washington, DC: APA; 1995. pp. 565–97.

36. Hughes CC. The culture bound syndromes and psychiatric diagnosis. In *Culture and Psychiatric Diagnosis: A DSM-IV Perspective* (eds Messiah J, Kleinman A and Faberge H). Washington, DC: APA; 1996. pp. 298–308.

37. Bhugra D, Jacob KS. Culture bound syndromes. In *Troublesome Disguises* (eds Bhugra D, Munro A). Oxford: Blackwell; 1997. pp. 296–334.

38. Wig NN. Problems of mental health in India. *J. Clin. Soc. Psychiatry* 1960; 17: 48–53.

39. Malhotra HK, Wig NN. Dhat syndrome: a culture-bound sex neurosis of the orient. *Arch. Sex. Behav* 1975; 4: 519–28.

40. Prakash O, Meena K. Association between Dhat and loss of energy – a possible psychopathology and psychotherapy. *Med. Hypotheses* 2008; 70: 898–9.

41. Ranjith G, Mohan R. Dhat syndrome as a functional somatic syndrome: developing a sociosomatic model. *Psychiatry* 2006; 69: 142–50.
42. Avasthi A, Gupta N. *Manual for Standardized Management of Single Males with Sexual Disorders.* Chandigarh: Marital and Psycho Sexual Clinic; 1997.
43. Prakash O, Sathyanarayana Rao TS. Sexuality research in India: an update. *Indian J. Psychiatry* 2010; 52: 260–3.
44. Abdul Salam KP, Sharma MP, Prakash O. Development of cognitive-behavioral therapy intervention for patients with Dhat syndrome. *Indian J. Psychiatry* 2012; 54: 367–74.
45. Chaturvedi SK, Chandra PS, Isaac MK and Sudarshan CY. Is there a female dhat syndrome? *NIMHANS Journal* 1993; 11(2): 89–93.
46. Patel V, Ramasundarahettige C, Vijayakumar L, Thakur JS, Gajalakshmi V and Gururaj G. Suicide mortality in India: a nationally representative survey. *The Lancet* 2012; 379(9834): 2343e2351.
47. Parkar SR, Nagarsekar BB, Weiss MG. Explaining suicide: identifying common themes and diverse perspectives in an urban Mumbai slum. *Soc. Sci. & Med.* 2012; http://dx.doi.org/10.1016/j.socscimed.2012.07.002
48. Manoranjitham SD, Rajkumar AP, Thangadurai P, Prasad J, Jayakara R, Jacob KS. Risk factors for suicide in rural south India. *Br. J. Psychiatry* 2010; 196(1): 26e30.
49. Nadkarni A, Dabholkar H, McCambridge J, Bhat B, Kumar S, Mohanraj R, Murthy P, Patel V. The explanatory models and coping strategies for alcohol use disorders: an exploratory qualitative study from India. *Asian J. Psychiatr.* 2013; 6(6): 521–7.
50. Trivedi JK. Importance of under graduate psychiatry training. *Indian J. Psychiatry* 1998; 40: 101–2.
51. Medical Council of India Salient Features of Postgraduate Medical Education Regulations, 2000 (amended up to May 2013). Available from: www.mcindia.org/RulesandRegulations/PGMedical EducationRegulations2000.aspx
52. Das M, Gupta N, Dutta K. Psychiatry training in India. *Psychiatry Bull.* 2002; 26: 70–2.
53. Murthy, SR. Mental health programme in the 11 five year plan. *Indian J. Medical Research* 2007; 125: 707–12.
54. Sundar, S. Traditional healing systems and modern music therapy in India. *Music Therapy Today* 2007. (Online) VIII (3). Available at: http://musictherapyworld.net
55. Sousa AD, Sousa JD. Music therapy in chronic schizophrenia. *J. Pakistan Psychiatric Soc.* 2010; 7(1): 13.
56. McCall MC, Ward A, Roberts NW, Heneghan C. Overview of systematic reviews: yoga as a therapeutic intervention for adults with acute and chronic health conditions. *Evid. Based Complement. Alternat. Med.* 2013; 2013: 945895.
57. Ward L, Stebbings S, Cherkin D, Baxter GD. Yoga for functional ability, pain and psychosocial outcomes in musculoskeletal conditions: a systematic review and meta-analysis. *Musculoskeletal Care* 2013; 11(4): 203–17.
58. Cramer H, Lauche R, Haller H, Dobos G. A systematic review and meta-analysis of yoga for low back pain. *Clin. J. Pain.* 2013; 29(5): 450–60.
59. Unutzer J, Klap R, Sturm R, Young AS, Marmon T, Shatkin J, Wells KB. Mental disorders and the use of alternative medicine: Results from a national survey. *Am. J. Psychiatry* 2000; 157(11): 1851–7.
60. Janakiramaiah N, Gangadhar BN, Naga Venkatesha Murthy PJ, Harish MG, Subbakrishna DK, Vedamurthachar A. Antidepressant efficacy of Sudarshan Kriya Yoga (SKY) in melancholia: a randomized comparison with electroconvulsive therapy (ECT) and imipramine. *J. Affect. Disord.* 2000; 57(1–3): 255–9.
61. Cramer H, Lauche R, Langhorst J, Dobos G. Yoga for depression: a systematic review and meta-analysis. *Depress. Anxiety* 2013; 30(11): 1068–83.
62. da Silva TL, Ravindran LN, Ravindran AV. Yoga in the treatment of mood and anxiety disorders: a review. *Asian J. Psychiatr.* 2009; 2(1): 6–16
63. Gangadhar BN, Nagendra HR, Jagadisha T, Subbakrishna DK, Shetty KT, Muralidhar D. Efficacy of yoga as an add-on treatment in schizophrenia. Final project report submitted to the Department of Ayurveda, Yoga, Unani, Siddha, and Homeopathy (AYUSH), Government of India; 2010.
64. Vancampfort D, Vansteelandt K, Scheewe T, Probst M, Knapen J, De Herdt A, De Hert M. Yoga in schizophrenia: a systematic review of randomised controlled trials. *Acta Psychiatr. Scand.* 2012; 126(1): 12–20.

65. Behere RV, Arasappa R, Jagannathan A, Varambally S, Venkatasubramanian G, Thirthalli J, Subbakrishna DK, Nagendra HR, Gangadhar BN. Effect of yoga therapy on facial emotion recognition deficits, symptoms and functioning in patients with schizophrenia. *Acta Psychiatr. Scand.* 2011; 123(2): 147–53.
66. Varambally S, Gangadhar BN. Yoga: a spiritual practice with therapeutic value in psychiatry. *Asian J. Psychiatry* 2012; 5: 186–9.

9

Mental health in Nepal

Mahendra Nepal, Shree Ram Ghimire,
Smriti Nepal and Bharat Kumar Goit

Introduction

Nepal is a small beautiful country; known as the land of Mount Everest and the birth place of Lord Buddha. It has a population of 26,494,504. A decade-long political conflict has been resolved and the country is now headed towards political stability following election of a Constitution Drafting Assembly. The population is predominantly rural and approximately a quarter of people still live below the poverty line. The majority of the population depends on agriculture, and the economy has not made progress due to the dependency of its GDP on India.

There has been significant progress in the health status of the population and in the major health indicators. This progress is reflected by increases in human resources and government and private health facilities, including medical colleges. However, only 6.51 percent of the total annual budget is spent on health and a negligible budget is given to mental health. Mental health is a part of the general health services which is neglected and given low priority.

There are no national epidemiological data on mental health illness, however studies have reported that depressive illness, anxiety disorder, schizophrenia, bipolar affective disorder, substance misuse and dementia are the major mental illnesses among the adult and geriatric population. Similarly, mental retardation, somatoform disorders, attention deficit hyperactivity disorder and disruptive behavior disorder are common psychiatric morbidity patterns among children and adolescents. Suicide was the leading individual cause of death for women of reproductive age in both the 1998 and 2008/9 Nepal Maternal Mortality and Morbidity Survey (MMM) studies. Substance use disorder is becoming a problem among young people and recent data show that the number of drug users has reached 91,543.

The majority of people have no concept of biological causes of mental illness and think that suffering is due to bad fortune, loss of control over self, or even being possessed by a holy spirit or black magic. Most do not seek treatment due to stigma and seek treatment from faith healers rather than doctors. Despite the strong discrimination and stigma attached to mental health, increases in numbers of mental health professionals (psychiatrists, clinical psychologists, psychiatric nurses, etc.), medical colleges with mental health facilities along with postgraduate programs in psychiatry, and community mental health programs of NGOs have brought positive hope.

There is no Mental Health Act and a separate National Mental Health Policy exists only on paper. The role of government is to prioritize this issue to protect the fundamental human rights of mentally ill people along with development of mental health manpower and mental health facilities. Affordable mental health services, and mental health prevention and promotion activities along with intersectoral collaboration is needed to combat stigma.

The country

Nepal lies on the southern slopes of the middle part of the Himalayan mountain range in South Asia in between the Tibet region of China to the North and India to the South. It is known as the land of Mount Everest and the birth place of Lord Buddha (Index Mundi, 2013). It has an area of 147,181 km²; it occupies 0.03 percent and 0.3 percent of the total land area of the world and of Asia, respectively. Nepal has an extreme topography and climate because it lies on the slopes of the Himalayan mountain range. The altitude ranges from 70 meters to 8,848 meters above sea level, and the climate varies from hot and humid tropical to cold and snowy arctic depending upon altitude. Geographically, Nepal is divided into three East to West ecological zones namely, the Northern Region (the Mountains), the Mid Region (the Hills) and the Southern Region (the Terai – flat land). For administrative purposes, the country is divided into five North–South administrative development regions, namely the Eastern, Central, Western, Mid-Western and Far-Western Development Regions which are further divided into 75 administrative districts. The regions are composed of smaller units, called Village Development Committees (VDC) and Municipalities, numbering 3,915 and 58, respectively. As the name indicates, the VDCs have rural locations whereas the municipalities are urban locations (Index Mundi, 2013; Geographia, 1997–2005).

Population size, growth and distribution

A recent census (June 22, 2011) found the total population of Nepal to be 26,494,504 (Central Bureau of Statistics (CBS), 2012). Increase of the population during the last decade was recorded as 3,343,081 with an annual average growth rate of 1.35 percent. Half (50.27 percent – 13,318,705) of the total population were found to live in the Terai region while the populations in the Hill and Mountain regions constitute 43 percent (11,394,007) and 6.73 percent (1,781,792) of the total population. The Central development region has the highest population (36.45 percent) and Far-Western region has the lowest (9.63 percent) among the five development regions.

Sex ratio

The sex ratio (number of males per 100 females) at the national level decreased from 99.8 in 2001 to 94.2 in 2011. In absolute numbers there are 796,422 more females than males in the country (CBS, 2012).

Population density

Population density (average number of people per km²) at national level was 180 in 2011 compared to 157 in 2001. The highest population density was found in Kathmandu district (4,416 persons per km²) and lowest (three persons per km²) in Manang district (CBS, 2012).

Caste/ethnicity

A total of 125 caste/ethnic groups were reported in the census of 2011. The Chhetris constituted the majority of the total population, i.e. 16.6 percent (4,398,053) followed by Hill-Brahmans, Magar, Tharu and other caste groups (CBS, 2012).

Mother tongue

There are a total of 123 languages spoken, according to the 2011 census. Nepali is spoken as the mother tongue by 44.6 percent (11,826,953) of the total population. Other languages commonly spoken are Maithili, Bhojpuri, Tharu, etc. (CBS, 2012).

Religion

Ten religious categories were identified in the 2011 census. Hinduism was the most commonly practiced religion with 81.3 percent (21,551,492) of the population following it. This was followed by Buddhism, Islam, Kirat, Christianity, etc. (CBS, 2012).

Disability

About 2 percent (513,321) of the total population were reported to have some kind of disability. Physical disability was the commonest disability (36.3 percent of the population with disability) followed by blindness/low vision, deafness/hard of hearing, etc. Disability due to mental conditions is low in prevalence according to the survey (CBS, 2012).

Literacy rate

The overall literacy rate (for the population aged five years and above) reportedly increased from 54.1 percent in 2001 to 65.9 percent in 2011. The male literacy rate was 75.1 percent compared to a female literacy rate of 57.4 percent. The highest literacy rate was reported in Kathmandu district (86.3 percent) (CBS, 2012).

Political system

The country has been in the process of drafting and adopting its constitution for the last five years, and the Constitution Drafting Assembly which also acts as a parliament is involved in this. Currently there is an interim constitution on the basis of which country is run.

The political system of Nepal functions within a framework of a republic with a multi-party system. Executive power is exercised by the Prime Minister and his cabinet, while legislative power is vested in the Constituent Assembly (Index Mundi, 2013). The President is the head of state whose role is to act as a ceremonial head and appoint the government and monitor it.

Until 1990, Nepal was an absolute monarchy run under the executive control of the king.

Economy of Nepal

Nepal was an isolated, agrarian society until the mid-twentieth century. It entered the modern era in 1951 without a minimum infrastructure of schools, hospitals, roads, telecommunications, electric power, industry or civil service (Dahal, 2012). The country has, however, made progress towards sustainable economic growth since then and is committed to a program of economic liberalization. Agriculture remains Nepal's principal economic activity, employing 80 percent of the population and providing 37 percent of GDP. Only 6.51 percent of the total budget is allocated to health (*Nepal News*, 2013).

Health System

Nepal is divided into five development regions, 14 zones and 75 districts for administrative purposes (United Nations Population Information Network (POPIN), 1994). The Department of Health Services, working under the Ministry of Health and Social Welfare, controls and coordinates health services and centers. The sub-health post is the first point of contact for basic health services. There is a network for referring patients from sub-health posts to health posts then to Primary Healthcare centers (PHCs), district hospitals, zonal hospitals, regional hospitals and finally to tertiary centers (POPIN, 1994). Nepal has achieved remarkable improvements in health, especially maternal and childhood mortality, over the last two decades. As a signatory to several international conventions such as the Declaration of Alma Ata, the International Conference on Population and Development and the Millennium Declaration (Dixit, 1995), Nepal has committed to improving the health of its people, using an approach that is rooted in primary health care, targeting the marginalized and excluded population (Ministry of Health and Population (MoHP), 2010). The government's approach is set out in key national health policies and strategies – including the Second Long Term Health Plan 1997–2017 (Ministry of Health and Population (MoHP), 2007), Health Sector Strategy 2004 (Ministry of Health, 2004) and Nepal Health Sector Programme (NHSP). The Government's commitment is reflected in the improvement of maternal and child health (MNCH) indicators observed during the last several decades and shown in Table 9.1 (National Planning Commission Secretariat, 2012; MoHP (Population Division) 2012).

Health manpower

There has been a significant increase in health manpower and health facilities (Table 9.2) in the past few years (National Planning Commission Secratariat, 2012; MoHP (Population Division, 2012).

Table 9.1 Maternal and child health indicators in Nepal

Indicators	2001	2006	2011
Crude birth rate	33.1	27.7	24.3
Crude death rate	9.6	8.3	–
Fertility rate (per woman)	4.1	3.1	2.6
Infant mortality rate	64	48	46
Mortality rate under five	91	61	54
Maternal mortality rate	–	281	–
Average life expectancy at birth (years)			
Total	60.4	64.1	–
Male	60.1	63.6	–
Female	60.7	64.5	–

Table 9.2 Health manpower in Nepal

	2010/11	2011/12
Doctors	11,431	12,571
Nurses	–	19,098
Auxiliary nurse midwives (ANM)	–	19,222

Table 9.3 Health facilities under the Ministry of Health and Population in Nepal

Facility	2008/9	2009/10	2010/11
Hospitals	100	117	95
Health centers	207	208	209
Health posts	676	675	676
Sub-health posts	3,114	3,127	3,129
Hospital beds (available)	5,644	5,600	5,644

Health facilities under the Ministry of Health and Population have increased, as shown in Table 9.3 (National Planning Commission Secretariat, 2012; MoHP (Population Division), 2012).

History of development of mental health services in Nepal

Modern mental health services were virtually unknown in Nepal until 1961 (Aich, 2010, p. S76). The first psychiatric outpatient service was started at Bir Hospital, Kathmandu in 1961. A five-bed inpatient unit was established in the same hospital in 1965. The psychiatry department of Bir Hospital was converted into a mental hospital in 1984 and was later (in 1985) shifted to its current location (Lagankhel, Patan) in Lalitpur district. It is the only government-run mental hospital in Nepal with a bed strength of 50. A 10-bed neuropsychiatric unit was established in the Royal Army Hospital in Kathmandu in 1972 (Nepal, 1999, p. 3).

The need for mental health services started increasing gradually. This demand was somewhat fulfilled by the establishment of the department of psychiatry at the first medical school of Nepal, namely the Institute of Medicine (IOM) under the Tribhuban University Teaching Hospital (TUTH), which also provided a base for teaching and training activities. Here a psychiatric outpatient service was started in February 1986, followed by the addition of a 12-bed psychiatric inpatient unit in December 1987. Eventually a de-addiction unit, with 10 beds, was added to the psychiatric inpatient unit; this made a total strength of 22 beds. Since 1997, clinical psychological services have been offered in this institution for the first time in Nepal. Furthermore, in 1997, postgraduate training in psychiatry was started (at IOM) with the intake of two students for a three-year residency scheme. In 1998 a two-year MPhil course in clinical psychology was started, and a Bachelor of Psychiatric Nursing course was started in 1999 (Aich, 2010, p. S76; Shyangwa *et al.*, 2003, p. 27).

The creation of the Mental Health Project by the Institute of Medicine in 1989 with initial sponsorship by Redd Barna (Save the Children's Fund, Norway) set up a new era in the development of mental health services in Nepal. It was a national level project supported by a number of agencies including the government of Nepal, the Ministries of Education and Health, the National Planning Commission, the United Mission to Nepal and several other agencies, and this project was instrumental in: introducing changes in curricula for all types of health workers including the undergraduate medical program (MBBS); providing training to large numbers of teachers and trainers of health courses; developing models of community mental health programs at the village, district, zonal and regional levels; drafting the National Mental Health Policy; drafting mental health legislation; conducting pilot projects in prevention and health promotion for children; providing assistance in developing training programs in psychiatry, clinical psychology, psychiatric nursing and other subjects; and conducting landmark research to generate data for planning and program development. The Mental Health Program of the United Mission to Nepal (MHP–UMN) provided invaluable and essential support and assistance in securing external financial and other resources (Mental Health Project (MHP), 2000–2003).

Similarly, in the BP Koirala Institute of Health Sciences (BPKIHS), Dharan, a joint venture between Nepal and India started with an outpatient psychiatric service in 1995 and eventually a 20-bed psychiatric ward in February 2000. The postgraduate psychiatry program (MD) was started in the same year with the enrollment of one postgraduate resident (Aich, 2010, p. S76; Nepal, 1999, p. 3; Shrestha, 1986, p. 97).

During the last one-and-half decades a number of private medical colleges have been set up in Nepal, with psychiatry facilities including postgraduate psychiatry programs. The institutes having psychiatry residency programs include: the Universal College of Medical Sciences, Bhairahawa; the National Medical College, Birgunj; the Manipal College of Medical Sciences, Pokhara; and the Nepal Medical College, Kathmandu (Aich, 2010, p. S76).

Thus, Nepal has taken a big step forward in the development of specialist human resources within the country, considering that previously it did not have any training programs in psychiatry within the country and doctors used to be sent to other countries for this.

Concept of mental illness among the general population

Nepal is a country of different and varied ethnicity, cultures and traditions, but when it comes to mental illness, all these cultures share very similar concepts.

These are based largely on a religio-magical belief system – on the concept of 'Karma' (suffering for sins and misdeeds of the past – of both present and past lives). Misconception, misperceptions and stigma regarding mental illness and health are widely prevalent in Nepalese society varying in intensity and nature in different population groups.

In Nepal, most of the people think that suffering from mental illness is equivalent to being mad, being unfit to remain in society and the family due to loss of self control, or being possessed by a holy spirit (black magic). Individuals with severe mental disorders, as well as their family members, are targets of stigma and discrimination to the point where they hesitate to come forward for appropriate treatment (Nepal, 1999, p. 3). Even patients with neurotic disorders do not like to consult mental health professionals because of the stigma associated with mental diseases. Most of the rural population believe that mental illness is the result of bad fortune and people visit local faith healers for a cure (Shyangwa et al., 2003, p. 27). There is no concept of biological causes of mental illness, even among the educated. Instead, mental illness is related to life stresses, family or social conflict and associated evil spirits (Acharya, 1998).

Mental health facts and figures

There are no national epidemiological data on mental illness; however, data from other South Asian developing countries with similar settings and contexts can help us estimate the situation reasonably well (Shyangwa et al., 2003, p. 27). Studies from neighboring countries, especially

India are considered quite appropriate and applicable. Similarly large multicenter international studies like those of Wang *et al.* (2007) are often quoted and used. This study involved 85,000 people in 17 different countries; it showed high prevalence of mental illnesses and reported that approximately two-thirds of mentally ill people were not receiving any treatment.

The estimation of the extent of psychiatric morbidity in Nepal was based mainly on clinical data from healthcare providers like health centers/hospitals and not from epidemiological field studies. Very few attempts have been made in Nepal to obtain epidemiological data on mental illness by field studies. The first epidemiological field survey was conducted in a village in Kathmandu valley in 1984 which reported the prevalence of mental illness to be around 14 percent.

A mental health prevalence survey done in two developing towns of the Western region of Nepal identified a high point prevalence (35 percent) of psychiatry morbidity (Upadhyaya and Pol, 2003, p. 328). Similarly, a recent epidemiological study in a rural community of Nepal (Baglung district) revealed an overall prevalence of 37.5 percent (Khatri *et al.*, 2013, p. 52). The study found mental illness to be more common in males (46.1 percent) than females (30.8 percent), possibly due to higher alcohol use among males. In contrast, a similar study done in the Western region of Nepal revealed higher rates in females (42 percent) than in males (28 percent) (Wang *et al.*, 2007, p. 841).

Another study of patients attending for free mental health service check-ups, conducted by Maryknoll Nepal, found depressive disorder (18.93 percent), bipolar affective disorder (16.09 percent) and schizophrenia (13.73 percent) as the most common mental illnesses (Sedhain, 2013, p. 30).

Similarly, a study among 4,761 new cases attending mental health services in different parts of Nepal (Bajhang, Dadheldhura, Doti, Achham, Surkhet, Dailekh, Salyan, Rolpa, Dhadhing, Okhaldhunga, Morang, Ilam and Palpa) revealed higher morbidity among males (59 percent) than females (41 percent) of which anxiety neurosis emerged as the most common (50 percent) followed by depression (24.88 percent) (Upadhyaya *et al.*, 2013, p. 14).

Thus different studies have concluded that depression is the commonest mental health problem in Nepal. This may be due to a number of factors, especially domestic conflict, poverty, unemployment, social and religious factors, etc.

One study conducted by Wright *et al.* (1989) to assess the prevalence of mental illness among the attenders at general and primary healthcare services in the Kathmandu Valley found between 30 and 40 percent of patients attending only because of a mental disorder with no physical health problem.

Some attempt to study child and adolescent mental illness has been made. A recent retrospective study carried out in a tertiary center of Nepal (IOM, TUTH) revealed mental retardation, somatoform disorders and attention deficit hyperactivity disorder together with disruptive behavior disorder as common psychiatric morbidity among children and adolescents (Tulachan *et al.*, 2011, p. 20). A similarly high prevalence of mental retardation was shown by Regmi *et al.* (1999, p. 26) and Shrestha (1986, p. 97), whereas somatoform disorder was the commonest disorder observed in the studies of Nepal *et al.* (1988, p. 71) and Pokhrel *et al.* (2001, p.116) in a pediatric group in a similar setting.

Mental illness is also common among geriatric populations; however, the prevalence is unknown. A study done by Pradhan in an old age sheltered home in Kathmandu found senior citizens to be suffering commonly from depression (89.1 percent) (Pradhan, 2011, p. 13). As the number of elderly people in Nepal is increasing, mental health disorders (including dementia) are a growing problem (Jha and Sapkota, 2013, p. 292). There has been no epidemiological survey of dementia in Nepal (Shakya, 2011). A preliminary survey done in a village of Lalitpur revealed that almost 50 percent of people aged over 60 were suffering from memory-related problems. Since the methodology of this survey is not available and the prevalence rate is too high to be accepted, no meaningful conclusions can be drawn (Jha and Sapkota, 2013, p. 292).

Fainting attacks and epilepsy

With a view to studying the impact of improved obstetric services on neuropsychiatric conditions of childhood (fainting attacks and epilepsy), a district-wide population study was conducted in Morang district by Nepal and his team. In this study, the prevalence of epilepsy was found to be seven per 1,000 population (Shyangwa *et al.*, 2003, p. 27). Interestingly, in this survey 9 percent of epileptic cases were being treated by traditional healers whereas 29 percent of them had consulted faith healers in the past (Nepal *et al.*, 1996, p. 17).

Suicide

Nepal is lacking in systematic, reliable and nationally representative data about suicide due to the poor quality of registration systems and because cases of suicide are often miscategorized by hospitals (Pradhan *et al.*, 2010). At present, police data are the only source of national-level suicide data. But there is underreporting of suicide in police data – possibly intentionally because the act of suicide is illegal in Nepal and is highly stigmatized. The lack of comprehensive regular data on suicide in Nepal makes it difficult to determine national and sub-national rates, to identify at-risk groups, to assess trends over time, and to monitor the impact of interventions (Bajracharya *et al.*, 2008, p. 44).

Suicide was the leading individual cause of death for women of reproductive age in 1998 and this climbed dramatically in 2008/9. The well-known study on maternal mortality in Nepal, namely the Nepal Maternal Mortality and Morbidity Survey (MMM) was carried out in 1998 and repeated in 2008/9; the surveys found the alarming trend of suicide as the single main cause of death among women of reproductive age (Family Health Division, 2010). The percentage of deaths attributable to suicide increased from 10 percent to 16 percent during that period. The rates give an indication of the severity of the problem; 22 per 100,000 in 1998 and 28 per 100,000 in 2008/9.

Suicide rates were higher in younger women (aged 10 to 24); 21 percent of suicides were among women aged 18 years and under, indicating youth is a factor to be investigated. The 2008/9 MMM study also suggests that in women there may be an increased risk between 15 and 34 years, a reduced risk between 35 and 44, and an increased risk again after 45 (Family Health Division, 2010). The 2008/9 MMM study indicated that suicide accounted for a far greater proportion of deaths among the unmarried than the married.

Females still remain psychologically and emotionally suppressed in our society which could be the reason for suicide being more common amongst them. According to the Metropolitan Police Range Office, in Hanuman dhoka, females comprised 90 percent of total child suicide cases in Kathmandu; all of those cases were by hanging (*ekantipur*, 2011). Among males, the problem is not as great as in females.

Patients attempting suicide by self-poisoning usually end up in the emergency departments of hospitals. They are admitted for management of medical complications and are subsequently referred to psychiatry for further evaluation. A cross-sectional study of 100 cases of self harm that came to the emergency department of TUTH, reported more females (71 percent) than males (29 percent) (Shakya *et al.*, 2010, p. 14). The 16–30 year age group comprised the largest proportion of females (76 percent) and Metacid (an organophosphorus compound) ingestion (29 percent) was found to be the most common means of self harm.

A recent study conducted at Dhulikhel Hospital, among self-poisoning cases brought in for psychiatric evaluation, revealed an almost equal gender distribution (Risal et al., 2013, p. 10). More than 90 percent had made a single attempt, using organophosphorus compounds. The most common psychosocial precipitants were depression (50 percent), family disputes (19 percent) and marital disharmony (17 percent).

Poisoning was the most common means of suicide among women of reproductive age in the 2008/9 MMM study (Pradhan et al., 2010); mainly through ingestion of pesticides which are readily available in most rural households in Nepal. It is interesting to note that the different studies from medical settings have found poisoning as the commonest cause of suicide (Pradhan et al., 2010; Shakya et al., 2010, p. 14; Risal et al., 2013, p. 10) whereas police data indicated hanging to be the commonest mode of suicide (ekantipur, 2011).

Substance abuse

In Nepal, drugs such as cannabis and alcohol have been traditionally used for centuries (Aryal, 2010). Use of these drugs was part of the cultural norm and did not create any major social problems. The arrival of 'hippie' youths from the West in the 1960s ushered in an era of modern international trends in drug use. Initially, cannabis was the main drug of abuse, but just like fashion, this kept shifting to different drugs at different times. The types of drugs used moved from cannabis to synthetic opiates and other chemical substances (Jhingan et al., 2003, p. 339). Moreover, the mode of drug use has also changed, from smoking/ingestion to injecting. The injecting of drugs has become very popular lately and is one of the major causes of HIV, and hepatitis B and C infections. Substance abuse has thus become a growing problem and drug control is a major challenge for the Nepalese government.

According to the World Health Organization, prevalence estimates for alcohol use disorders (among females and males over 15 years of age) were 0.48 percent and 3.80 percent, respectively (Atlas of Substance Use Disorders, 2010). Few studies have been carried out on harmful use of alcohol in Nepal. The study by the Demographic and Health Survey of Nepal revealed that 67 percent of the males between 15 and 60 years of age consumed alcohol (Ministry of Health, 2002). The largest percentage (73.3 percent) were in the 25–29 year age group. The study also found that consumption of alcohol is greater in urban areas (75 percent) than rural areas (66.7 percent).

Another community study in the eastern part of Nepal (Dharan), of 2,344 adults, found a prevalence of alcohol dependence of 25.8 percent which peaked at 45–54 years (Jhingan et al., 2003, p. 339). Dependence was common among those with lower levels of education, widowers, divorcees and those of the Matawli community; the extent of dependence was influenced by socio-cultural sanctions.

A study using a two-stage representative sample of 1,400 households in the Kathmandu Metropolitan city showed that 22 percent of males and 9 percent of women aged 12 years and over use alcohol, and the prevalence of alcohol dependence in the general population was 4.5 percent by CAGE and 5.5 percent by Brief-MAST questionnaires (Shrestha et al., 2001). The study shows the ratios of dependent men to women in the general population as 5:1 and 4:1 by CAGE and Brief-MAST, respectively. Similarly, alcohol dependence among alcohol users was 14.7 percent by CAGE and 17.7 percent by Brief-MAST. Males are 5.6 times and 3.78 times more alcohol dependent than females from CAGE and Brief-MAST, respectively.

Alcohol use among children in Nepal is not uncommon. A national survey, in 2000, among 426 children between 10 and 17 years of age found that 21.8 percent of boys and 11.2 percent of girls had consumed alcohol in the last 12 months (Dhital, 2000). The median age of initiation was 13 years; cultural practices accounted for initiation in 60 percent of them.

Alcohol problems are more widespread than is seen in the clinical setting (Regmi *et al.*, 1998). Most often, people with alcohol dependence do not seek treatment unless major complications or consequences arise (Shakya *et al.*, 2008, p. 27). A study of help-seeking behavior in patients with alcohol dependence, in a tertiary care hospital in the eastern part of Nepal, found that the main reason for delay in seeking help is lack of awareness of the problems and consequences of drinking (Shakya *et al.*, 2011a, p. 15). Moreover, alcohol abuse and related problems do not come to the attention of doctors; they are largely tolerated and considered as a moral problem of conduct rather than a health problem and so are treated by local 'quacks' and faith healers.

Prevalence estimates for drug use disorders (among females and males over 15 years of age) were 0.02 and 0.15 percent, respectively (Atlas of Substance Use Disorders, 2010). A recent survey of hard drug users, that covered 17 municipalities from 15 districts spread over five development regions of Nepal revealed that the majority of users start taking drugs at the age of 15–19 years (53.4 percent) (Aryal, 2010). The study found that majority (72 percent) of drug abusers are in the 15–29 year age group. The types of drugs used are marijuana (86.9 percent), chemical drugs (86 percent), 'brown sugar' (60.5 percent), opium (7.1 percent), and Dendrite (2.6 percent). The mode of administration is injection (61.9 percent) and oral (38.6 percent). Among needle users, approximately one third (29 percent) share needles with other drug users.

Recently the Government of Nepal has reported the number of drug users as 91,543; out of which 85,204 are males and 6,330 are females (Himalayan News Service, 2013). These statistics were made public by the Ministry of Home Affairs on the occasion of International Day against Drug Abuse and Illicit Trafficking. 2008 data released by the government had reported the number of drug users as 46,309 (Himalayan News Service, 2013). This shows that drug users are increasing in number at an alarming rate despite numerous awareness programs and police crackdowns on drug traffickers. Unemployed people top the chart of drug users with 50.1 percent followed by the employed (28.7 percent) and students (21.2 percent). Students, especially of grades 6–10, and the group who have taken their SLC (School Leaving Certificate) examinations and/or pre-university examinations, together account for the largest number of drug users (Himalayan News Service, 2013). The most commonly consumed drug was marijuana followed by hashish, controlled pharmaceutical drugs and other hard drugs (heroin and cocaine). Stress, family disputes, curiosity and failure in studies have, among others, been the reasons given for drug use (Himalayan News Service, 2013).

There are numerous rehabilitation and drug treatment centers run by NGOs/INGIOs; these have certainly made an attempt to fill the gap in services and facilities; however, due to lack of proper monitoring by government, the quality of such services is questionable (Shakya 2013). Moreover, the majority of them have turned out to be commercial ventures.

Impact of armed conflict

The decade-long civil unrest had major impacts on mental health. In a study by Shakya *et al.* (2011b), among a clinical sample of 50 subjects, it was found that the conflict had affected more than half directly, physically and/or psychologically (Shakya *et al.*, 2011b). The majority of them had biological/somatic symptoms besides anxiety and psychotic symptoms. In a study among internally displaced persons during armed conflicts, 80.7 percent of males were found to suffer from anxiety and 80.3 percent from depression (90.3 percent and 88.5 percent, respectively, in females) (Thapa and Hauff, 2005, p. 672).

A prospective study carried out on mental health before (2000) and after exposure (2007) to direct political violence during the People's War in Nepal, using Nepali versions of the Beck Depression Inventory and Beck Anxiety Inventory, reflected the direct impact of war on mental health and presented it as a strong risk factor (Kohrt *et al.*, 2012, p. 268). The study revealed that depression increased from 30.9 to 40.6 percent, and anxiety increased from 26.2 to 47.7 percent. Similarly, post-conflict post-traumatic stress disorder (PTSD) was found to be 14.1 percent. This is an international landmark study that could compare post-conflict data with data from the pre-conflict phase. This could give a prospective perspective.

Another study showed that the more violent or inhuman the experience, the worse the impact on mental health (Mollica, 2001, p. 1213). Integration of mental health services into primary health care can be the only cost-effective, large-scale measure to provide care and support to such people.

Mental health care systems

There is no separate mental health department or unit in the Ministry of Health in Nepal. Mental health is looked after by the general Department of Health Services and the only mental hospital provides expertise to the Department or the Ministry in planning or policy-making processes.

Apart from the central mental hospital, some zonal and regional hospitals have psychiatric services with outpatient (OPD) facilities but those units often lack inpatient facilities. Presently, only about 11 psychiatrists work full time in the government sector (Center for Mental Health and Counseling – Nepal (CMC–Nepal), 2013). There is a gross lack of coordination between the Ministry of Health and private medical institutes, NGOs/INGOs and other mental health services. Most of the private medical colleges have both inpatient and outpatient mental health facilities; however, some of the private hospitals have only outpatient facilities.

Mental health services provided can be described under three subheadings, namely:

1. The public mental health system;
2. The private mental health system;
3. Services provided by non-govermental organizations (NGOs)/international non-govern-mental organizations (INGOs).

Public mental health system

The public mental health system comprises services provided by the mental hospital and some regional/zonal hospitals of the Ministry of Health and teaching hospitals of the medical schools in both government and private sectors; and the total number of such providers is 18. Only a few of them also have inpatient psychiatric facilities – others primarily provide outpatient services. Only the psychiatry departments of Tribhuvan University Teaching Hospital (TUTH, Kathmandu) and of BP Koirala Institute of Health Sciences (BPKIHS) provide comprehensive psychiatric services including psychiatry, clinical psychology, psychiatric nursing and other services, the rest provide only psychiatric services.

Around five of these are located in the Kathmandu Valley – the rest are based in various regional areas of Nepal. They provide invaluable specialist mental health services in the regions outside the capital. Some, which are based near the Nepal–India border, have a significant number of clients from the other side of the border.

Some offer a more comprehensive range of services including psychology, nursing and other services. A few also run outreach clinics/services; the majority only offer hospital-based care. As mentioned earlier, only a few have inpatient facilities, among these, the mental hospital has highest number of beds (around 50); TUTH has a total of 22 beds. Only a few provide a 24-hour emergency psychiatric service. TUTH has been a pioneer in this kind of service; otherwise such facilities have been made available mainly by the private sector providers.

The service provided by the mental hospital is free or costs a minimal fee – and it has the capacity to provide services at no or minimum cost to poor patients. Other institutions usually charge a fee which is less than what is charged in the private sector and often they also have limited provision of free services. Apart from providing services, these institutions also act as bases for teaching and learning activities for a number of academic programs and provide a base for research. Thus, these institutions provide the bulk of care to a large number of Nepalese people and act as the backbone of the mental health service in the country.

Private mental health care system

The private mental health care system consists of private clinics run by psychiatrists who (except for few) also work in the public system. Very few have inpatient facilities, and these are limited largely to the urban areas, numbering around half a dozen.

People from affluent, mid- or high socioeconomic strata and those who want to avoid stigma tend to use these services for conditions of mild to moderate severity. The cost of treatment is borne by the patient and family – so if the cost increases because of severity or chronicity of illness, patients are transferred to public sector facilities.

Kathmandu Valley has around half a dozen private inpatient facilities and more than a dozen privately run clinics. With the increase in the number of psychiatrists in the last decade, such facilities have also spread to the regional centers.

There is no mental health insurance scheme in the country either in the public or the private sectors.

Services provided by NGOs/INGOs

Many NGOs/INGOs are providing mental health services, independently, at the community level (Devkota, 2013). They play a key role especially in mental health promotion and counseling. Some of them provide curative services as well. There are no clear data regarding the numbers of NGOs involved in mental health nor regarding the fields of their involvement. A few of the NGOs working in the area are the Transcultural Psychosocial Organization (TPO) Nepal, the Center for Mental Health and Counseling – Nepal (CMC-Nepal), Sahara Paramarsha Kendra, Antardrishti, Antarang, Koshish Nepal (Devkota, 2013), the Center for Victims of Torture, Nepal (CVICT), Maryknoll Nepal, Terre des Hommes Nepal, Autism Care Nepal, the Alzheimer's Disease and Related Dementias Society (ARDS), Saint Xavier's Social Services Center with Drug Rehabilitation Center, etc.

The Transcultural Psychosocial Organization (TPO) Nepal, which is one of the leading psychosocial organizations, works with children and families in conflict-affected and vulnerable communities. It works by developing sustainable, culturally appropriate, community-based psychosocial support systems (Transcultural Psychosocial Organization (TPO) Nepal, 2010).

The Center for Mental Health and Counseling – Nepal (CMC–Nepal), which was started by the United Mission to Nepal, is a national level NGO (Himalayan News Service, 2013) and is a development of the previous Mental Health Program of the United Mission to Nepal (MHP–UMN) which was established in 1983 with the first community mental health program in Lalitpur district. It has been a pioneer organization, initiating landmark work and research in the field of psychiatry, initially on its own but later in collaboration with the Institute of Medicine, the mental hospital and other national institutions.

The UMN–MHP has played a vital role in securing financial support, scarce specialist manpower and other support from overseas donors and institutions, without which many of the big developments of recent times would not have been possible. It acts as a catalyst in initiating several key national level activities, e.g. development of community service models for villages, districts, zones and regions; drafting of the National Mental Health Policy and mental health legislation (in collaboration with the Mental Health Project (MHP) of IOM and the mental hospital).

The absence of such support has been increasingly felt and observed at national level.

Currently, CMC–Nepal works on preventive, health promotional and curative aspects of mental health, with the aim of providing mental health services in the community. It also supports other organizations in their psychosocial programs.

Autism Care Nepal is the only organization in Nepal which is active in the field of care of autistic children and providing support to their families; it is run by passionate parents who care for autistic children (Autism Care Nepal, 2008–2010). It provides support and information services to persons with autism and people who work with autistic children. It aims to educate, raise awareness and act for the rights of autistic children throughout Nepal.

Maryknoll Nepal is a non-profit, non-governmental voluntary social organization whose main aim is to provide services to homeless mentally ill persons, and achieve the release of all the chronically mentally ill patients locked in jails like the central jail in Kathmandu and Dhulikhel jail in Kavre (Maryknoll Nepal, 2013). In the absence of traditional mental hospitals, mentally ill persons who could not be kept at home used to be kept in jails; this is not ethical but at least used to provide them with shelter and food. Maryknoll Nepal emphasizes the provision of care, treatment and rehabilitation to the mentally ill, within their own families and communities. It also provides outreach care services in different parts of the country.

Redd Barna (Save the Children Fund of Norway) has played a key role in development of mental health in Nepal since the 1980s through their support of the Mental Health Project (MHP) of the Institute of Medicine (IOM) and other institutions. It has supported national NGOs in the area of comprehensive child care.

The Center for Victims of Torture, Nepal (CVICT) provides psychosocial services to victims of torture (Center for Victims of Torture, 2013).

Koshish is a non-profit, national NGO working to improve the quality of mental health policies and programs, and at the same time challenge existing discriminatory attitudes towards people affected by mental illness. Koshish has been working informally and voluntarily on mental health issues since 2004. During these years it has become involved in the rehabilitation of numerous people affected by mental illness (Devkota, 2013).

The Alzheimer's Disease and Related Dementias Society (ARDS) is a non-profit organization established in 2012 with the aims of raising awareness of dementia, supporting people with dementia and their caregivers, and providing dementia training to doctors and nurses (Alzheimer's Disease and Related Dementias Society (ARDS), 2012).

There are a number of other similar organizations working mainly in the Kathmandu Valley in areas like drug abuse prevention, treatment and rehabilitation; care of intellectually disabled children and support to their families; suicide prevention; domestic violence, etc., and these have been contributing to raising awareness of such issues.

Role of traditional healers

Owing to a strong belief in traditional healing, the first point of contact for the majority of mental health patients is the readily available traditional healers rather than health professionals. This practice is more common in rural areas, especially among illiterate people and some ethnic groups but also not uncommon in urban areas. There is a lack of adequate data and information about this aspect of mental health care due to lack of research. However, experts believe that achievement of mental health goals is virtually impossible without involving traditional healers in Nepal.

In many communities, local faith healers are considered to be 'Janne' (persons with special knowledge of physical, mental and spiritual care) and are consulted by people for all types of problems – physical, mental, social or spiritual. Thus, they act as gatekeepers for the majority of psychiatric patients in Nepal. Without their approval, referral or participation, treatment may either not be provided or delayed or inappropriately organized. Often, mentally ill people are referred by faith healers to local paramedics, who refer them to doctors and then to psychiatrists. Commonly referred problems include acute psychosis, conversion disorder, alcohol and drug dependence, and depression (Regmi et al., 2004, p. 142). Various studies have reported very high rates (70 to 90 percent) of consultation with traditional healers by mentally ill persons. There are around one million traditional healers of all types in Nepal and they tend to provide some sort of psychosocial care to people, and form the bulk of providers of some form of counseling especially in rural settings. Not only counseling, but other aspects of mental health care in the traditional way are provided by them too.

The MHP of IOM carried out a pioneering pilot project to involve traditional healers in the mental health care system in Morang, Kaski, and other field districts by giving them three days training in modern mental health approaches for identification of five target conditions and referring patients to nearby health institutions for provision of medications and to raise awareness. An elaborate training methodology and manual have been developed (Mental Health Project (MHP), 2000–2003).

The current number of mental health professionals is inadequate to rapidly bring awareness of mental health and illnesses. In such a situation, one probable alternative could be the utilization of the skills of traditional healers. WHO states that 'It is essential to understand and respect the spiritual aspect of mental health as defined by both individuals and cultures' (World Health Organization (WHO), 2004). Mental well-being, for many people, is linked to their relationship with their concept of God and they believe traditional healers are the ones to help them overcome their problems (Regmi et al., 2004).

Prevention and promotional activities

Prevention and promotional activities are limited in both extent and type of program, especially in general mental health. In areas like drug abuse prevention, a large number of organizations mainly in the NGO sector are actively working mainly in urban areas and some of them were established in the 1970s. Experts agree that they have been effective and useful, depending on the resources available. However, no systematic study has been done to assess their efficacy longitudinally and since the programs tend to be fragmented and regional in nature, that makes it difficult to assess their impact in overall prevention.

The MHP of IOM had conducted three pilot projects to prevent the development of behavioral and mental problems among children from poor socioeconomic and untouchable caste groups. Results were promising and some of the approaches have been adopted and replicated by CMC–Nepal in other areas such as school mental health programs, prevention and health promotion programs for children, etc. Awareness-raising campaigns to increase awareness about mental illness and health, and reduce stigma, are the main activities conducted by the government, the mental hospital, CMC–Nepal and other NGOs. The Psychiatrists' Association of Nepal (PAN) marks Annual World Mental Health Day with such activities.

Previously, mental health programs were organized with the financial support of WHO. They used mass media (radio and television) to generate awareness of mental health and to reduce the stigma attached to it (Upadhyaya, 2013, p. 2). Impact evaluation was never conducted and the programs were stopped as they were not deemed cost effective. Now, mental health promotion activities are being conducted by NGOs in their own ways.

Because of lack of adequate budgets and programs for mental health (due to a low level of awareness and knowledge about its importance amongst government and policy-makers) mental health promotion is lagging in Nepal (World Health Organization (WHO), 2007).

Mental health policy

The main initiative and thrust towards drafting and making the government adopt a Mental Health Policy came from the Mental Health Project (MHP) of the Institute of Medicine and the United Mission to Nepal.

In 1997, the government of Nepal adopted a national Mental Health Policy and included mental health as an element in primary health care. The key components of the policy include: (1) to ensure the availability and accessibility of minimum mental health services for all; (2) to prepare human resources in the area of mental health; (3) to protect the fundamental human rights of the mentally ill; and (4) to improve awareness about mental health (National Mental Health Policy, 1996).

But mental health still continues to be of low priority on the national health agenda. Despite being adopted with the very active advocacy of the MHP, PAN and others, the government has never shown any interest in formally accepting it and acknowledging the need to have a policy document. It somehow has not been on the agenda for cooperation with WHO in Nepal, although WHO has always declared it a priority area of work and advocated this in other member countries. Therefore, the policy has never formally been implemented, although parts of activities mentioned in it have been done by committed professionals, NGOs and others.

There is an essential drug list for different levels of health institutions. Health institutions with specialists have more drugs available than primary health clinics where there are only limited drugs available from the essential drugs list. Unfortunately, the provision of medicines for common mental illness is not free (Upadhyaya, 2013, p. 2). The emergency/disaster preparedness plan for mental health is not adequate and lacks detail both in government and NGO sectors, whereas the plan in general health is much more elaborate.

Mental health legislation

There is no separate mental health legislation or act at national level.

Few mentally ill patients reach health facilities for treatment. Families of patients often resort to locking them in rooms or chaining them up when they become hard to manage and/or are abandoned. The Nepali Civil Code 1963/64 assumes state responsibility for treatment of mentally ill people (Devkota, 2013). The legal definition of mental illness is not clear and the language of the legislation refers to the mentally ill as someone with a broken mind or madness. This attitude is reflected in day-to-day practice where mentally ill people are described as 'mad' (Upadhyaya, 2011).

A draft of mental health legislation developed by the MHP of the IOM was first submitted in the year 2000 and a revised draft in 2007. Unfortunately, it was not processed in a timely manner and enough attention and due priority was never given to it by the government and Ministry of Health.

The second draft was reviewed in 2011 and a five-member committee was formed to update the draft and to submit it to Ministry of Health and Population (Regmi *et al.*, 2004). It still has not been passed and Nepal does not yet have modern and proper legislation.

Training, education and human resource development

There has been a transformational and very significant development in the area of human resources in Nepal over the past two decades (Dixit, 1998, p. 61). The basic training of psychiatrists and psychiatric nurses is now fairly thorough: three years for psychiatrists (after undergraduate training in medicine) and two years for psychiatric nurses (Jha and Adhikari, 2009, p. 185).

Since 1997, Nepal has established psychiatry, clinical psychology and psychiatric nurse training programs at the Institute of Medicine, Tribhuvan University in Kathmandu. First, a postgraduate program (MD) in psychiatry was started in 1997 with support from the United Mission to Nepal and other institutions of Nepal, India, Pakistan and overseas. This was followed by a postgraduate program (MPhil) in clinical psychology and Bachelors in Nursing (BN) in psychiatric nursing in 1998, at IOM. The first nationally trained psychiatrist passed in 2000, and since then a number of other institutions have started such programs increasing the available number of specialists in the country. Since 2000, an MD in psychiatry has also been running in BPKIHS, Dharan.

IOM and colleges under Tribhuvan University (TU) have extensive teaching programs in psychiatry. The psychiatry unit in the MBBS curriculum is a separate and must-pass unit along with general medicine; it is run by the Department of Psychiatry with external examiners in university examinations, etc.

Medical undergraduates receive 45 hours of theory and two weeks clinical posting in psychiatry. Their exam now includes psychiatry with an emphasis on the clinical component (Tribhuvan University Medical Education Department, 1994). Apart from TU-affiliated colleges, other colleges do not have similar programs.

At present there are a number of private medical colleges in Nepal with postgraduate psychiatry programs (Aich, 2010, p. S76), the Ministry of Health has started a postgraduate residency program in psychiatry under the National Academy of Medical Sciences (NAMS, Bir-Hospital) in the mental hospital in Lalitpur.

Postgraduate study in psychiatry is by full-time residency programs for three years (Regmi *et al.*, 2004, p. 142). Postgraduates are trained thoroughly in clinical, academic and research areas. They also need to submit a thesis before a final-year examination. The postgraduate training program currently incorporates training in psychometric tests, neuroradiology, neurology, EEGs, clinical psychology and rural psychiatry. It also incorporates training in treatments such as pharmacotherapy, cognitive therapy, behavioral therapy as well as a variety of psychosocial skills (Aich, 2010, p. S76).

Doctors and other primary health care workers are given short-term in-service training courses as part of their mental health training in different areas and regions.

There is no provision for continuing medical education for people working at specialist level (Upadhyaya, 2013, p. 2). The basic training of the different kinds of traditional care practitioners, religious healers and alternative/complementary healers is non-structured and individually planned. Mental health orientation programs have been organized for school teachers, police personnel, jailers, students and teachers, and community and religious workers in the past.

Although much has been achieved in this area in Nepal in recent times, the country still faces a lack of manpower in the field of specialist mental health care and this is one of the major problems in provision of care in the country, especially in rural and regional Nepal.

There are no official figures on employment by governmental, non-governmental and private healthcare in the various urban and rural settings of the country. However, in 1980, Nepal had two psychiatrists, two neurologists and no psychiatric nurses, psychiatric social workers or clinical psychologists (Jha, 2007, p. 348).

By 2000, this had grown to 27 psychiatrists, seven in the private sector, 12 in the universities and eight in public mental health care. There were no child psychiatrists or psycho-geriatricians, four neurologists, no psychiatric social workers, five psychiatric nurses, one occupational therapist and five clinical psychologists (Regmi, 2000).

According to a report by the World Health Organization Assessment Instrument for Mental Health Systems, the breakdown according to profession is: 32 psychiatrists (0.129 per 100,000 population), six psychologists (0.024 per 100,000 population), 16 other medical doctors, unspecialized in psychiatry (0.0645 per 100,000 population), 68 nurses (0.274 per 100,000 population), no social workers and no occupational therapists (World Health Organization (WHO) and Ministry of Health and Population (MoHP), 2006). In 2010, there was one child psychiatrist, 54 psychiatrists, 10 clinical psychologists and 28 mental health nurses (Upadhyaya, 2013, p. 2).

Now, there are 65 psychiatrists including one child psychiatrist (only about 11 work under MoHP; others are in TUTH, BPKIHS, private medical colleges and private hospitals, and abroad), more than 48 psychiatric nurses, 14 clinical psychologists, no psychiatric social workers and only four occupational therapists (in CMC–Nepal). This represents remarkable progress in supply of specialist manpower, but the majority of mental health professionals currently work in urban areas. There are no data on the distribution of traditional health practitioners.

Main issues

The key mental health issue in Nepal, at present, is the implementation of the National Mental Health Policy and legislation. The National Mental Health Policy was adopted by the Ministry of Health in 1997 but it exists only in files. No further plans have been made to achieve the goals of the policy. Lack of separate mental health legislation is also a major issue in provision of care, especially to severely ill persons and their families, and therefore the whole of society. Lack of a coordinating body to oversee the implementation and coordination of policy at the government level and also for public education and awareness campaigns on mental health and mental disorders hampers any systematic development of mental health (*ekantipur*, 2011). The human rights of mentally ill persons are not being properly addressed. Therefore, the Ministry of Health needs urgently to initiate actions to address these major hindrances to implementation of the policy and the development of mental health services.

There are other issues that prevent successful implementation of mental health services, these are: lower priority in comparison with physical health needs; the stigma associated with mental disorders resulting in failure to seek appropriate care; inadequate funding of mental health care; lack of trained manpower; scarcity of public-health perspectives in mental health leadership; lack of consumer and pro-patient movements.

Lack of expertise in community mental health among specialists in both mental health and public health and lack of adequate resources allocated to this area are the main stumbling blocks to further development. So these need to be addressed urgently too.

Future directions

Although, in the last three decades, tremendous progress has been made in mental health services in Nepal, there is still a long way to go.

Despite the deeply rooted discrimination and stigma attached to the field, many young doctors and other professionals are choosing to be trained in the different mental health disciplines (Regmi et al., 2004, p. 142). This is a very positive indication. Mental health services, which were rudimentary to begin with, were further fragmented by the armed conflict of the recent past (Thapa and Hauff, 2005, p. 672).

The way for the government to increase mental health awareness is by providing adequate services in all regions of the country. This can be done by integrating mental health services into primary health care (World Health Organization (WHO) and World Organization of Family Doctors, 2008). Integrating mental health services into primary health care is a successful option which helps to provide effective mental health care in countries which have inadequate resources to address the burden of mental disorders properly (Becker and Kleinman, 2013, p. 66). In addition, this provides opportunities for people who generally prefer to contact primary care centers rather than institutes dealing solely with mental illness because of the social stigma attached. This will thus result in early detection, treatment and support of mentally ill patients and their families. However, on the other hand there are difficulties and impracticalities of integration of mental health services into primary health care in a low-resource country like Nepal.

There are some alternative options to fill this gap. The first is training general practitioners (GPs) and primary care workers to enhance their skills in screening for and detecting symptoms of mental illness (Jacob, 2011, p. 195). They can provide patient education and counseling services, and referral to psychiatrists as and when required. This will help to reduce the burden of illness detection that is placed on psychiatrists. Transferring the role to GPs also increases the chances of detecting more cases of mental illness, especially in rural areas (Chandrashekhar et al., 1981, p. 174). But here the issue of retention of GPs and trained health workers in rural areas arises. In such a situation, the government can take an active role and implement policies after adequate consultation to improve retention of GPs in rural Nepal.

Another option is to designate other mental health practitioners, such as psychologists, psychiatric social workers and psychiatric nurses, to detect mental disorders. This option is recommended by WHO as helpful where there is a scarcity of specially trained medical doctors (World Health Organization (WHO), 2004). However, there are constraints on this option as the numbers of other mental health practitioners are minimal and inadequate to provide services to the affected.

Community mental health services are limited to a few places in Nepal. The development of a national community mental health program is an important and urgent issue for the Ministry of Health to address (Shyangwa and Jha, 2008, p. 36).

WHO describes community-based care as an approach which provides services close to home, including general hospital care for acute admissions, and long-term residential facilities in the community; treatment and care specific to the diagnosis and needs of each individual; partnership with carers and meeting their needs; and legislation to support the above aspects of care. A balance of community-based and hospital-based services has been shown to be the most effective form of comprehensive mental health care (World Health Organization (WHO), 2001). Evidence suggests that, in low-income and middle-income countries, support for primary care services to enable them to identify and treat people with mental disorders, with training, assistance and supervision by available specialist mental health staff, is the best way to extend mental health care to the population (Saxena et al., 2007). Health service evaluations have shown that community-based care models, such as community-based rehabilitation and community outreach programs in India, are able to reach out to people in rural and impoverished communities, producing tangible benefits in terms of improved clinical outcomes, reduced levels of disability and reduced family care-giving burdens (Chatterjee et al., 2003, p. 57; Murthy, 2004, p. 75).

Similar results may be obtained in the context of Nepal. Taking basic and free mental health care to the doorstep of every member of our society will realize the vision of health as a fundamental right.

There is a need for interdisciplinary research training programs to develop research skills to conduct evaluations of mental health programs. WHO recommends collaboration between the mental health services of well-resourced and poorly-resourced countries to share experience and provide international training (World Health Organization (WHO), 2004). This can be a very positive initiative if international organizations like WHO can assist in the initial process of collaboration development.

Use of the media

The media is not only a powerful source of information for the general public but also an extremely powerful tool to bring about social changes within a short span of time and thus can be a powerful agent of change. In the context of Nepal, the use of the media as a social marketing strategy can help to promote mental health awareness. It is important to acknowledge that the power of the media, if used correctly, can be beneficial in mental health promotion and prevention activities. The use of local radio, loudspeakers, etc., are effective strategies to promote community awareness, challenge stigma and raise awareness about mental health issues. The media thus acts as a tool for advocacy and strengthening community capacity. Significant positive changes in knowledge and attitudes towards mental health have been found in UK, US and Norwegian evaluations of media campaigns (Jané-Llopis *et al.*, 2005, p. 9). The enormous power of the mass media should be harnessed to benefit the people in Nepal.

Conclusion

Despite many lacunae and scarcities in this field, mental health in Nepal has progressed in leaps and bounds and its expansion and scope have been ever widening. Nepal has a scarcity of mental health workers but there has been remarkable and visible progress in the last two decades.

The fight against mental illness is a complex task that requires a well-coordinated multisectoral approach. Both government and non-state agencies (such as NGOs/INGIOs, civil society organizations) need to work together to integrate various strategies, involving awareness raising and preventive measures, and targeting of at-risk groups, and functioning at the individual, family, community and societal levels. Mental health promotional and preventive programs need to be locally relevant, culturally appropriate and cost effective, and require social and public health approaches. In addition, government leadership on mental health is a key to success.

References

Acharya, AK (1998), 'Knowledge, attitude and practice of mental illness in a village population', Tribhuvan University, Kathmandu, Nepal.

Aich, TK (2010), 'Contribution of Indian psychiatry in the development of psychiatry in Nepal', *Indian Journal of Psychiatry*, 52(supplement 1), S76–S79, viewed 7 October 2013, www.ncbi.nlm.nih.gov/pmc/articles/PMC3146204/?tool=pmcentrez&report=abstract

Alzheimer's Disease and Related Dementias Society (ARDS) (2012), Nepal, viewed 1 October 2013, www.ardsnepal.org/

Aryal, SP (2010), 'Survey on hard drug users in Nepal: A practice for policy analysis and advocacy', paper presented at consultative meeting, Bangkok, 13–14 December 2010.

Atlas of Substance Use Disorders (2010), *Resources for the prevention and treatment of substance use disorders (SUD)*, World Health Organization (WHO), Geneva.

Autism Care Nepal (2008–2010), viewed 10 October 2013, www.autismnepal.org/

Bajracharya, MR, Manandhar, K and Deo KK. (2008), 'Age and gender distribution in deliberate self-poisoning cases', *Post Graduate Medical Journal of Nepal Academy of Medical Sciences*, 8(1), 44–9, viewed 10 October 2013, www.pmjn.org.np/index.php/pmjn/article/view/36/31

Becker, AE and Kleinman, A (2013), 'Global health: mental health and the global agenda', *The New England Journal of Medicine*, 369(1), 66–73.

Center for Mental Health and Counseling – Nepal (CMC–Nepal) (2013), Kathmandu, viewed 1 October 2013, www.cmcnepal.org.np/

Center for Victims of Torture (CVICT) (2013), Kathmandu, viewed 1 October 2013, www.cvict.org.np/

Central Bureau of Statistics (CBS) (2012), *Nepal in figures*, Government of Nepal, Kathmandu, Nepal, viewed 3 October 2013, http://cbs.gov.np/wp-content/uploads/2014/Nepal%20in%20figure/Nepal%20In%20Figures%202013_English.pdf

Chandrashekhar, CR, Isaac, MK, Kapur, RL and Sarathy, RP (1981), 'Management of priority mental disorders in the community', *Indian Journal of Psychiatry*, 23(2), 174–80.

Chatterjee, S, Patel, V and Chatterjee, A (2003), 'Evaluation of a community based rehabilitation for chronic schizophrenia in India', *British Journal of Psychiatry*, 182(1), 57–62.

Dahal, MK (2012), *Nepalese economy: development vs underdevelopment,* Telegraphnepal.com, viewed 3 October 2013, www.telegraphnepal.com/national/2012–10–08/nepalese-economy:-development-vs-underdevelopment.html

Devkota, M (2013), 'Mental health in Nepal: the voices of Koshish', *American Psychological Association*, Washington DC, viewed 3 October 2013, www.apa.org/international/pi/2011/07/nepal.aspx

Dhital, R (2000), *Alcohol and young people in Nepal*, CWIN, Kathmandu, Nepal, viewed 13 October 2013, http://apapaonline.org/data/National_Data/Cambodia/Nepal/Alcohol_and_Youth_Nepal.pdf

Dixit, H (1995), *Nepal's quest for health*, Kathmandu Book Publishing (Pvt.) Limited, Kathmandu.

Dixit, H (1998), 'Training doctors in Nepal', *Human Resources for Health Development Journal*, 2(1), 61–8.

ekantipur (2011), '9 out of 10 teenage suicides by girls, say police', *ekantipur*, 23 December, viewed 10 October 2013, www.ekantipur.com/2011/12/23/capital/9-of-10-teenage-suicides-by-girls-say-police/345996.html

Family Health Division (2010) Department of Health Services, 'Nepal maternal mortality and morbidity study 2008/2009', Ministry of Health, Government of Nepal, viewed 9 October 2013, www.dpiap.org/resources/pdf/nepal_maternal_mortality_2011_04_22.pdf

Geographia (1997–2005), 'Nepal', *Geographia*, viewed 3 October 2013, www.geographia.com/nepal/

Himalayan News Service (2013), 'Statistics paint scary picture of drug use', *The Himalayan Times*, 26 June, viewed 8 October 2013, www.thehimalayantimes.com/fullTodays.php?headline=Statistics+paint+scary+picture+of+drug+use+&NewsID=381620

Index Mundi (2013), *Nepal government profile 2013*, viewed 3 October 2013, www.indexmundi.com/nepal/government_profile.html

Jacob, KS (2011), 'Repackaging mental health programs in low- and middle-income countries', *Indian Journal of Psychiatry*, 53, 195–8.

Jané-Llopis, E, Barry, M, Hosman, C and Patel, V (2005), 'Mental health promotion works: a review', *Promotion and Education*, supplement, 9–25, 61, 67.

Jha, A (2007), 'Nepalese psychiatrists' struggle for evolution', *Psychiatric Bulletin*, 31, 348–50.

Jha, A and Adhikari, SR (2009), 'Mental health services in New Nepal – observations, objections and outlook for the future', *Journal of Nepal Medical Association*, 48(174), 185–90.

Jha, A and Sapkota, N (2013), 'Dementia assessment and management protocol for doctors in Nepal', *Journal of Nepal Medical Association*, 52(189), 292–8.

Jhingan, HP, Shyangwa, P, Sharma, A, Prasad, KM and Khandelwal, SK (2003), 'Prevalence of alcohol dependence in a town in Nepal as assessed by the CAGE questionnaire', *Addiction*, 98(3), 339–43.

Khatri, JB, Poudel, BM, Thapa, P, Godar, ST, Tirkey, S, Ramesh, K and Chakrabortty, PK (2013), 'An epidemiological study of psychiatric cases in a rural community of Nepal', *Nepal Journal of Medical Sciences*, 2(1), 52–6, viewed 8 October 2013, http://nepjol.info/index.php/NJMS/article/view/7654

Kohrt, BA, Hruschka, DJ, Worthman, CM, Kunz, RD, Baldwin, JL and Upadhyaya, N. (2012), 'Political violence and mental health in Nepal: prospective study', *British Journal of Psychiatry*, 201,268–75, viewed 9 October 2013, www.ncbi.nlm.nih.gov/pmc/articles/PMC3461445/

Maryknoll Nepal (2013), viewed 1 October 2013, www.maryknollnepal.org.np/

Mental Health Project (MHP) (2000–2003), *Annual report of mental health project*, Institute of Medicine (IOM), Kathmandu, Nepal.

Ministry of Health (2002), *Demographic and health survey*, Kathmandu, Nepal.

Ministry of Health (2004), *Health sector strategy: an agenda for reform*, His Majesty's Government, Nepal, viewed 7 October 2013, www.ministerial-leadership.org/sites/default/files/resources_and_tools/Health%20Sector%20Strategy_An%20Agenda%20for%20Reform.pdf

Ministry of Health and Population (MoHP) (2007), Health Sector Reform Unit, *Second long term health plan 1997–2017: Perspective plan for health sector development*, Government of Nepal, Kathmandu, Nepal, viewed 7 October 2013, http://mohp.gov.np/english/publication/second_long_term_health_plan_1997_2017.php

Ministry of Health and Population (MoHP) (2010), *Nepal health sector programme–2: Implementation plan*, Government of Nepal, Kathmandu, Nepal, viewed 7 October 2013, www.nhssp.org.np/health_policy/Consolidated%20NHSP-2%20IP%20092812%20QA.pdf

Ministry of Health and Population (MoHP) (Population Division) (2012), *Nepal demographic and health survey 2011*, Government of Nepal, Kathmandu, Nepal, viewed 7 October 2013, http://dhsprogram.com/pubs/pdf/FR257/FR257[13April2012].pdf

Mollica, RF (2001), 'Assessment of trauma in primary care', *Journal of the American Medical Association*, 285(9), 1213.

Murthy, RS (2004), 'The National Mental Health Programme: progress and problems', *Mental Health – An Indian Perspective (1946–2003)*, Directorate General of Health Services (Ministry of Health and Family Welfare), New Delhi, pp. 75–91.

National Mental Health Policy (1996), Director General of Health, Nepal, viewed 13 October 2013, http://mhpolicy.files.wordpress.com/2011/06/mental-health-policy.pdf

National Planning Commission Secretariat (2012), Central Bureau of Statistics (CBS), *National population and housing census 2011 (National Report)*, Government of Nepal, Kathmandu, Nepal, viewed 7 October 2013, http://cbs.gov.np/wp-content/uploads/2012/11/National%20Report.pdf

Nepal, MK (1999), 'Mental health in Nepal', *Nepalese Journal of Psychiatry*, 1, 3–4.

Nepal, MK, Sharma, P and Gurung, CK (1988), 'The first child psychiatric clinic: an initial appraisal', *NEPAS*, 7(1), 71–5.

Nepal, MK, Sharma, VD and Shrestha, PM (1996), 'Epilepsy prevalence, a case study of Morang district', *Proceedings of EPICADEC and Department of Psychiatry, Institute of Medicine*, pp. 17–23.

Nepal News (2013), *Government presents budget worth Rs 517.24 billion*, nepalnews.com, viewed 7 October 2013, www.nepalnews.com/archive/2013/jul/jul14/news16.php

Pokhrel, A, Ojha, SP, Koirala, NR, Regmi, SK, Pradhan, SN and Sharma, VD. (2001), 'A profile of children and adolescents referred by paediatricians to the child guidance clinic of Tribhuwan University Teaching Hospital', *Nepalese Journal of Psychiatry*, 2, 116–22.

Pradhan, A, Suvedi, BK, Barnett, S, Sharma, S, Puri, M, Poudel, P, Rai Chitrakar, S, Pratap, NKC and Hulton, L (2010), *Nepal Maternal Mortality and Morbidity Study 2008/2009*. Family Health Division, Department of Health Services, Ministry of Health and Population, Government of Nepal, Kathmandu.

Pradhan, SN (2011), 'Depression in elderly', *Journal of Psychiatrists' Association of Nepal*, 1(1), 13–14.

Regmi, SK (2000), 'Mental health in Nepal: past, present and future', paper presented at Second International Conference of the Bangladesh Association of Psychiatrists, Dhaka, 28–29 February.

Regmi, SK, Khalid, A and Pokhrel, A (1998), 'Psychiatric morbidity profile of patients attending psychiatry OPD, TUTH', The souvenir of 1st National Conference of Psychiatrists' Association of Nepal, Nepal.

Regmi, SK, Khalid, A, Nepal, MK and Pokhrel, A (1999), 'A study of sociodemographic characteristics and diagnostic profile in psychiatric outpatients', *Nepalese Journal of Psychiatry*, 1(1), 26–33.

Regmi, SK, Pokhrel, A, Ojha, SP, Pradhan, SN and Chapagain, G (2004), 'Nepal mental health country profile', *International Review of Psychiatry*, 16(1–2), 142–9.

Risal, A, Sharma, PP and Karki, R (2013), 'Psychiatric illnesses among the patients admitted for self-poisoning in a tertiary care hospital of Nepal', *Journal of Advances in Internal Medicine*, 2(3), 10–13.

Saxena, S, Thornicroft, G, Knapp, M. and Whiteford, H (2007), 'Global Mental Health 2: Resources for mental health: scarcity, inequity, and inefficiency', *The Lancet*, 370(9590), 878–89.

Sedhain, CP (2013), 'Study of psychiatric morbidity of patients attending free mental health check up camp, Simra, Bara, Nepal', *Journal of Psychiatrists' Association of Nepal*, 2(1), 30–4, viewed 8 October 2013, www.nepjol.info/index.php/JPAN/article/view/8572/6968

Shakya, DR (2011), 'Dementia: forget me not', *ekantipur,* 4 December, viewed 10 October 2013, www. ekantipur.com/the-kathmandu-post/2011/12/04/health-and-living/dementia-forget-me-not/228973. html

Shakya, DR (2013), 'Substance use disorder: a neglect area', *Advocating Psychiatry in Nepal*, Nepal.

Shakya, DR, Shyangwa, PM and Sen, B (2008), 'Physical diseases in cases admitted for alcohol dependence', *Health Renaissance*, 5(1), 27–31.

Shakya, YL, Acharya, R, Gupta, MP, Banjara, MR and Prasad, PN (2010), 'Factors determining self-harm', *Journal of Institute of Medicine*, 32(3), 14–17, viewed 10 October 2013, http://webcache.googleuser content.com/search?q=cache:Zty-68RbAUAJ:www.researchgate.net/profile/Ramesh_Aacharya/ publication/239938942_Factors_determining_self-harm/file/e0b4951c387b6648b0.pdf+&cd= 1&hl=en&ct=clnk&gl=au

Shakya, DR, Shyangwa, PM and Sen, B (2011a), 'Help seeking behavior in patients with alcohol dependence in tertiary care hospital in eastern Nepal', *Journal of Psychiatrists' Association of Nepal*, 1(1), 15–19.

Shakya, DR, Lamichhane, N, Shyangwa, PM and Shakya, R (2011b), 'Nepalese psychiatric patients with armed-conflict related stressors', *Health Renaissance*, 9(2), 67–72.

Shrestha, DM (1986), 'Neuropsychiatric problems in children attending a general psychiatric clinic in Nepal', *Nepal Paediatric Society Journal*, 5, 97–101.

Shrestha, NM, Shrestha, DM, Karmacharya, K and Sharma A (2001), *A study of prevalence of alcohol use and suicide in Kathmandu Metropolitan City*, WHO South-East Asia Regional Office, New Delhi.

Shyangwa, PM and Jha, A (2008), 'Nepal: trying to reach out to the community', *International Psychiatry*, 5(2), 36–8.

Shyangwa, PM, Singh, S and Khandelwal, SK (2003), 'Knowledge and attitudes about mental illness among nursing staff', *Journal of Nepal Medical Association*, 42, 27–31, viewed 8 October 2013, http://jnma.com.np/jnma/index.php/jnma/article/viewFile/713/1419

Thapa, SB and Hauff, E (2005), 'Psychological distress among displaced persons during an armed conflict in Nepal', *Social Psychiatry and Psychiatric Epidemiology*, 40(8), 672–9.

Transcultural Psychosocial Organization (TPO) Nepal (2010), viewed 10 October 2013, www. tponepal.org/

Tribhuvan University Medical Education Department (1994), Tribhuvan University Institute of Medicine Curriculum for MBBS, Tribhuvan University, Kathmandu, Nepal.

Tulachan, P, Chapagain, M, Kunwar, AR and Sharma, VD (2011), 'Psychiatric morbidity pattern in a child and adolescent guidance clinic', *Journal of Psychiatrists' Association of Nepal*, 1(1), 20–3

United Nations Population Information Network (POPIN) (1994), *Report of the International Conference on Population and Development (ICPD)*, United Nation Population Division, viewed 7 October 2013, www.un.org/popin/icpd/conference/offeng/poa.html

Upadhyaya, KD (2011), Presidential Address, *Journal of Psychiatrists' Association of Nepal*, 1(1), 1–4.

Upadhyaya, KD (2013), 'National mental health policy 1996, what has been achieved: A review', *Journal of Psychiatrists' Association of Nepal*, 2(1), 2–6.

Upadhyaya, KD and Pol, K (2003), 'A mental health prevalence survey in two developing towns of western region', *Journal of Nepal Medical Association*, 42, 328–30, viewed 8 October 2013, www.jnma.com. np/jnma/index.php/jnma/article/download/610/1345

Upadhyaya, KD, Nakarmi, B, Prajapati, B and Timilsina, M (2013), 'Morbidity profile of patients attending the centres for mental health service provided jointly by the Government of Nepal and community mental health service of community mental health and counseling – Nepal (CMC–Nepal)', *Journal of Psychiatrists' Association of Nepal*, 2(1), 14–19, viewed 8 October 2013, http://webcache.google usercontent.com/search?q=cache:f00KrblbklcJ:www.nepjol.info/index.php/JPAN/article/download/ 8569/6965+&cd=1&hl=en&ct=clnk&gl=au

Wang, PS, Aguilar-Gaxiola, S and Alonso, J. (2007), 'Use of mental health services for anxiety, mood, and substance disorders in 17 countries in the WHO world mental health surveys', *The Lancet*, 370(9590), 841–50, viewed 8 October 2013, www.sciencedirect.com.elibrary.jcu.edu.au/science/article/pii/ S0140673607614147

World Health Organization (WHO) (2001), *Mental health, human rights and legislation: WHO's framework*, viewed 28 September 2013, http://wfmh.com/wp-content/uploads/2013/12/fact_sheet_mnh_hr_ leg_2105.pdf

World Health Organization (WHO) (2004), *Promoting mental health: concepts, emerging evidence, practice*, World Health Organization, Geneva.

World Health Organization (WHO) (2007), *Policy papers on health Nepal*, World Health Organization, Nepal (country office), viewed 1 October 2013, http://www.nep.searo.who.int/LinkFiles/Health_ Information_PPH.pdf

World Health Organization (WHO) and Ministry of Health and Population (MoHP) (2006), *WHO–AIMS report on mental health system in Nepal*, World Health Organization (country office), Nepal.

World Health Organization (WHO) and World Organization of Family Doctors (2008), *Integrating mental health into primary care: a global perspective*, World Health Organization, Geneva.

Wright, C, Nepal, MK, Bruce-Jones, WD (1989), Mental health patients in primary health care services in Nepal, *Asia Pacific Journal of Public Health*, 3(3), 224–30.

10

Mental health in Pakistan

Rizwan Taj

Introduction

Pakistan is a sovereign state in South Asia. It is bordered by Afghanistan and Iran to the west, India to the east, China to the far northeast, and has a 1,046-kilometre (650 mile) coastline along the Arabian Sea and the Gulf of Oman to the south. It is a federal parliamentary republic consisting of four provinces and four federal territories. With a population of about 193,238,868 (July 2013 estimate), it is the sixth most populous country in the world, ethnically and linguistically diverse, with a semi-industrialized economy. Terrorism, poverty, illiteracy and corruption are major challenges.

The median age is 22.2, with 34 per cent of the population under the age of 15, and only 4.3 per cent over the age of 65. Urbanization is growing at the rate of 3 per cent a year and 36.2 per cent of the population lives in urban areas. The five major cities of Karachi, Lahore, Faisalabad, Rawalpindi and Islamabad have populations of 13.12 million, 7.13 million, 2.84 million, 2.02 million and 0.8 million respectively (2009). The overall population is growing at a rate of 1.52 per cent a year (2013 estimate), with a birth rate of 23.76 births per 1,000 (2013 estimate). Ethnically, the population consists of Punjabi 44.68 per cent, Pashtun (Pathan) 15.42 per cent, Sindhi 14.1 per cent, Sariaki 8.38 per cent, Muhajirs 7.57 per cent, Balochi 3.57 per cent and others 6.28 per cent. Religious groupings include Muslim (official) 96.4 per cent (Sunni 75 per cent, Shia 20 per cent) and others (including Christian and Hindu) 5 per cent. The main languages spoken are Punjabi 48 per cent, Sindhi 12 per cent, Saraiki (a Punjabi variant) 10 per cent, Pashtu 8 per cent, Urdu (official) 8 per cent, Balochi 3 per cent, Hindko 2 per cent, Brahui 1 per cent, English (official lingua franca of the Pakistani elite and most government ministries), Burushaski and other 8 per cent.

Literacy, defined as the proportion of the population aged 15 and over who can read and write, is relatively poor with considerable gender differences (68.6 per cent male and 40.3 per cent female) (2009 estimate) and is the focus of considerable government effort to improve this. At present, 2.7 per cent of GDP is spent on education. Males spend an average of eight years in school and females seven years (2011).

Progress on the Millennium Development Goals has been slower than anticipated. Infant mortality is 59.35 deaths per 1,000 live births (2013 estimate), the total fertility rate is 2.96

children born per woman (2013 estimate), maternal mortality is 260 deaths per 100,000 live births (2008), 30.9 per cent of children under the age of five years are underweight, and there are an estimated 98,000 people living with HIV/AIDS (0.1 per cent prevalence, 2009) and 5,800 annual deaths from AIDS (2009). There is a high risk of infectious diseases, especially from food or waterborne diseases (bacterial diarrhoea, hepatitis A and E and typhoid fever); vector borne diseases (dengue fever and malaria); and animal contact disease (rabies). Health expenditure is 2.5 per cent of GDP (2011). There are 0.813 physicians (2009) and 0.6 beds per 1,000 population (2010).

Psychiatric epidemiology in Pakistan

Mental health is the most neglected field in Pakistan where 10–15 per cent of the population, i.e. more than 14 million, suffer from mild to moderate psychiatric illness, the majority of whom are women.

Pakistan has a democratically elected government which has considerable recent challenges to tackle, including terrorism and internal displacement. Mental health legislation to protect the human rights of people with mental illness was passed in 2001.

The specialist mental health infrastructure is limited. For a population of 190 million, there are 520 psychiatrists and there are fewer than 3,000 psychiatric inpatient beds. There are a number of psychology graduates but very few are clinically trained. There are only a handful of psychiatric nurses working in hospital settings and no community psychiatric nurses at all.

The psychiatrists are mostly based in tertiary-level provincial hospitals, which generally have departments of psychiatry. There are also three long-stay facilities for mental health. Thus, while specialist care is generally available in provincial hospitals, there are hardly any districts with specialist staff or facilities, and most district psychiatric posts lie empty. This infrastructure does not meet the population needs for mental health care.

The incidence and prevalence of mental illness have both increased against the background of growing insecurity, terrorism, economic problems, political uncertainty, unemployment and disruption of the social fabric. Almost 39 per cent of individuals below the poverty line is an alarming factor worth noting. Many people are now presenting to psychiatrists probably because of growing awareness through the good work of the media.

Major mental disorders in Pakistan are depression (6 per cent), schizophrenia (1.5 per cent) and epilepsy (1–2 per cent).[2]

In addition, there is a serious problem of substance misuse and drug addiction. About four million[3] drug addicts have been estimated in the last national survey in Pakistan, with a growing number of injectable drug users in the urban population creating a public health predicament.

Drug use in Pakistan

According to United Nations Office on Drugs and Crime (UNODC) technical summary report 2012 on drug use in Pakistan, annual prevalence is estimated to be 5.8 per cent, or 6.45 million of the population in Pakistan aged between 15 and 64 used drugs in 2012.[4] Cannabis is the most commonly used drug with an annual prevalence of 3.6 per cent or approximately four million people. Cannabis is followed by sedatives and tranquilizers, such as benzodiazepines, heroin, opium and other opiates. Proportionately, more men use drugs in Pakistan than women, although prevalence estimates for women are likely underestimates. The proportions are 8.5 per cent and 2.9 per cent, respectively. Drug use patterns vary considerably between men and women. Women are more likely to consume amphetamines and painkillers, with 92 per cent of female users regularly misusing painkillers, and tranquilizers and sedatives. In comparison, only 48 per cent of male users also misuse these substances. Men are more likely to use cannabis than women, at 44 per cent and less than one per cent respectively.

High levels of opiate use have been found with 0.9 per cent or just more than one million users of whom 0.7 per cent use heroin and 0.3 per cent use opium annually. Levels of use of opiates are highest as a proportion of the population in provinces that border cultivation areas in Afghanistan.

The highest prevalence of any drug use is seen in Khyber Pakhtunkhwa where 11 per cent of the population use illicit substances. The provinces of Sindh and Punjab reveal levels of use of 6.5 and 4.8 per cent respectively.

There are an estimated 420,000 People Who Inject Drugs (PWID) in Pakistan. Heroin is most likely to be administered via injection, although users also report injecting painkillers, amphetamines, and tranquilizers with average age of first injection being 26.[4]

Synthetic drugs in the form of amphetamine-type stimulants (ATS) have emerged as a concern with 0.1 per cent found to use amphetamines and 0.02 per cent using methamphetamine. While the levels of annual use of ATS are low, the findings are nonetheless noteworthy because it is the first time a research study has reported related data for Pakistan.

Non-medical use of prescription drugs has been found in a sizable population of men and women, although is it significant that more women use sedatives and tranquilizers than men.

Suicide

Suicide has become a major health problem in Pakistan but despite this, there are no official data available and exact rates are not known. Rates for men are consistently higher than for women: the highest rates for men were between the ages of 20 and 40 in Larkana.[5]

Suicide and attempted suicide are understudied subjects in Pakistan, an Islamic country where they are considered criminal offenses. National suicide statistics are not compiled nor are suicide mortality statistics reported to the World Health Organization (WHO). A two-year analysis of all such reports in a major newspaper in Pakistan showed 306 suicides reported from 35 cities.[6] Men outnumbered women by 2:1. While there were more single than married men, the trend was reversed in women. The majority of victims were under 30 years of age and 'domestic problems' was the most common reason stated. More than half the subjects used organophosphate insecticides, while psychotropics and analgesics were used infrequently.[6]

Deliberate self-harm

Modes of deliberate self-harm (DSH) have been found to vary in different regions of Pakistan. However, self-poisoning has been found to be the most common method. Benzodiazepine, bleach, bathroom cleanser, organophosphorus compounds, rat poison, louse powder and Dettol are commonly used.

Although it is hard to get proper estimates, according to a study conducted in a tertiary care hospital in Karachi, females (59 per cent) outnumbered males (41 per cent) with the age group ranging from 12 to 76 years, and 69 per cent were under the age of 30 years. Married women (32 per cent) form the largest group followed by single women (25 per cent), single men (24 per cent) and married men (16 per cent).[7] The number of divorced and widowed individuals in both groups was negligible.

Family disputes, interpersonal conflicts with the opposite sex, marital problems, chronic illness and financial problems are the most common precipitating factors in various studies. Legal, social and economic discrimination, chronically poor physical health and being unmarried are other common risk factors for deliberate self-harm.

Depression in Pakistan

Epidemiological studies from Pakistan have given conflicting findings. Besides a very high prevalence of depression in different studies, rates from Northern Pakistan are very different from the big urban cities. There are five community-based studies[8–12] reporting prevalence estimates for depression and anxiety from various regions of Pakistan (see Table 10.1). These studies give variable prevalence estimates of depression; from as high as 66 per cent in women from rural areas to 10 per cent in men from urban areas. The mean overall point prevalence is 33.62 per cent ($n = 2658$),[12] which means that on average every third Pakistani is expected to be suffering from depression and anxiety. All of the studies carried out in Pakistan were cross-sectional in design. This marked difference in prevalence could also be due to systematic error in centre-based sampling methodology.

Table 10.1 Prevalence of depression from community studies in Pakistan

Location	Male (%)	Female (%)
North Pakistan[8]	15	46
Rural Punjab[9]	25	66
Urban Punjab[10]	10	25
Semi-urban Karachi[11]	18.1	42.2
Urban Karachi[12]	25.5	57.5

Globally, depression affects 20 per cent of people, while in Pakistan it is more serious, estimated at 34 per cent.[12] Around 35.7 per cent of citizens of Karachi are affected with this mental illness, while 43 per cent from Quetta and 53.4 per cent from Lahore are also affected.[12]

Sociodemographic factors associated with increased prevalence of anxiety and depressive disorders include female sex, middle age and low level of education. Loss of husband (being widowed, separated or divorced), increasing duration of marriage, and being a housewife are also positively associated.

Socioeconomic adversity and relationship problems are major risk factors for anxiety and depressive disorders in Pakistan.

Mental health literacy

Mental health patients are stigmatized as social outcasts in a very different manner from people facing other illnesses, they are often perceived as deviants and their condition is treated as a shameful secret by their families. In a number of cases, family members are offended by the suggestion of seeking outside help, as talking about personal and intimate problems is a cultural taboo.

Unawareness about many mental illness and monetary constraints are the major hurdles to the development of mental health services. Most people with mental illnesses therefore have no access to psychiatric services, of which they are unaware. Either they turn to traditional healers or they live with their disabling psychiatric disorders. Moreover, available facilities are under-utilized as a result of the social stigma associated with psychiatric labeling.[13]

In a study it was found that the knowledge of the general practitioners about depression was inadequate.[14] This not only leads to under-diagnosis of people suffering from depression, which in turn becomes a reason for longer duration and greater severity of illness, but also leads to over-prescription of benzodiazepines to patients with depression for their complaints of insomnia.

Mental health legislation

The Constitution of Pakistan guarantees basic rights and liberties to all citizens of the state. Article 25 of the Constitution stipulates equality of all citizens before the law.[15]

It is such an unfortunate thing that the legislators of this country never realized that issues relating to mental health deserve attention. For 54 years the only law in Pakistan dealing with mental health issues was the Lunacy Act of 1912.

The Disabled Persons Ordinance was promulgated in 1981 to provide for the employment, rehabilitation and welfare of disabled persons.[16]

It provided for the formation of a national council which was entrusted with the following functions:

1. Formulate policy for the employment, rehabilitation and welfare of disabled persons.
2. Evaluate, assess and coordinate the execution of the policy by the provincial council.
3. Have overall responsibility for the achievement of the purposes of this Ordinance.

The Mental Health Ordinance, 2001, was promulgated on the 20th February, 2001.[17] The legislation also provided for the establishment of a Mental Health Authority which was given an ambitious mandate. It is evident that the authority is primarily tasked with providing advice to the government on mental health policies and legislation. It is also involved in service planning, service management and coordination, and in monitoring and quality assessment of mental health services. The Mental Health Ordinance, 2001, espoused various legislative provisions to protect and provide support for users, which was a step in the right direction.

The first Federal Mental Health Authority was formed in 2001 but lapsed in 2005 without achieving any significant progress in the implementation of the Ordinance. This authority was reconstituted in December 2008.

The National Policy for Persons with Disabilities was formulated in 2002. Its goal was the empowerment of persons with disabilities, for the realization of their full potential in all spheres of life.

A disaster/emergency preparedness plan for mental health exists and was last revised in 2006.

Although mental health legislation to protect the human rights of people with mental illness was passed in 2001, implementation has been very slow and received a setback when the federal Mental Health Authority was dissolved, following federal devolution to the provinces. Sind Assembly passed the Sind Mental Health Act, 2013, which has provided for the establishment of a Mental Health Authority.

Currently there is no legislation to protect the rights of mentally impaired persons in Punjab, Khyber Pakhtunkhwa and Baluchistan. There is an urgent need to recreate the Authority and extend the implementation process.

Mental health policy

The health sector has been accorded a low priority by successive governments. The health budget constitutes a mere 3.9 per cent of GDP whereas per capita expenditure on health by the government is US$21. Just 0.4 per cent of health care expenditures by the government health department are devoted to mental health. Of all the expenditures on mental health, 11 per cent is devoted to mental hospitals. 5 per cent of the population has free access (at least 80 per cent covered) to essential psychotropic medicines. For those that pay out-of-pocket, the cost is 7 per cent of the one-day minimum daily wage in the local currency. None of the mental disorders are covered by social insurance schemes. The per day cost of antipsychotic medication is US$2 per day, and the per day cost of antidepressant medication is US$5 per day.[2]

Pakistan's mental health policy was last revised in 2003. Its salient features include developing community mental health services, downsizing large mental hospitals, developing a mental health component in primary healthcare, human resources, involvement of users and family, advocacy and promotion, human rights protection of users, equity of access to mental health services across different groups, and strengthening the financing and monitoring system. This plan also catered for reforming mental hospitals to provide more comprehensive care. Additionally a budget, a timeframe and specific goals have been identified in the last mental health plan.

The role of international organizations such as World Health Organization (WHO) and their impact on the country has been minimal as they have focused only on one centre which is the WHO Collaborating Centre for Mental Health at Benazir Bhutto Hospital, Rawalpindi. This approach, especially post-devolution, should be modified with provincial collaboration centres, so that the impact of the mental health service in the provinces and periphery can be enhanced.

Current psychiatric services in Pakistan

The specialist mental health infrastructure is inadequate. A very limited number of hospitals have psychiatric wards and according to the WHO's *Mental Health Atlas* (2011) there are only 419 certified psychiatrists (now increased to 520) and 480 psychologists in Pakistan. For a population of 190 million, there are less than 3,000 psychiatric inpatient beds. There are a number of psychology graduates but very few are clinically trained. There are fewer than 50 psychiatric nurses working in hospital settings and no community psychiatric nurses at all. The psychiatrists are mostly based in tertiary-level provincial hospitals, which generally have departments of psychiatry. Thus, while specialist care is generally available in provincial hospitals, there are hardly any districts with specialist staff or facilities, and most district psychiatric posts lie empty. This infrastructure therefore does not meet the population needs for mental health care.

At the time of independence there were two mental hospitals in Pakistan. One was the mental hospital in Lahore (Punjab Institute of Medical Health) and the other one was the Sir Cowas Jee mental hospital in Hyderabad. Subsequently mental hospitals in Peshawar and Dhodial were established in 1950 and 1963, respectively. No mental rehabilitation facility was available till 1970. Fountain House was established by the Lahore Mental Health Association in 1971.

There are four major psychiatric hospitals in the country which are integrated with mental health outpatient facilities. Six hundred and twenty-four community-based psychiatric inpatient units are available in the country providing a total of 1.926 beds per 100,000 population. Just 1 per cent of these beds are reserved for children and adolescents. Of the admissions to such inpatient units, 75 per cent are female whereas 18 per cent are children/adolescents. The number of beds has risen by 4 per cent in the last five years.[2]

There are 3,729 outpatient mental health facilities in the country of which 1 per cent are for children and adolescents only. These facilities treat 343.34 users per 100,000 population. Of all users treated in outpatient facilities 69 per cent are female whereas 46 per cent are children or adolescents.

The percentage of females treated in various facilities is much higher than that of men. They account for 74 per cent of the patients treated in mental hospitals, 69 per cent of those treated in outpatient facilities and 75 per cent of the patients treated in psychiatric inpatient units. This gender difference in prevalence of psychiatric illnesses could be because of gender discrimination and the underprivileged status of females in the country resulting in more social stressors and more frequent relapses and chronic illnesses.

Regarding services, community psychiatric services are still at a basic level, while general psychiatric services are not up to the mark in the public sector and very costly in the private sector, which is not within the reach of majority of people. Though the trend is now changing in the field of research, there is very little input so far.

Despite the alarming situation of mental illness in Pakistan, there is not a single academic degree programme in neuroscience nor a world class research and treatment centre for psychiatric disorders in Pakistan.

There are no specialized forensic facilities or psychiatrists in our country. There are no rehabilitation programmes in place for those proven not guilty on account of mental illnesses. In Pakistan, the Pakistan Medical and Dental Council (PMDC) is the sole body for proper licensing of physicians. All physicians need to be registered with this central body. The problem lies in the implementation of rules. There are a large number of psychiatric hospitals claiming to deliver psychiatric care with no qualified psychiatrists on their panels. There are reports of abuse of psychiatric patients. In some centres patients are chained and beaten brutally.

Human resources

The total number of people working in mental health facilities or private practice per 100,000 population is 203.07. In Pakistan there are a total of 342 psychiatrists (0.20 per 100,000), 478 psychologists (0.28 per 100,000), 3,145 social workers (1.87 per 100,000) and 22 occupational therapists (0.01 per 100,000).

Of the psychiatrists, 45 per cent work for government-administered mental health facilities, 51 per cent work for NGOs/for-profit mental health facilities/private practice and 4 per cent work for both the sectors (Figure 10.1).

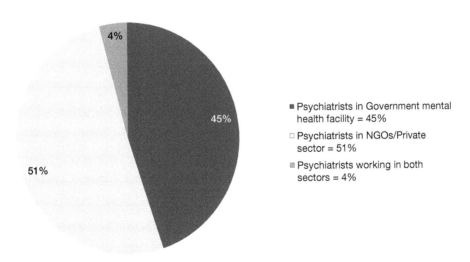

■ Psychiatrists in Government mental health facility = 45%

□ Psychiatrists in NGOs/Private sector = 51%

▨ Psychiatrists working in both sectors = 4%

Figure 10.1 Percentage of psychiatrists in government and private sector work in Pakistan

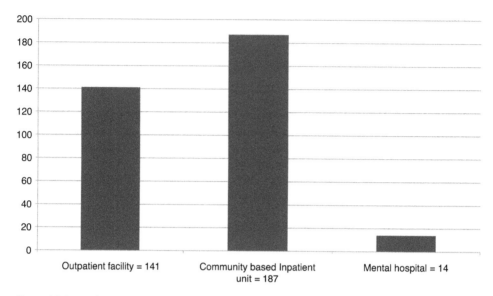

Figure 10.2 Psychiatrists working in different facilities in Pakistan (total: 342)

In terms of facilities, 141 psychiatrists work in outpatient facilities, 187 in community-based psychiatric inpatient units and 14 in mental hospitals (Figure 10.2).

The number of professionals who graduated in 2013 from academic and educational institutions per 100,000 is as follows: 2.1 medical doctors (not specialized in psychiatry); 1.5 nurses (not specialized in psychiatry); 0.002 psychiatrists; 0.07 psychologists with at least one year of training in mental health care; 0.008 nurses with at least one year of training in mental health care; 0.005 social workers with at least one year of training in mental health care; 0.002 occupational therapists with at least one year of training in mental health care. Around 20 per cent of psychiatrists emigrate to other countries within five years of completion of their training.[2]

Decentralization of mental health services

In the current situation of mental health services in Pakistan, psychosocial interventions and mental health awareness raising cannot be delivered by professionals alone. So there is need for inter-sectoral collaboration and a multifaceted and a multiprofessional approach in implementing mental health care in the community.

Previous work shows that the school mental health programme as a part of community mental health programme in Pakistan succeeded especially well in improving the awareness of mental health, not only of school teachers and school children but also of the whole community.[18]

In Pakistan, a huge public sector programme for training and deploying 'lady health workers' (LHWs) has been in place since 1994 and has been expanded to cover over 70 per cent of the rural population with a work force exceeding 90,000.[19]

Recently, efforts have been made to integrate mental health into primary care in rural areas of Pakistan. A number of innovative programmes to develop indigenous models of care like the 'Community Mental Health Programme' and 'Schools Mental Health Programme' have been developed. These programmes have been found to be effective in reducing stigma and increasing awareness of mental illness amongst adults and children living in rural areas.

With the support and technical guidance of a UK partner, over 300 psychiatrists, LHWs, school and college teachers, and media professionals have received mental health training since 2012.[20]

Integrated mental health services

The World Health Organization (WHO) has established a collaboration centre in Rawalpindi. The WHO has provided consultation services and initiatives on many projects to low- and middle-income countries. These have been implemented with variable success. The management of five common mental illnesses in primary health care is one of the options. The illnesses include depressive disorder, psychosis, substance abuse, mental retardation and epilepsy.

The role of non-governmental organizations

Non-governmental organizations (NGOs) working for the promotion of mental health in Pakistan have been evolving in recent decades, but have not kept pace with the demand for more and better services. Their role is, in any case, limited to sporadic public awareness programmes, gender discrimination issues, and social and cultural activities. They have no comprehensive strategy for the promotion of mental health issues

There are 18 NGOs in the country involved in individual assistance activities such as counselling, housing or support groups.

Paediatric mental health in Pakistan

Children comprise 43 per cent of the Pakistani population and there are estimated to be more than 78,786,000 individuals (according to a recent estimate) below the age of 18 years.[21]

The changing economic structure of the country has led to rapid urbanization, attracting young people from the countryside to the cities in search of jobs, thereby undermining the traditional role and structure of the family. Rapid urbanization has been shown to increase behavioural and emotional problems in children in developing countries.[22]

For developing countries like Pakistan, UNICEF estimates that one in five children suffer from chronic malnutrition and a similar number have diets deficient in one or another essential nutrient. This leads not only to physical but also cognitive and behavioural abnormalities. Other environmental hazards that produce mental retardation are also more widespread. The rate of serious mental retardation is 1.5 per cent, which is amongst the highest in developing countries.[23] Of about half a million children with epilepsy, 94 per cent are untreated[24] or maltreated by the traditional healers.

Though country-wide surveys are not available in the literature, estimates gauge the prevalence of childhood mental disabilities in Pakistan to be around 17 per cent (8 per cent mental retardation and 9 per cent behavioural, emotional and pervasive developmental disturbances).

A general lack of education and awareness in our population makes Pakistani parents poor candidates for screening for childhood mental disabilities. There is a dearth of local studies exploring the ability of Pakistani school teachers and general practitioners (GPs) to identify developmental and intellectual defects among children.

The enigma of child mental health is as obscure as mental health in general. It is commonplace to be asked whether children develop mental illness. In Pakistan, there are very few psychiatrists trained in child mental health. The number of child and adolescent psychiatrists is 0.01 per cent of the number of general adult psychiatrists. At present in Pakistan, there are no formal services to meet the needs of the vast majority of children.

The first indoor child psychiatry unit in Pakistan has established in Mayo Hospital, Lahore, in 2013. The practice of child psychiatry is limited to few tertiary care centres. Attention deficit hyperactivity disorder (ADHD) forms the bulk of cases seen in the office of a child psychiatrist. This is followed by depressive and anxiety disorders. Although the diagnosis of ADHD is as common as one in 20 children in the United States, the prevalence estimates from Pakistan cannot be overlooked; a tertiary care centre-based study reported a frequency estimate of 34 per cent.[25] This further emphasizes the need to develop child and adolescent psychiatric services in Pakistan.

Undergraduate psychiatric education

Undergraduate psychiatric education is in the doldrums, which is evidenced by the very low weight is given to the subject at undergraduate level. The Pakistan Medical and Dental Council has taken a positive step by introducing the subject of behavioural sciences in the early academic years, though there is a dearth of trained behavioural scientists to cater to this need appropriately. Exaggerated claims are being made for the high quality of postgraduate education in psychiatry. But keeping in mind the very few training slots, huge numbers of patients in public sector hospitals, large number of trainees, inadequate number of trained teachers, personal biases and fallacies in the exam system, there remains a question about the quality of postgraduate education.[26]

Explanatory models of illness

Explanatory models (EMs) are defined as 'the notions about an episode of sickness and its treatment that are employed by all those engaged in the clinical process' (Kleinman:[27] 105). Explanatory models are presented as conceptual tools to understand how different cultural and social contexts affect the ways that people negotiate their experiences with illness. These include beliefs about causes of illness, which in turn can influence illness-related behaviours, use of services and patient satisfaction.

Qualitative literature from Pakistan indicates that people with common mental disorders (CMDs) when closely questioned about the onset, see the origins of their problems in their social world.[28,29] There is some evidence that prevalence of CMDs is influenced by social factors such as population density, poverty, societal violence and terrorism.[30] Other risk factors include being divorced or widowed, conflict with in-laws, financial strain and the status of being a housewife rather than employed.

In Pakistan, the majority of the psychiatric patients go to traditional faith healers and religious healers who believe that mental illness is caused by supernatural forces such as spirit possession, evil eyes, magic or testing by God.

Role of faith healers in mental health in Pakistan

It appears that in the last century, modern medicine has purposefully shied away from the role of seemingly extremely variable factors like religion and spirituality in healing. Predominantly Muslim countries have witnessed this change in focus to a lesser extent, presumably as a result of religious and cultural factors.

A survey, carried out at two leading high-volume public hospitals in Islamabad showed that the patients wanted their physicians to pay due reverence to prayer (*Dua*). Similarly, for most patients, the religious inclination of the physician was perceived as an essential factor in the overall effectiveness of treatment.[31]

In addition to lack of awareness, cultural beliefs and insufficient mental health services, this may be a reason why people consult faith healers for treatment of mental illnesses.

The involvement of traditional faith healers in community mental health reform is critical. It is widely perceived by members of the community, reinforced by the beliefs of traditional faith healers, that mental illness is caused by supernatural forces such as spirit possession or testing by God, as mentioned above. Religious healers are usually the first group of practitioners sought out by families of the mentally ill. Pakistani people have strong faith in religious healers and the Quranic texts used by them, which places these healers in a powerful position to help people solve their psychosocial problems.[32] The traditional healers use talismans and give them to the families of the patients.

Although native faith healers are found in all parts of Pakistan, where they practise in harmony with the cultural value system, their practice is poorly understood. In a study that investigated mental disorders among attenders at faith healers, it was found that the classification used by faith healers was based on the mystic cause of disorders: *saya* (27 per cent), *jinn* possession (16 per cent) or *churail* possession (14 per cent). *Jinn* or *churail* are considered supernatural creatures. *Jinn/churail* possession disorders are usually the name used by the faith healers for dissociative disorders, specifically for trance and possession disorders. Sixty-one percent of attenders were given a research diagnosis of mental disorder: major depressive episode (24 per cent), generalized anxiety disorder (15 per cent) or epilepsy (9 per cent).

There was little agreement between the faith healers' classification and DSM diagnosis. Faith healers use powerful techniques of suggestion and cultural psychotherapeutic procedures. Faith healers are a major source of care for people with mental health problems in Pakistan, particularly for women and those with little education.[33]

Further research should assess methods of collaboration that will permit people with mental health problems to access effective and culturally appropriate treatment.

References

1. Pakistan Demographic Profile 2013. Index mundi. www.indexmudi.com.
2. WHO–AIMS report 2009, published by WHO and Ministry of Health, Islamabad.
3. Khalily TM. Personality characteristics of addicts and non-addicts determined through Rorschach findings. *Pak. J. Psych.* 2009; 40(1):3–15.
4. United Nations Office on Drugs and Crime (UNODC) technical summary report 2012.
5. Khan MM, Naqvi H, Thaver D, Prince M. Epidemiology of suicide in Pakistan: determining rates in six cities. *Arch. Suicide Res.* 2008; 12(2):155–60.
6. Khan MM *et al.* The pattern of suicide in Pakistan. *Crises* 2000; 21(1):31–5.
7. Khan M.M *et al.* Deliberate self harm in Pakistan. *Psychiatr. Bull.* 1996; 20:367–8.
8. Mumford DB, Nazir M, Jilani FU, Baig IY. Stress and psychiatric disorder in Hindukush: a community survey of a mountain village. *Br. J. Psychiatry* 1996; 168:299–307.
9. Mumford DB, Saeed K, Ahmad I, Latif S, Mubbashar MH. Stress and psychiatric disorder in rural Punjab: a community survey. *Br. J. Psychiatry* 1997; 170:473–8.
10. Mumford DB, Minhas FA, Akhtar I, Akhtar S, Mubbashar MH. Stress and psychiatric disorder in urban Rawalpindi: a community survey. *Br. J. Psychiatry* 2000; 177:557–62.
11. Ali BS, Amanullah S. Prevalence of anxiety and depression in an urban squatter settlement of Karachi. *J. Coll. Physicians Sur. Pak.* 2000; 10:4–6.
12. Mirza I, Jenkins R. Risk factors, prevalence, and treatment of anxiety and depressive disorders in Pakistan: systematic review. *BMJ* 2004; 328:794–7.

13. Mubbashar MH. Development of mental services in Pakistan. *Intern. Psych.* 2003; 1:11–14.
14. Gadit A, Vahidy A. Knowledge of depression among general practitioners. *J. Coll. Physicians Sur. Pak.* 1997; 6:249–55.
15. Constitution of Pakistan, 1973.
16. Disabled Persons Ordinance, 1981.
17. Mental Health Ordinance.
18. Rehemn A *et al.* Randomized trial of impact of school mental health program in rural RWP, Pakistan. *The Lancet* 1998; 352: 1022–5.
19. Ahmed F. Health system strengthening using primary health care approach. Panel D: Societal partnership and local development to improve health. Topic: Community empowerment through micro-credit scheme to improve community health. Paper presented at: Revitalizing Primary Health Care, 6–8 August 2008, Jakarta, Indonesia.
20. www.thet.org/hps/resources/case-studies/health-partnerships/mental-health/integrating-mental-health-into-primary-care-in-rural-areas-of-pakistan#sthash.YQf1iIAG.dpuf
21. UNICEF Statistics (Internet), cited 6 March 2010.
22. Rahim SIA *et al.* Effects of rapid urbanization on child behavior and health in a part of Khartoum, Sudan. II, Psychosocial influences on behavior. *Soc. Sci. Med.* 1986; 22:723–30.
23. Stein Z *et al.* Serious mental retardation in developing countries: an epidemiologic approach. *Ann. N. Y. Acad. Sci.* 1986; 477:8–21.
24. Shorvon SD, Farmer PJ. Epilepsy in developing countries: a review of epidemiologic, sociocultural and treatment aspects. *Epilepsia* 1988; 29: S36–54.
25. Syed EU, Naqvi H, Hussein SA. Frequency, clinical characteristics and co-morbidities of attention deficit hyperactivity disorder presenting to a child psychiatric clinic at a university hospital in Pakistan. *J. Pak. Psychiatr. Soc.* 2006; 3:74–7.
26. Gadit AA. State of mental health in Pakistan. *JPMA* July 2001.
27. Kleinman A. *Patients and Healers in the Context of Culture: An Exploration of the Borderland between Anthropology, Medicine, and Psychiatry*. Berkeley and Los Angeles, California: University of California Press, 1980.
28. Rabbani R. Views about women's mental health: study in a squatter settlement of Karachi. *J. Pak. Med. Assoc.* 1999; 49:139–42.
29. Tareen E. The Perception of Social Support and the Experience of Depression in Pakistani Women. PhD Thesis, University of Essex, 2000.
30. Naeem S, Ali BS, Iqbal A, Mubeen S, Gul A. What probably made a difference? A qualitative study of anxious and depressed women who exhibited different levels of change after counseling. *J. Pak. Med. Assoc.* 2003; 53: 242–7.
31. Ahmed W, Choudhry AM, Alam AY, Kaisar F. Muslim patients perceptions of faith-based healing and religious inclination of treating physicians. *Pakistan Heart Journal* 2007; 40(3–4):61–5.
32. Karim S, Saeed K, Rana MH, Mubbashar MH, Jenkins R. Pakistan mental health country profile. *Int. Rev. Psychiatry* 2004; 16:83–92.
33. Saeed K, Gater R. The prevalence, classification and treatment of mental disorders among attenders of native faith healers in rural Pakistan. *Soc. Psychiatry Epidemiol.* 2000; 35(10):480–5.

11

Mental health services in Sri Lanka

Harischandra Gambheera

Country profile

Sri Lanka is a small island in the Indian Ocean off the southern coast of the Indian subcontinent with a land area of 65,610 square kilometres. It had been known as Ceylon until it obtained complete independence from its British rulers in 1972. Sri Lanka is a densely populated country with approximately 20 million inhabitants (Department of Census and Statistics, 2012). The documented history of Sri Lanka goes as far back as 3,000 years (Geiger, 1912). Sri Lanka is a culturally diverse country and is home to many ethnic groups, including Sinhalese, Sri Lankan Tamils, Indian Tamils, Burghers, Moors, etc. There is also an indigenous tribe known as Vedda living mainly in Bintenne. Two provinces of the country, north and eastern, were in the shadows, under the influence of the 30 years long ethnic conflict which completely ended in August 2009. The adverse consequences of the long war were not only limited to the north and east of the country, for it hindered the development of the entire country.

Conflicts and wars have a significant effect on epidemiology of psychiatric disorders. The trauma, loss of loved ones, loss of livelihood and refugee state resulting from wars and conflicts increase psychiatric morbidity. Many researchers all over the world have found a drastic increase of post-traumatic stress disorder (PTSD), depression, somatization, and substance use disorders (Fazel *et al.*, 2005). The war that lasted for thirty years in the north and east of Sri Lanka had a major impact on the epidemiology of psychiatric disorders in the entire country and hindered the development of already compromised psychiatric services, with greatest impact in the war-affected areas.

Sri Lanka is also a land that is frequently affected by natural disasters such as floods and droughts affecting the lives and livelihoods of its people. The Tsunami that impacted more than two thirds of Sri Lankan shores, killing more than 35,000 people, had a major impact on psychiatric morbidity, so much so that the prevalence of PTSD, depression and other psychiatric disorders were increased even after two years (Hollifield *et al.*, 2008). However, the intervention of WHO and other relief agencies in this disaster was helpful not only in the aftermath of the Tsunami but also in producing a long-lasting effect in developing community psychiatric services.

Psychiatric epidemiology

Only a few epidemiological studies have been carried out in Sri Lanka and there is a dearth of psychiatric epidemiological data available. The surveys done neither cover the entire gamut of psychiatric diagnoses nor are the samples representative of the national population. A survey by Wijesinghe *et al.* (1978), in a semi-urban population found that the six-month prevalence for all psychiatric disorders was 45.5 per 1,000, with psychoses amounting to 6.9 (males 5.5; females 8.4) per 1,000, and neuroses to 25.2 (males 9.9; females 40.6) per 1,000. The prevalence rate of schizophrenia in this study was 3.8 per 1,000 and alcoholism amongst males over 25 years was 28.7 per 1,000. The rate of mental retardation detected was 4.8 per 1,000 population. The treatment gap in Sri Lanka is very significant and the great majority of patients detected in the survey (94.5 per cent) have never received any form of psychiatric treatment.

Suicide

Even though the numbers of suicides are gradually coming down over the years, Sri Lanka is known to have very high suicide rates for males, outnumbering female suicide rates. According to the data available to the Sri Lanka Police, deaths registered as suicides for the year 2011 number 3,770 (16.85/100,000, male 2,939, female 831) (Sri Lanka Police, 2011). In an epidemiological study on intentional self-poisoning done in rural Sri Lanka, Eddleston *et al.*, (1998) found that many patients were young with a median age of 25 years, and of the 198 people who died, 156 were men. Over half of female deaths were in those under 25 years old; male deaths were spread more evenly across age groups.

Deliberate self-harm is a common public health problem in the developing world with a worldwide incidence of three million cases and 220,000 deaths each year (Jayaratnam, 1990). Like in any other developing country, deliberate self-harm is a common problem in Sri Lanka and more common amongst young people. Most of the surveys carried out in Sri Lanka have been conducted in rural agricultural areas and have found that the commonest poisons used were agricultural pesticides, yellow oleander (*Thevetia peruviana*) seeds, and medicinal or domestic substances (Eddleston *et al.*, 1998).

Suicidal intention in patients taking poison is low and most of the youngsters use the method of self-poisoning as a means of conflict resolution. The stated conflicts or difficulties are usually extremely trivial and insignificant, such as firm advice by parents or the death of a pet. Self-poisoning is a learned behaviour as a method of conflict resolution and more than 90 per cent of the patients had heard about people killing themselves by poisoning (Eddleston *et al.*, 1998). The most common poisons used were highly lethal pesticides such as paraquat and organophosphates, with case fatality rates exceeding 60 per cent. Therefore, the death rate was high in self-poisoning irrespective of the desire to die of the patients.

Many suicide prevention steps, such as reducing access to poisons in domestic environments (Hawton *et al.*, 2009), improving medical care following ingestion and decriminalization of attempted suicide have been introduced.

Depression

Major depressive disorder is a common mental illness and is the third leading cause of the global disease burden (World Health Organization, 2008) with a lifetime prevalence of 16.2 per cent (Kessler *et al.*, 2003). There are few studies of the epidemiology of depression and culture-specific presentations of depression in Sri Lanka. The study samples are not representative of the national population and the results would not be valid for the entire Sri Lankan population. Ball *et al.* (2010) report that the lifetime depression rate is 6.6 per cent in a survey conducted in the urban population in Colombo, Sri Lanka, in 2010. Depression was commoner in women as in other studies; the lifetime rate of depression was 4.8 per cent in men and 8.1 per cent in women.

Though major depression is a common mental illness the life-time prevalence varies significantly across cultures (World Health Organization, 2004). Epidemiological studies in Asian populations are rare and use varying diagnostic criteria. However, studies indicate that rates of depression in Asia Pacific, whilst lower, are comparable to those in western countries (Chiu, 2004). The prevalence of depression varies not only across cultures but also across time (Klerman and Weissman, 1989). Depression, which was the fourth leading cause of the global disease burden in 2000, will be the second leading cause in 2020. Socio-cultural factors rather than hereditary factors may be responsible for such an increase in prevalence

Countries in South Asia are undergoing rapid urbanization leading to many changes in societies and standards of living. Urbanization brings about a unique set of phenomena, both advantageous and disadvantageous, resulting in many societal changes. Though it has a great positive impact on the economy its adverse effect on mental health is significant. Researchers point out that certain changes secondary to urbanization, such as an increased population resulting in over-crowding, unemployment and poverty; increased crime and pollution; cultural changes leading to conflicts, estrangement and isolation; child employment; and disintegration of families, adversely affect lifestyles and mental health (Trivedi *et al.*, 2008; Turan and Besirli, 2008). Urbanization affects the entire population with a greater effect on the vulnerable groups of society – the elderly, children and adolescents, and women. The effects of urbanization on mental health are reflected in increased rates of sociopathy, substance abuse, alcoholism, crime, delinquency and vandalism (Trivedi *et al.*, 2008). It is clear that urbanization and its adverse accompaniments increase not only psychiatric conditions that are the direct effect of urbanization (such as sociopathy, crime and substance abuse) but also psychoses and depression that are determined predominantly by genetic inheritance. Even though Sri Lanka is not experiencing rapid urbanization in comparison with other Asian countries, there is a significant increase in the urban population, partly secondary to migration and partly due to expansion of cities. The urban lifestyle has also expanded into the rural society of Sri Lanka with development in the recent past, and that urbanization and associated societal changes may have significant impacts on mental health and the levels of psychiatric disorders.

It has been well established that there is a cultural variation in clinical presentation of different psychiatric syndromes. Non-westerners are prone to somatize their distress, and some somatic symptoms serve as cultural idioms of distress in many ethnocultural groups. Such manifestations may be misinterpreted leading to inappropriate diagnoses and treatment procedures (Laurence and Kirmayer, 2001). There are many studies that conclude that cultural factors influence the manner in which a given population may interpret and conceptualize their experience of depression (Chang *et al.*, 2008). This important factor that may have an impact on the prevalence of depression has been taken into consideration by a group of researchers at the University of Peradeniya, Sri Lanka, who have developed a new scale called the Peradeniya Depression Scale (PDS) using cultural idioms (Abeysinghe *et al.*, 2012). Abeyasinghe *et al.* use culture-specific idioms under five categories of symptoms, related to biological symptoms, somatic symptoms, depressed affect, depressed cognition and symptoms related to depressive behaviour. The somatic symptoms used in the PDS representing psychological distress were burning sensation of the body, headache, chest discomfort, aching pain/limb discomfort, abdominal fullness and feeling faint.

Historic therapeutic interventions

The Veddas living in the Bintenne jungles in Sri Lanka are considered to be remnants of an old tribe of aborigines who lived before the arrival of King Vijaya from Vanga Country, India, 2,500 years ago (Siriweera, 2012). Even though there is no reliable written history about King Vijaya, and when and where he arrived in Sri Lanka, there is evidence to suggest there were several aboriginal tribes in Sri Lanka before he colonized the country (Uragoda, 1987). It is believed that some of the tribes assimilated into Sinhala Buddhist culture while one of the tribes, called Yakka, remained isolated in the jungles. Veddas are considered to be remnants of the Yakka tribe.

The Veddas believed that diseases were sent by evil spirits and it was necessary to make an offering in order that the disease might be removed (Seligmann *et al.*, 1911). Veddas practice devil dances called *Kirikoraha* in order to send away the evil spirits that they considered the causes of all sickness. There is no evidence to believe that they attributed their illness to any organic cause or that they used any medicine for any of their ailments. They trusted entirely to incantations to propitiate evil spirits. In fact, there is no evidence that they divided their illnesses into categories such as physical and mental. This situation continued until the mid-nineteenth century.

The beliefs and practices of medicine that prevailed amongst the native tribes would have mixed with the Ayurvedic system of medicine inherited from India approximately 2,500 years ago, together with Buddhism, as some of the tribes were assimilated into Sinhala Buddhist culture.

According to *Susrutha Samhita* there are eight categories of the Ayurvedic system of medicine, and black magic and/or mysticism (*butavidya*) is one of them that deals with illnesses caused by demons and mental illnesses (Galmangoda, 2003). Like in the Vedda community there was no clear distinct division between physical and mental illnesses recognised in Ayurveda, instead they were interconnected. Illnesses caused by malignant spirits, a bad astrological period, evil charms and illnesses caused by enraged deities were included in this category.

The Ayurvedic system of medicine holds that imbalance of three humours: bile (*pita*), phlegm (*semha*) and air (*vata*) causes illness of the mind in addition to the effects of supernatural causes such as malignant spirits. Therefore, medicinal herbs and other kinds of medicines are used externally or internally as therapeutic agents for the treatment of mental illness in the Ayurvedic system of medicine, in addition to incantations (*manthra*), devil dances (*tovil*) and rituals of appeasement (*Shanthikarma*) (Jinadasa, 2010).

Communication experts believe that patients' perceptions during repeated rituals can cause relatively permanent changes in cognition so that the illnesses secondary to abnormality in the cognitive process could be improved by rituals of appeasement (Etugala, 1998). It appears that there is some form of psychotherapeutic intervention involved in these processes.

Mental health literacy

Mental health literacy means knowledge and belief about mental disorders which aid their recognition, management or prevention (Jorm, 2000). A study done by the author on the effect of the media on mental health in an urban population in Colombo revealed that mental health literacy is poor, and knowledge about illness-specific symptoms was very poor, as well as knowledge about diagnosis. Most of the caregivers who participated in the study did not have a good understanding of the modern allopathic treatment methods available in hospitals, and almost everybody sought relief through traditional rituals and the Ayurveda system of medicine in the early stages of the illness.

The evolution of modern psychiatric services in Sri Lanka

The concept of mental illness is an ancient one found in Ayurvedic medicine that prevailed in Sri Lanka and India for over 2,000 years. Organic and supernatural causes were considered as aetiological factors in mental illnesses and the treatment methods were based on those causative factors (Neki, 1973). Both Buddhism and Ayurveda originated in India and were introduced to Sri Lanka in the pre-Christian era (Anon., 1984). Doubtless, there would have been methods of treatment that prevailed and were practised by the native Sri Lankan tribes. Ayurveda inherited from India would have mixed with the local tradition of medicine practised by native tribes in Sri Lanka.

After the British colonized Sri Lanka in 1796, they recognized the need for a modern western system of approach to mental illness, and in 1839 Governor Mackenzie introduced an ordinance to establish lunatic asylums (Carpenter, 1988). Mentally ill patients were housed in a leprosy asylum in Hendala during this period (Uragoda, 1987). Building of a separate asylum in Borella close to the city of Colombo was started in 1846 (Wambeek and Carpenter, 1988) and patients from Hendala leprosy asylum were transferred to the lunatic asylum in Borella in 1847. As this hospital was overcrowded, soon many mentally ill people were imprisoned in jails throughout the island. The asylum provided protection and occupational therapy as the main mode of treatment. The Borella asylum became increasingly overcrowded over the years and was an extremely unhealthy environment for inhabitation by the mentally ill. Even though the need existed for a long time, the addition of new accommodation or building a new asylum were delayed by many barriers under the British colonial administration. After much debate, steps were taken to build a new asylum in Cinnamon Gardens, Colombo. The new asylum, which was opened in 1884, became overcrowded within a period of one year (Carpenter, 1988).

At the beginning of the twentieth century the overcrowding was so great that the asylum was occupied by double the number of persons it was intended to accommodate. Together with the overcrowding, the standards of all other facilities enjoyed by the inmates had gone down drastically and the need for a new and bigger asylum arose. As a result, a foundation stone was laid 1918 at Angoda to build a new asylum with facilities to accommodate 1,800 patients. Although it was meant to reduce the problems faced by the patients at the Cinnamon Gardens asylum, the colonial government spent an inordinately long period of time building this new asylum.

Mental Hospital Angoda was opened in 1926, eight years after laying the foundation stone, providing facilities for 1,728 patients. The environment and the treatment regime at Angoda were no different from the previous asylum, as the new asylum was also overcrowded and new treatment modalities were not available. Several committees and commissions were appointed to make recommendations to improve mental health services in Sri Lanka but only part of the proposals made by Professor Mapother were slowly implemented. Professor Edward Mapother, who had a good understanding of mental hospitals in Britain and India, had come from England to conduct a comprehensive survey of the Angoda asylum and to make recommendations to the Colonial government. It is worth noting here how he described the Angoda asylum.

The floor, roof and walls of each cell consist alike of drab cement without any attempt at colouring or decoration. High up in one wall is a small window with stout iron bars. In the floor is a large hole into which the patient may pass his motion and urine. These cells are incompletely divided from one another by a partition which does not reach the roof so that the noise and stink from any one cell may reach at least all the others of the same row. Into these empty cells I was informed that the most noisy and troublesome patients in the hospital were turned at night completely naked. The doors of the cell contain no observation window, and considering the violent character of many of these patients there is every ground for believing that the doors are rarely opened in the night by the solitary attendant on duty. It needs little imagination to picture the suffering of any patient in an early stage of bodily illness passing a night under such conditions, a situation which must frequently arise. I am told that the noise proceeding from this building is like that on a bad night in a menagerie.

Mapother, 1938

Decentralization of mental health services

Following his observations Professor Mapother made extensive recommendations including starting a specialist medical service, decentralization of psychiatric services, amending the Ceylon Lunacy Ordinance, etc. The Mapother report was a landmark study of the mental health treatment system of Ceylon resulting in several drastic changes in the system. Decentralization of the centralized psychiatric services was one of his principal recommendations. The psychiatric services started moving away from the Angoda asylum, and the building of another mental hospital was started ten years later in Mulleriyawa only a few kilometres away from Angoda. The 1,000-bed mental hospital was opened at Mulleriyawa 20 years after Mapother's recommendation. A branch of Angoda Hospital was opened in Pelawatta 30 miles south of Colombo in 1944, providing non-custodial care to 60 patients transferred from Angoda. The Pelawatta Hospital with a large amount of land for cultivation was converted to a rehabilitation hospital for chronically mentally ill people.

Professor Mapother reported that the many problems faced by inmates of the Angoda asylum were basically due to overcrowding: 'The relation to this overcrowding to sickness and mortality is obvious since at Angoda a large proportion of all deaths is due to tuberculosis or dysentery' (Mapother, 1938). The number of medical officers employed was inadequate to meet the demands of overcrowding and he recommended increasing the number in order to meet the ever-increasing need. Professor Mapother also pointed out that there was a lack of programmes and specific treatments tailored for psychiatric disorders for the inmates due to inadequacy of the medical officers and lack of training and specialization. He recommended creation of a specialized service for medical officers devoted to psychiatry to rectify these deficiencies. He proposed further educational opportunities for medical officers in India or in England. As per his suggestion several medical officers were sent abroad for training and the first Ceylonese psychiatrist started treating patients in 1940.

As a response to Professor Mapother's recommendation, the first outpatient clinic was started in Colombo General Hospital in 1943 and the first child guidance clinic was established in General Hospital Colombo in 1947. Further to these, the first 24-bed acute psychiatric unit outside the asylum at Angoda was opened at the General Hospital Colombo in 1949. The unit remains even today, under the clinical supervision of the Department of Psychological Medicine, Faculty of Medicine and University of Colombo. The decision was made to expand the services outside the district of Colombo and both inpatient facilities and outpatient clinics were opened at Galle Kandy and Jaffna in 1962.

Treatment modalities such as occupational therapy, recreational therapy and rehabilitation (with training and enrolment of occupational therapists, psychiatric social workers and psychiatric nurses) were the main therapies. The treatment modalities were revolutionized with the introduction of psychotropic medications into the psychiatric services in 1965 (Carpenter, 1988).

Mental health legislation

The first mental health legislation introduced in India was the Lunacy Act 1858 (Somasundram, 1987), and in Sri Lanka the first legislation was the Mental Disease Ordinance 1873 (Sri Lanka Government, 1873). They provided guidelines for setting up mental asylums and procedural checks for admission and treatment of patients with a view 'to segregate those who by reasons of insanity were troublesome and dangerous to the other fellow citizens'. In the initial stages, the primary objectives of the asylums were to provide services to the colonial government's own people but not the native people of the Indian subcontinent. The Lunacy Act 1845 and the County Asylum Act 1845 were in force in the United Kingdom, governing mental health services and giving legal rights to incarcerate mentally ill patients during the period mental health legislation was introduced in India and Sri Lanka.

Even though occupational therapy and other ethical treatments had been introduced, asylums in India and Sri Lanka remained primarily designed for custodial care and detention rather than treatment. Amendments were brought about in 1940 and 1956 to the initial ordinance, with no significant change in the basic structure

Sri Lanka was privileged to have mental health legislation as far back as in 1873, but the unfortunate fact is that the same laws are in force even 140 years later. The management of major psychiatric illnesses has been revolutionized with the advancement of new pharmaco-therapies and the majority of patients could be managed in the community. This paradigm shift from managing mentally ill people in asylums to managing them in the community warrants major changes in mental health legislation. Despite drastic changes in the management of major mental illnesses and appropriate changes in legislations elsewhere in the world, the mental health legislation drafted in 1873 still remains in force in Sri Lanka.

Several committees were appointed by several consecutive governments at the request of the Sri Lanka College of Psychiatrists to draft a new Mental Health Act over the last three decades. However, none of those drafts were enacted by the Parliament, and it appears that there is a major obstacle preventing any of them going through the Parliament of Sri Lanka.

Mental health policy of Sri Lanka

A mental health policy drafted by a committee under the leadership of the Sri Lanka College of Psychiatrists was approved by the government of Sri Lanka for the first time in 2005 (Ministry of Health Care and Nutrition, 2005). The basic objective of the policy is to decentralize the psychiatric services that have been centralized in large mental hospitals in Colombo and to establish a community mental health service. According to the policy of Sri Lanka, the district has been considered as the basic service unit. A minimum of one Acute Psychiatric Inpatient Unit (APIU) should be based in a District General Hospital, which is the largest inpatient establishment in a district. Apart from the acute inpatient unit there should be a rehabilitation unit based in each district. All the districts in the island are divided into a number of health administrative areas known as Medical Officer of Health (MOH) areas, depending on the population. There is a small district hospital situated in each of these MOH areas. The policy is to establish Primary Community Mental Health Centres (PCMHC) in every district hospital in each MOH area.

A community mental health team comprising a Medical Officer of Mental Health (MOMH), Community Psychiatric Nurses (CPN) and a Community Support Officer (CSO) will be attached to each PCMHC. A medical officer who has successfully completed the Diploma training programme conducted by the Postgraduate Institute of Medicine will be appointed as the Medical Officer of Mental Health in the community team. A medical officer with brief training in psychiatry has been appointed to each MOH area till he/she is replaced by a medical officer with a postgraduate Diploma in Psychiatry. The MOMH is supposed to work in close collaboration with the District Psychiatrist, and his duties include awareness raising, early detection of cases and appropriate referral, providing continuing care, and maintaining a database of persons with mental disorders facilitating the provision of continuing care. Other duties include conducting programmes for suicide prevention, to reducing substance abuse and promoting school mental health. The main objective of this list of duties is to reduce the treatment gap which still remains high.

Modern-day psychiatry in Sri Lanka

Introducing mental health care into primary health care settings is a practical and accepted mode of bridging the treatment gap in low- and middle-income countries, with resultant better health outcomes (World Health Organization, 2008). Mental health services in Sri Lanka rely on a dedicated primary community psychiatric team. In implementation of the Mental Health Policy there should be at least one APIU per district with the acceptable variation depending on the population of the district. Apart from the primary community mental health care team there should be a rehabilitation centre and continuing care unit in each administrative district in order to provide a comprehensive community psychiatric service. Sri Lanka has 25 districts and the population of these varies from 2,584,000 (Colombo) to 105,000 (Mannar). Densely populated districts may need more than one APIU or a larger number of beds to meet the needs of the people.

Every administrative district is divided into several health administrative areas with a population of approximately 50,000–60,000 and each administrative area is manned by a team of primary care public health professionals headed by an MOH. As stipulated in the Mental Health Policy of Sri Lanka a community mental health team comprised of an MOMH, CPNs and a CSO is appointed to a hospital in each MOH area. Though the policy has not been implemented for the entire country, the Ministry of Health is in the process of implementation, with slow progress. While the Ministry of Health has already completed appointing psychiatrists to all the districts in the island it has failed to build APIUs in all districts and fulfil the need for primary community mental health centres in each MOH area.

National Institute of Mental Health

As a response to the recommendations of Professor Mapother in 1938 and with the implementation of Mental Health Policy 2005, the psychiatric services were decentralized. With the establishment of APIUs and outpatient clinics in every district, overcrowding and the work load in Angoda Hospital were reduced significantly. With the decentralization of psychiatric services, downsizing of the Angoda Mental Hospital would be inevitable. Therefore it was proposed that the Angoda Mental Hospital, with over 1,000 psychiatric beds, be upgraded to a National Institute of Mental Health (NIMH) and further structural and administrative changes be made in order to serve the proposed objectives.

Establishment of an NIMH was a proposal of national importance included in the Health Policy of Sri Lanka. This NIMH would be the nerve centre, providing clinical care for patients from the western province of Sri Lanka, and offering specialized services such as perinatal mental health, learning disability, old age, child and adolescent mental health, and forensic services. Training and research in the national interest with planning of mental health services were the main objectives of establishing an NIMH. There is a well-equipped training centre with three large lecture theatres, a modern library with a reading room and a postgraduate training laboratory. The facilities of the training centre have been adequate to host several international conferences such as the World Congress of Asian Psychiatry and the SAARC Psychiatric Conference.

NIMH is a well-equipped hospital with all required modern facilities, comprised of eight psychiatric units managed by multidisciplinary teams headed by psychiatrists, a medical unit manned by a physician and laboratory facilities managed by a haematologist and a microbiologist. It is the main centre for both undergraduate and postgraduate training in psychiatry on the island and all postgraduate examinations are conducted there.

A centre for research was established and regular training programmes are being conducted to enhance the research culture in the institution. The Ethical Review Committee that meets monthly is functioning at its full capacity to fulfil the need of young researchers to improve the quality of psychiatric research. The UNESCO Bioethics Unit was established in NIMH in 2011, and various courses are conducted at the institute as well as outside the institute for various training programmes and conferences. A regular publication on bioethics, *Ethic Bulletin* is published and circulated biannually.

Undergraduate training

Introduction of psychiatry as a final-year specialty in most medical schools in the island is an important step in the training and competence of all primary care doctors in psychiatry. Previously, as in most medical schools in the region, psychiatry was taught in the third and fourth years with all other medical subspecialties, with little emphasis on its importance. Teaching and assessment was minimal, and most medical graduates could qualify with little or no knowledge of psychiatry. The current programmes in all the leading medical schools in Sri Lanka have up to eight weeks or more of full-time exposure to different aspects of psychiatry and mental health, and the undergraduates are assessed extensively on a par with the other final-year specialties – medicine, surgery, obstetrics and gynaecology, and paediatrics.

Postgraduate training

The Post Graduate Institute of Medicine (PGIM) of the University of Colombo was established in 1980 and conducts a five-year course leading to an MD in psychiatry. Doctors who are recruited for the training programme after passing a selection exam have to undergo three years of training in general adult psychiatry with limited training in child and adolescent psychiatry, forensic psychiatry and neurology before they sit an MD in Psychiatry examination. Successful candidates in the MD examination need a further two years of training in two approved centres in Sri Lanka or/and abroad before they can be certified as specialists in psychiatry. Provisions are available for trainees who so wish, to be Board certified as child and adolescent psychiatrists and forensic psychiatrists after passing the MD exam.

Currently, there are certified specialists in psychiatry in almost all the districts of Sri Lanka, based at the District General Hospitals. A large proportion of the senior registrars sent for overseas training however, have never returned to Sri Lanka (Mabbashar and Humayan, 1999). Thus the psychiatrist per population ratio has remained low at 1:500,000 to 1:1,000,000 on most occasions. Against this backdrop it was decided to train middle grade doctors with limited competency who would be less attractive for recruitment by high-income countries. These doctors were offered a Diploma in Psychiatry by the PGIM, and are usefully serving in PCMHCs in district hospitals and covering the duties of psychiatrists in places where there are no specialist psychiatrists.

Training of allied specialists

As envisaged in the National Mental Health Policy, the training of other mental health professionals has to now take priority in Sri Lanka. Foremost is the need to train psychiatric nurses and psychiatric social workers with a particular focus on the community. These professionals can play a critical role in timely, effective and appropriate services for those with mental disorders (World Health Organization, 2005). Accordingly, nurses and psychiatric social workers are being trained at NIMH. Unlike in the west, the ratio of psychiatric beds to the population has always been low in South Asian countries. Mental hospitals have not been widespread and most patients have been cared for in the community by their families (Farooq and Minhas, 2001). Therefore, a paradigm shift from institutional to community care is obvious and necessary. Services in the community have to concentrate on strengthening families to care for those with mental disorders (Linsley, 2001).

References

Abeyasinghe, R., Thennakoon, S. and Rajapakse, T. (2012). The development and validation of the Peradeniya Depression Scale (PDS) – A culturally relevant tool for screening of depression in Sri Lanka. *J. Affect. Disorders,* 142, 143–9.

Anon. (1984). *Desiya Cikista Sangrahaya.* Colombo: Department of Ayurveda.

Ball, H. *et al.* (2010). Epidemiology and symptomatology of depression in Sri Lanka: A cross-sectional population-based survey in Colombo District. *J. Affect. Disorders,* 123, 188–96.

Carpenter, J. (1988). *The History of Mental Health Care in Sri Lanka.* Colombo: Marga Publications.

Chang, S. *et al.* (2008). Cross-national difference in the prevalence of depression caused by the diagnostic threshold. *J. Affect. Disorders,* 106(1–2), 159–67.

Chiu, E. (2004). Epidemiology of depression in the Asia Pacific region. *Australas Psychiatry,* 12(supp), 4–10.

Department of Census and Statistics (2012). Colombo, Sri Lanka.

Eddleston, M., Rezvi Sheriff, M. and Hawton, K. (1998). Deliberate self harm in Sri Lanka: an overlooked tragedy in the developing world. *BMJ,* 11(317), 133–5.

Etugala, A. (1998). *Sanjananaya and Sannivedanayap* (Perception and Communication), Colombo, p. 40.

Farooq, S. and Minhas, F. (2001). Community psychiatry in developing countries – a misnomer? *World Health Psych, Bull.,* 25, 226–7.

Fazel, M., Wheeler, J. and Danesh, J. (2005). Prevalence of serious mental disorder in 7000 refugees resettled in western countries: a systematic review. *Lancet,* 365, 1309–14.

Galmangoda, S. (2003). *Ayurveda Adyayana.* Colombo: University of Kelaniya, Sri Lanka.

Geiger, W. (1912). *Mahawansa* (Great Chronicle of Sri Lanka), Oxford: Oxford University Press.

Hawton, K. *et al.* (2009). Evaluation of acceptability and use of lockable storage devices for pesticides in Sri Lanka that might assist in prevention of self-poisoning. *BMC Public Health,* 9, 69.

Hollifield, M. *et al.* (2008). Symptoms and coping in Sri Lanka 20–21 months after 2004 Tsunami. *Br. J. Psych.,* 193, 39–44.

Jayaratnam, J. (1990). Acute pesticide poisoning: a major global health problem. *World Health Stat.,* 43(3), 139–44.

Jinadasa, M. (2010), *Bali Communication,* Colombo, p.58.

Jorm, A. (2000). Mental health literacy, public knowledge and beliefs about mental disorders. *Br. J. Psych.,* 177, 396–401.

Kessler, R. *et al.* (2003). National comorbidity survey replication, the epidemiology of major depressive disorder: results from the National Comorbidity Survey Replication (NCS–R). *JAMA,* 289(23), 3095–105.

Klerman, G. and Weissman, M. (1989). Increasing rates of depression, *JAMA,* 261 (15), 2229–35.

Laurence, J. and Kirmayer, M. (2001). Cultural variations in the clinical presentation of depression and anxiety: implications for diagnosis and treatment. *J. Clin. Psychiatry,* 62(suppl 13), 22–8.

Linsley, K. (2001). Training implications of community-oriented psychiatry. *Advances in Psychiatric Treatment,* 7, 208–15.

Mabbashar, M. and Humayun, A. (1999). Training psychiatrists in Britain to work in developing countries. *Advances in Psych. Treatment,* 5, 443–6.

Mapother, E. (1938). Ceylon Sessional Paper XIII. *Report on present arrangements for treatment of mental disorders in Ceylon and suggestion for reorganization.* Colombo: Ceylon Government Press.

Ministry of Health Care and Nutrition (2005). The Mental Health Policy of Sri Lanka: 2005–2015. Colombo.

Neki, J. (1973). Psychiatry in South-East Asia. *Br. J. Psych.,* 123, 257–69.

Seligmann, C., Gabriel, C. and Seligmann, B. (1911). *The Veddas.* s.l. Cambridge: Cambridge University Press.

Siriweera, W. (2012). *History of Sri Lanka.* Colombo: s.n.

Somasundaram, O. (1987). The Indian Lunacy Act, 1912: the historical background. *Indian J. Psychiatry,* 29(1), 3–14.

Sri Lanka Government (1873). *Mental Disease Ordinance.* Colombo: Government Press.

Sri Lanka Police (2011). Available at: www.police.lk (accessed 9 November 2013).

Trivedi, J., Sareen, H. and Dhyani, M. (2008). Rapid urbanization – its impact on mental health: a South Asian perspective. *Indian J. Psychiatry,* 50(3), 161–5.

Turan, M. and Besirli, A. (2008). Impacts of urbanization process on mental health. *Anatolian J. Psychiatry,* 9, 238–43.

Uragoda, G. (1987). *A History of Medicine in Sri Lanka.* Colombo: Sri Lanka Medical Association.

Wambeek, J. and Carpenter, J. (1988). Report on the lunatic asylum of Borella (1866). In: *The History of Mental Health Care in Sri Lanka.* Colombo: Colombo National Archives, p. 26.

Wijesinghe, C., Dissanayake, S. and Dissanayake, P. (1978). Survey of psychiatric morbidity in a semi-urban population in Sri Lanka. *Acta Psychiatr.,* 58(5) 413–41.

World Health Organization (2004). World Mental Health Survey Consortium. Geneva: World Health Organization.

World Health Organization (2005). *Atlas: Psychiatric Education and Training across the World.* Geneva: World Health Organization.

World Health Organization (2008). *Integrating Mental Health into Primary Care: a Global Perspective.* Geneva: World Health Organization.

Additional resources

Dogra, N. and Karim, K. (2005). Diversity training for psychiatrists. *Advances in Psychiatric Treatment,* 11, 159–67.

World Health Organization (2007). *Atlas: Nurses in Mental Health 2007.* Geneva: World Health Organization.

Section 3
Greater China

Overview

Yueqin Huang

China is the third largest country in the world, located in the east of Asia, the west of the Pacific Rim. The mainland has a 20,000-kilometer continental border and an 18,000-kilometer coastline, and an area of 9.6 million square kilometers. This geographic location has obvious advantages: the southeast monsoon benefits agricultural production and the marine industry in many ways. It also promotes international communication, especially relationships with the West and Central Asia and Europe. The Taiwan Strait is a 180-kilometer-wide strait separating the island of Taiwan from the Asian mainland. Taiwan forms an important communication link from southeast Asia to northeast Asia in the Asia-Pacific region.

China has thirty-one provincial-level administrative provinces and regions, excluding Taiwan, Hong Kong and Macao. According to the data from the sixth China Population Census in 2010, the population of the mainland was 1.34 billion, of whom 51.27 percent were male, and the sex ratio was 1.05.

Mental health is not only a major global public health issue but also a serious social issue, as well as a legal issue. As a medical issue, it requires professional medical diagnosis and judgment. As a social issue, it requires certain restrictions and proper regulation of voluntary and compulsory admissions, and as a legal issue, it requires proper judicial procedures concerning human rights violations. The Mental Health Ordinance of Hong Kong and the Mental Health Act of Taiwan were enacted in 1962 and 1990, respectively. Legislation in mainland China started relatively late. The Mental Health Law of the People's Republic of China (PRC), put into effect as of May 1, 2013, and a chapter of the Criminal Procedure Law Amendment of the PRC, put into effect as of January 1, 2013, have largely protected the legitimate rights of those with mental illness.

Prevalence and characteristics of mental disorders are changing with social and economic development in China. Lifestyle and stress may play an important role in the changes. In China, the first psychiatric epidemiological study was carried out by Tsung-yi Lin in Taiwan from 1946 to 1948 on all households and all 19,931 residents in three communities. The earliest psychiatric epidemiological study in mainland China was in 1980, and in Hong Kong in 1984. There have since been many regional epidemiological surveys in China. In the past ten years, there have been achievements in epidemiological studies of mental disorders in China because of improved methodology and the government paying more attention to mental health. Better designs, measurements and evaluations as well as more advanced instruments have been used, to obtain better systematic data on mental disorders in China. At the beginning of the 2000s, China took part in the WHO World Mental Health (WHO–WMH) Survey Initiative. The survey was carried out in urban Beijing and Shanghai. From then onward, there have been a number of regional epidemiological studies funded by governments, such as in Beijing, Zhejiang, Hebei, Hong Kong and Taiwan. These epidemiological surveys of mental disorders in China provide useful evidence of the effects of biological, genetic, social, economic and demographic factors on mental disorders. This will be of real benefit to medical and social researchers as well as government officials and policy-makers.

The mental health service in China has developed from a relatively weak basis. Taking the mainland as an example, before 1949, the total number of psychiatrists was no more than 60 and there were only about 1,000 beds for the psychiatric service in mainland China. After 1949, the government gradually put more emphasis on mental health services. In recent years, the authorities have realized the importance and urgency of establishing an advanced and comprehensive network for the mental health services, and they have drawn up a series of plans to improve the current situation. These national plans have played important roles in the construction and development of the mental health service system. Meanwhile, the administrations in Hong Kong and Taiwan have also set up a series of medical health care insurance plans, and programs to improve the mental health systems, and they have demonstrated great success.

In summary, the many Chinese traditions, values, beliefs and changes have over time influenced the prevalence of mental disorders and management of mental health services in China. The need for psychiatric care has been rising significantly over the past few years. The complex and diverse service needs of people with serious mental illness also require continued attention and innovative approaches. Not only does the public display increasing awareness of adult psychiatric problems, but attention to childhood psychiatric conditions, substance abuse disorders and neurocognitive disorders has also been increasing dramatically. This is both a challenge and an opportunity for mental health professionals, individuals with mental disorders and their caregivers, and policy-makers.

12

Mental health in mainland China

Yueqin Huang, Hong Wang and Zhaorui Liu

Country/location geography

China is the third largest country in the world (after Russia and Canada), covering an area of 9.6 million square kilometers. It lies at the eastern end of Asia, on the west of the Pacific Rim. With a 20,000-kilometer border, China has 14 neighbors, including Russia, India, Myanmar and North Korea. It has an 18,000-kilometer coastline to the east, along the Bo Sea, Huang Sea, East Sea and South Sea; nearby countries across the sea include Japan, Korea and the Philippines. This geographic location has obvious advantages for China's maritime industry; in addition, the southeast monsoon greatly benefits agricultural production. China's location also promotes international communication, especially with the West and Central Asia and Europe.

Mainland China (i.e. excluding Taiwan, Hong Kong and Macao) has 31 provincial-level administrative regions. According to the data from the sixth China Population Census in 2010, the population of mainland of China was 1.34 billion, of whom 51.27 percent were male, and the sex ratio was 1.05 (this ratio varies slightly by age group). Those aged 14 and younger accounted for 16.60 percent of the population, while those aged 15 to 59 and 60 and above accounted for 70.14 percent and 13.26 percent, respectively. The last age group had increased by 2.93 percent compared with the 2000 census, so it is evident that China's population is gradually aging. Mainland China has more rural residents than urban residents (50.32 percent and 49.68 percent, respectively), although economic development has been narrowing this gap over the years.

China is a multi-ethnic country. The various ethnic folk cultures have a long, rich and colorful, history. Among the 56 ethnic groups in total, Han is the majority group, accounting for 91.51 percent of the population (The State Council of the People's Republic of China, 2001, 2012). Most of the minorities live in the southwestern, northwestern and northeastern areas of the mainland.

Across China, the distribution of both the population and economic resources is uneven, with a greater concentration of both in the east than in the west. A consequence of this is that the prevalence of physical and mental disorders varies widely by region.

Mental health policy

Mental health is not only a major global public health issue but also a serious social issue, as well as a legal issue, which needs to be addressed properly. As a medical issue, it requires professional medical diagnosis and judgment. As a social issue, it requires certain restrictions and the proper regulation of voluntary and compulsory admissions. As a legal issue it requires proper judicial procedures concerning human rights violations. In recent years, China has made remarkable progress in the protection of human rights in the field of mental health. The Mental Health Law of the People's Republic of China (PRC), put into effect as of May 1, 2013, and the Criminal Procedure Law Amendment of the PRC, put into effect as of January 1, 2013, have largely protected the legitimate rights of those with a mental illness.

The Chinese Mental Health Law, after 28 years of efforts, has filled a gap in the field of mental health legislation and will definitely have a broad and far-reaching influence on mental health promotion in China. The lead-up to the legislation can be divided into three periods. First, in the 1980s there was no experience of mental health legislation in China, and where issues did arise reference had to be made to the United Kingdom Mental Health Act of 1983 and some declarations on human rights from the United Nations. The second period was in the 1990s. While other countries around the world were advancing their mental health legislation, China was a latecomer in this field, mainly because of the urgent needs of economic development, which meant that the construction of a legal framework for the business world became the top priority for the legislature. Additionally, a lack of resources, the unsatisfactory status of the social security and public health systems, and the imbalance in development between urban and rural areas to a certain extent also slowed the process of establishing mental health legislation. The third period was one of accelerated advance, which started from the early twenty-first century. A high-level seminar on mental health organized by the WHO in Beijing and a high-level legislative mobilization meeting on mental health in Shanghai held in 1999 promoted this process. After 11 separate drafts, proposed legislation was released for comment. The Ministry of Health of China drew attention to this draft legislation in its Chinese Mental Health Work Plan (2002–2010), which pointed out that the pace of progress on the Mental Health Law should be increased. Finally, in the twenty-ninth session of the Standing Committee of the Eleventh National People's Congress, on October 26, 2012, the Mental Health Law was passed (Xie, 2013).

This law is composed of 85 articles, in seven chapters (The Mental Health Law of the People's Republic of China, 2012). It provides multi-level, comprehensive regulations on prevention, diagnosis, treatment, rehabilitation and legal liability. Articles 4 and 5 clearly state that the human dignity and personal safety of patients with a mental disorder are inviolable; they have the right to own their property without any arbitrary deprivation; the whole of society should show respect, understanding and concern to people with mental disorders; no one shall discriminate against, insult or abuse those with mental disorders, or restrict their personal freedom illegally. These articles will help promote universal respect for, and observance of, patients' human rights and equal social status.

The three fundamental principles stemming from this law are: treatment should be voluntary whenever possible; patients' rights and interests come first; and involuntary treatment should be applied only where there is danger or harmful behavior. The principle of voluntary treatment applies to all the steps of medical care, from outpatient clinical consultation and admission through to treatment and discharge. Voluntary discharge makes it possible for patients treated involuntarily to go through the discharge formalities themselves. In the past, the hospitals in mainland China permitted only those who arranged the involuntary admission of a patient to collect the patient from the hospital on discharge; if they did not want to collect the patient, the hospital would not let the patient discharge him/herself. Under the new law, hospitals can allow such patients, when they are sufficiently recovered, to go through the discharge formalities themselves. For patients who lack the capacity to handle the discharge procedures themselves, their legal guardians have a responsibility to undertake it on their behalf; if they refuse to do so, they will be guilty of abandonment and shall be punishable by law. Meanwhile, the new standard on compulsory treatment is essentially a 'potential damage offence' standard, which is stricter than in many other countries in the world. Under this new standard, a patient can be forced to receive treatment only because he or she has done harm or represents a real danger to others or society. It is believed that this legislation can better protect the interests of patients and avoid the abuse of compulsory treatment.

Article 18 of the Mental Health Law states that administrative staff in places such as prisons, detention centers and enforced isolation rehabilitation units should provide relevant information on mental health knowledge to prisoners and those in custody, pay attention to their mental health status and provide psychological counseling when necessary. Again, this strongly communicates to the authorities and to society as a whole that the interests and human rights of these vulnerable groups should be protected, with no discrimination, since they are at higher risk of mental disorders.

At the same time, the Criminal Procedure Law Amendment of the PRC, which came into effect on January 1, 2013, has a separate chapter on patients with a mental disorder who break the Criminal Law, namely, 'compulsory medical treatment procedures for those mental patients exempted from investigation of criminal responsibility by law enforcement'. This legislation is aimed at ensuring a balance between public safety and individual freedom, and protecting the legitimate rights of patients with mental disorders. The new law has made it clear that the People's Court has the sole authority to determine the application of compulsory treatment; those patients and their families who disagree with the determination can appeal to a superior People's Court. It also provides two ways to lift this measure. First, the medical center should regularly re-examine patients to see if they can be discharged, and make reports to the People's Court for further review of the case. Second, the patients and families have the right to apply to the People's Court for termination of the compulsory treatment. Further, the Criminal Procedure Law Amendment restricts which treatments may be used compulsorily. Thus compulsory treatment is now more standardized, and unreasonable infringements of the freedom of people with a mental disorder or disability can be better prevented. This judicial oversight of compulsory medical treatment should guarantee justice and the acceptability of compulsory medical decisions.

Since both the Mental Health Law and the Criminal Procedure Law Amendment have only recently been put into practice, it is not yet clear how judicial practice will better protect the interests of patients with mental disorders in China. On the whole, we expect medical institutions and the judicial system to solve a series of practical problems, and research on this is in progress.

Psychiatric epidemiology

It is widely known that China is currently the most populous country in the world. In the new century, the prevalence and characteristics of mental disorder are found to be changing with social and economic development in China, presumably as a result of the parallel changes in lifestyles and an increase in levels of stress.

The epidemiological study of mental disorders in China has progressed markedly, because of improved methodology and government interest in the mental health of the population. Most epidemiological researchers in the 1980s and 1990s in China were clinical psychiatrists. Nowadays, more epidemiologists, statisticians, social scientists and economists participate in psychiatric epidemiological studies on mental disorders. ICD-10 and DSM-IV are commonly used in clinical practice and research. Although in the early to middle parts of the last century, non-structured questionnaires were used by psychiatrists in such research, often making comparisons difficult, this has changed in the past decade. Now, fully structured or semi-structured interview assessments are used in accordance with strict epidemiological principles which yield more valid and reliable epidemiological data. In data analysis, modern epidemiological and statistical principles and methods are coupled with univariate and multivariate analysis. Better designs, measurements and evaluations as well as advanced instruments have been used to obtain more systematic data on mental disorders in China since 2000.

At present, the Ministry of Health in China mandates the use of ICD-10 in clinical practice. The American Psychiatric Association's DSM-IV is more commonly used in research. For classification of mental disorders, there are two kinds of disorders: psychotic and non-psychotic disorders. The former include schizophrenia, affective disorder, paranoid disorder, reactive psychosis and brain organic mental disorders. The latter include anxiety disorder, personality disorder, substance use disorder, eating disorder, somatic disorder, mental retardation, reactive state and emotional response.

The World Health Organization's Composite International Diagnostic Interview (WMH–CIDI) (Kessler and Ustun, 2004) is administered by trained lay interviewers, to offer a panoramic, fully structured diagnostic assessment based on DSM-IV and ICD-10. Diagnoses of mental disorders are based upon the WMH–CIDI assessment and computerized diagnostic algorithms. The Chinese version of the WMH-CIDI was derived using standard protocols of iterative translation, back-translation and harmonization, conducted by panels of bilingual experts. A clinical reappraisal shows good evidence of the CIDI's validity in the context of Chinese culture (Huang et al., 2008). The Structured Clinical Interview for DSM (SCID) is a semi-structured clinical assessment instrument used by trained psychiatrists. In the past decade, psychiatric doctors and nurses as interviewers have routinely used the SCID in psychiatric epidemiological surveys.

In China, there have been two large-scale epidemiological surveys of mental disorders in the past 30 years. The first was conducted in 1982 in 12 regions (Twelve Collaborating Units of Epidemiological Survey on Mental Disorders, 1986a, b), and the second was done in 1993 in seven regions (Zhang et al., 1998).

The 1982 11-region survey, sponsored by the Ministry of Health of China and supported by the World Health Organization, was completed through a large-scale collaborative effort of the 12 participating psychiatric study centers. Those units were chosen to represent the country's different geographical regions and socio-cultural groups. Each study center investigated 500 rural and 500 urban samples of households, to give a total sample of 12,000 households with 51,982 persons (38,136 of them over the age of 15 years). The members of the survey team in each of the 12 centers consisted of both senior and junior psychiatrists, general medical doctors, psychiatric nurses and medical assistants. The survey instruments included the Psychosis Screening Schedule (ten items), the PSE-9 Neurosis Screening Schedule (12 items), the PSE-9 (Chinese version), the Social Disability Screening Schedule (SDSS), the Household and Socio-demographic Information Schedule, the General Psychiatric Interview Schedule and Summary Form, and the Assessment Schedule for Children (ASC-40). Individuals aged fifteen and over who were given a positive rating on either one of the two diagnosis ratings in the Psychosis Screening Schedule were regarded as possible cases. They were seen individually for a further clinical assessment using the criteria and definition of the ICD-9. The survey found that the overall point prevalence of all mental disorders in the 12 study areas was 1.05 percent and that the lifetime prevalence was 1.27 percent. The point prevalence of schizophrenia was estimated as 4.75 per thousand in the population, and the lifetime prevalence was 5.69 per thousand. The point prevalence of schizophrenia in urban areas was 6.06 per thousand, and that in rural areas was 3.42 per thousand. The point prevalence of manic-depressive psychosis was 0.37 per thousand and the lifetime prevalence was 0.76 per thousand.

One-fifth of all survey respondents were screened for neurosis, which was estimated to have an overall prevalence of 2.22 percent, including the neurasthenic (1.30 percent), hysterical (0.36 percent), depressive (0.31 percent), anxiety (0.15 percent), phobic (0.06 percent), obsessive and compulsive (0.03 percent) and hypochondriacal (0.02 percent) subtypes. According to the government's requirements, the survey was focused on the prevalence of psychotic disorders, but it also covered moderate and severe mental retardation. The survey analyzed the correlates of mental disorders and found, most notably, that schizophrenia was associated with substantial social disability (Cooper and Sartorius, 1996). Despite the low prevalence rates, the results of the survey were important for planning and developing national mental health services in China. Further, carrying out the survey was instrumental in introducing the methodology of modern epidemiological psychiatry in community settings to Chinese psychiatrists.

Under the leadership of the Ministry of Health, the seven-region epidemiological survey of mental disorders was completed in 1993 in seven of the same 12 regions examined in 1982. Like the 1982 survey, this survey was supported by the WHO. The study methods and procedures were similar, but several new instruments were added, including the Negative Symptom Assessment Scale, the Wechsler Intelligence Scale for Children (WISC), the Adult Intelligence Disability Assessment Instrument, the Chinese Classification of Mental Disorders-Second Version (CCMD-2), ICD-10 and the instruments as well as tables used in the International Collaboration Research for Schizophrenia. As in the 1982 survey, each participating center studied 500 rural and 500 urban households. The final total sample was therefore 7,000 households, with 23,333 persons.

The survey found that the overall point prevalence of mental disorders (excluding neurosis by original design of the survey) in the seven study areas was 1.12 percent and the lifetime prevalence was 1.35 percent. Of all the mental disorders, the prevalence of schizophrenia was the highest, with a point prevalence of 5.31 per thousand and a lifetime prevalence of 6.55 per thousand. The prevalence of mental retardation was 2.70 per thousand, which was the second most prevalent disorder studied. Manic-depressive psychosis was ranked the third in prevalence, with a point prevalence of 0.52 per thousand and lifetime prevalence of 0.83 per thousand. The prevalence of alcohol dependence (0.68 per thousand) was significantly higher than in the earlier 12-region survey. The prevalence of Alzheimer's disease was 0.36 per thousand. The results informed policy-making.

Since this survey, there have been many smaller, regional epidemiological studies in China. Two provincial surveys of mental disorders were carried out in 1984 and 1994 in Shandong province by the Shandong Center for Mental Health. The surveys used the same instruments and procedures as in the two large-scale surveys described above. The sample of the 1984 Shandong survey comprised 29,492 households, with a total of 118,998 persons (88,822 over the age of 15 years). The 1994 sample comprised 26,460 households with 84,767 persons (67,901 over the age of 15 years). The 1984 survey found that the overall lifetime prevalence of all mental disorders in Shandong province was 0.98 percent, while the point prevalence was 0.91 percent. The 1994 survey, in comparison, found overall lifetime and point prevalence rates of all mental disorders of 1.32 percent and 1.22 percent, respectively. Thus, both lifetime and point prevalence rates were higher than in the 1984 survey. The prevalence of alcohol dependence had increased to 0.98 per thousand and the prevalence of neurosis had increased to 0.89 per thousand. There was no statistical difference in the prevalence rates of organic psychosis between the 1984 and 1994 surveys (Weng *et al.*, 1998).

In 1996, an epidemiological survey of mental disorders was carried out in Shenzhen city, using the same instruments and procedures as in the two large-scale surveys in 1982 and 1993. The Shenzhen survey investigated a rural and an urban sample of 500 households each, totaling 3,807 persons. The overall point prevalence of all mental disorders (except neurosis) among persons aged 15 years or above was estimated at 1.48 percent, while lifetime prevalence was estimated at 1.62 percent. The prevalence of schizophrenia (4.72 per thousand) was the highest among all of the mental disorders, followed by substance-related disorders (4.38 per thousand), organic psychosis (4.05 per thousand), moderate and severe mental retardation (2.36 per thousand), and mood disorders (0.34 per thousand) (Cheng *et al.*, 1999). Using CIDI-3.1, 7,134 people in Shenzhen were interviewed in 2005. The lifetime prevalence of all mental disorders was reported to be 21.17 percent. The highest prevalence rate was that for depressive disorder (6.71 percent), followed by obsessive-compulsive disorder (4.18 percent), psychotic disorder (1.46 percent), mania (1.14 percent), phobia disorder (0.92 percent), bipolar disorder (0.91 percent), general anxiety disorder (0.39 percent) and panic disorder (0.38 percent) (Zhang *et al.*, 2006).

At the beginning of the 2000s, China took part in the WHO's World Mental Health (WMH) Survey Initiative (www.hcp.med.harvard.edu/wmh). The survey was carried out in urban Beijing and Shanghai. Standardized methods of sampling, training, field procedures and measures were adopted. The aim was to re-examine the Chinese epidemiology of mental disorders in a cross-national context, and to generate a sample of respondents who could participate in further methodological research after the survey to refine the interview methods in preparation for a national survey. The survey used the WHO–CIDI 3.0 to include DSM-IV-defined anxiety, mood, impulse-control and substance use disorders. CIDI organic exclusion rules were applied in making all diagnoses. The CIDI was translated into Chinese and back-translated using a standard WHO protocol. An expert panel of three academic psychiatrists (Yucun Shen, Mingyuan Zhang and Shuran Li) and a survey methodologist (Mingming Shen) from the Research Center for Contemporary China in Beijing evaluated its content validity, tested it with Chinese patients, and revised it taking account of the cross-cultural equivalence of items. The subjects were urban dwellers who met four criteria: (1) aged 18 to 70 years, (2) living in a family household, (3) having formally registered in a non-agricultural household, and (4) residing within the urban districts of Beijing and Shanghai. Neighborhood committees (NCs) are established community organizations in urban China that were used as the pre-selected primary sampling units. The sampling team first approached 50 NCs in each city to check their actual conditions against the official demographic data. Forty-seven of these NCs in Beijing and 44 of them in Shanghai were chosen for the survey. According to the pre-decided sampling interval and random starting points, the desired number of households was sampled from the household registration list in each NC. In Beijing there were 4,024 eligible individuals who comprised the final master sample of respondents, while 3,856 respondents were chosen in Shanghai. The desired sample size was 2,500 completed interviews in each city. The actual sample size was 2,633 in Beijing, and 2,568 in Shanghai. The response rates were 74.8 percent and 74.6 percent, respectively. Weights were applied to the data to adjust for discrepancies between the sample and population census data on the cross-classification of key socio-demographic variables. Following a standard on-site training procedure, the field managers conducted a one-day training session for field samplers in those two cities and a seven-day training program for the interviewers. The demographic distribution of the weighted sample in Beijing was similar to that in Shanghai. The demographic distribution of the combined and weighted sample was similar to the population on post-stratification variables after being weighted. The disorders with highest estimated 12-month prevalence rates were major depressive disorder (2.0 percent), specific phobia (1.9 percent) and intermittent explosive disorder (1.7 percent). In the diagnostic class of disorder, impulse-control disorders were estimated to be the most prevalent (3.1 percent), followed by anxiety disorders (2.7 percent), mood disorders (2.2 percent) and substance use disorders (1.6 percent). The twelve-month prevalence estimate of any disorder was 7.0 percent in the total sample; of these disorders, 13.9 percent were classified as serious, 32.6 percent as moderate and 53.5 percent as mild. The distribution of severity across classes of disorder was different from the distribution of prevalence, with mood disorders having the highest proportion of cases classified as serious (21.4 percent) and impulse-control disorders the lowest (5.6 percent). Individual disorders within each class with the highest proportion of 'serious' cases were bipolar I–II disorders (100.0 percent) among the mood disorders, alcohol dependence (54.6 percent) among the substance disorders, social phobia (24 percent) among the anxiety disorders and intermittent explosive disorder (4.9 percent) among the impulse-control disorders. Inter-city comparison showed that the 12-month prevalence rates of most disorders were not significantly different except for social phobia (Beijing, 0 percent; Shanghai, 0.3 percent); intermittent explosive disorder (Beijing, 2.6 percent; Shanghai, 0.6 percent); alcohol abuse/dependence (Beijing, 2.5 percent; Shanghai, 0.4 percent); and alcohol dependence (Beijing, 0.8 percent; Shanghai, 0.3 percent) (Shen *et al.*, 2006).

Since 2001, there have been some regional epidemiological studies funded by local governments. In Zhejiang province, 14,639 people who were 15 years of age or older were investigated using SCID, and the adjusted prevalence of all mental disorders was estimated at 17.3 percent (Shi *et al.*, 2005). In Hebei province, 24,000 people who were 18 years of age or older were investigated, and a prevalence rate of all mental disorders of 16.24 percent was reported (Li *et al.*, 2007). In Kunming city, 5,033 rural and urban residents were interviewed using CIDI-2.1, and the 12-month prevalence was found to be 6.41 percent (Yang *et al.*, 2009). Using CIDI-3.0, the adjusted prevalence rate of mood disorders, psychotic disorders, anxiety disorders and substance use disorders, combined, in Guangzhou city was reported in 2006 to be 4.33 percent, and the lifetime prevalence to be 15.76 percent (Zhao *et al.*, 2009).

With the support of a national research grant under the Eleventh Five Year Plan, an epidemiological survey was recently carried out in Beijing. It investigated the prevalence, comorbidity and onset of mood disorders, anxiety disorder and substance use disorder in a cross-sectional study of 3,387 residents aged 16 years and over in Beijing using multi-stage stratified sampling, in 2010.

The CIDI-3.0 Computer-Assisted Personal Interview (CAPI) was administered by face-to-face interview for DSM-IV diagnoses in both urban and rural community settings. There were 2,469 respondents (a 72.9 percent response rate). The 30-day prevalence rate and adjusted prevalence rate of mood disorders were 0.81 percent and 0.87 percent, respectively; the 12-month prevalence rate and adjusted prevalence rate of mood disorders were 3.32 percent and 3.40 percent, respectively; and the lifetime prevalence rate and adjusted prevalence rates of mood disorders were 7.21 percent and 6.55 percent, respectively. The adjusted 30-day, 12-month and lifetime prevalence rates in males and females were 0.80 percent vs 0.76 percent, 3.28 percent vs 2.83 percent, and 5.86 percent vs 5.89 percent, respectively. The 30-day prevalence rate and adjusted prevalence rate of anxiety disorders were 3.16 percent and 3.08 percent, respectively; the 12-month prevalence rate and adjusted prevalence rate of anxiety disorders were 3.93 percent and 3.90 percent, respectively; and the lifetime prevalence rate and adjusted prevalence rate were 5.95 percent and 6.37 percent, respectively. The adjusted 30-day, 12-month and lifetime prevalence rates in males and females were 2.18 percent vs 3.17 percent, 2.69 percent vs 4.18

percent, and 4.57 percent vs 6.55 percent respectively. The 30-day prevalence rate and adjusted prevalence rate of substance use disorders were found to be 0.33 percent and 0.37 percent, respectively; the 12-month prevalence rate and adjusted prevalence rate of substance use disorders were 1.15 percent and 1.92 percent, respectively; and the lifetime prevalence rate and adjusted prevalence rate of substance use disorders were 5.30 percent and 5.58 percent, respectively. The adjusted 30-day, 12-month and lifetime prevalence rates of substance use disorders in males and females were 0.63 percent vs 0.16 percent, 3.63 percent vs 0.16 percent, and 11.14 percent vs 0.61 percent, respectively (Table 12.1). There was comorbidity among the mood disorders, anxiety disorders and substance use disorders. In China, the median age at onset for anxiety disorders is found to be 15 years, followed by 28 years for substance use disorders and 38 years for mood disorders (Liu et al., 2013).

Because of various methodological differences, the findings of the above studies cannot be readily compared with those from recent epidemiological studies conducted in Western communities. Some of the results, such as those involving schizophrenia, are quite similar to those in overseas studies using similar methods of assessment, while other results, most notably those involving the prevalence of neurotic and mood disorders, are markedly different. The consistency of results in psychotic disorders supports the view that biological causes are dominant in these disorders and that the biological vulnerability is relatively uniform throughout the world. The variability in the prevalence estimates of non-psychotic disorders, in comparison, argues that cultural factors that differ across cultures play a more important role.

Because both the DSM and ICD diagnostic systems were developed by American and European psychiatrists and based on Western cultures, the diagnostic categories in these systems might not be valid cross-culturally. Also, the evolving nature of the diagnosis and classification of mental disorders makes it difficult to compare results across surveys carried out using different methodologies and diagnostic criteria. Nonetheless, genuine differences exist in the cross-national distribution of mental disorders relating to genetic and environmental etiological factors. Debates about these issues have created both enthusiasm and controversy among psychiatrists, psychologists, neurologists, epidemiologists, sociologists and anthropologists, as well as among governmental officials and policy-makers in many countries (Kleinman, 2004).

Many researchers have reservations about the survey findings, because these epidemiological studies of Chinese people do not indicate that mental disorders are as rare as they were in surveys conducted in the last century. Two kinds of explanation, albeit empirically little examined and themselves debated, have been offered for the low prevalence estimates in the surveys. The first kind stress the methodological factors that lead to downward bias in estimates, including errors in sampling, stigma-induced under-reporting and culturally shaped reporting of symptoms, such as somatization. The second kind emphasize substantive processes that cause the prevalence to be genuinely low, such as a resilient family system and a cultural tradition of withstanding hardship that buffers Chinese people against mental disorders (Lee, 2002).

In summary, epidemiological surveys on mental disorder in China provide evidence of the relationship between biological, genetic, social, economic and demographic effects on mental disorders. Their results will be of value to medical and social researchers as well as governmental officials and policy-makers (Huang, 2013).

Mental health systems

The mental health service in mainland China has developed from a very weak base. In the late nineteenth century, some pioneers thought it was necessary to absorb Western advanced technologies to promote the socioeconomic development of China. As part of this process,

Table 12.1 Prevalence of DSM-IV disorders in 2,469 respondents in Beijing (percent)

Type of disorder	30-day prevalence			12-month prevalence			Lifetime prevalence		
	Total U/A	Male U/A	Female U/A	Total U/A	Male U/A	Female U/A	Total U/A	Male U/A	Female U/A
Mood disorders	0.81/0.87	0.83/0.80	0.80/0.76	3.32/3.40	3.10/3.28	3.46/2.83	7.21/ 6.55	6.10/5.86	7.92/ 5.89
Anxiety disorders	3.16/3.08	2.48/2.18	3.60/3.17	3.93/3.90	3.00/2.69	4.79/4.18	5.95/ 6.37	4.55/4.57	6.80/ 6.55
Substance use disorders	0.33/0.37	0.60/0.63	0.14/0.16	1.15/1.92	2.60/3.63	0.14/0.16	5.30/ 5.58	12.19/11.14	0.49/ 0.61
Any disorder	4.08/3.81	3.10/2.82	4.26/3.84	6.56/6.69	5.38/5.28	7.32/6.46	11.62/11.30	9.72/9.26	12.85/10.79

Abbreviations: U, unadjusted prevalence; A, adjusted prevalence.

Western medicine was introduced to China, especially through Guangzhou, a harbor communicating with Western countries in that period. In 1872, John G. Kerr, a doctor working at a hospital in Guangzhou, suggested the local government establish an asylum for lunatics, but it was not until 1897 that an asylum was built in Guangzhou (the first in China), which had only 30 beds, with the help of Kerr, who bought the land in 1891. Five other asylums were established in the next half century, in Beijing (1906), Suzhou (1923), Shanghai (1935), Chengdu (1939) and Nanjing (1947). Before 1949, the total number of psychiatrists was no more than 60 and there were only about 1,000 beds for psychiatric services.

After 1949, the new Chinese government gradually put more emphasis on mental health services. The Ministry of Health held the first national conference on the prevention and treatment of mental disorder in Nanjing in June 1958. At that time, there were 49 psychiatric medical institutions and about 11,000 beds for psychiatric services in the whole country. Only 21 provinces had a psychiatric medical service. The Second National Mental Health Conference was held in Shanghai in 1986, which was also led by the Ministry of Health. The numbers of psychiatric hospitals and beds had increased to 348 and 60,000, respectively (Xu, 1995). Both conferences agreed that there was an urgent need to integrate the three systems of health, civil affairs and public security, and to establish a coordination group to arrange services for patients with mental disorders.

In recent years, with increasing social and economic development, the authorities have realized the urgent need to establish an advanced and comprehensive mental health service network. In 2002, the Ministry of Health, Ministry of Civil Affairs, Ministry of Public Security and China Disabled Persons Federation signed the joint Chinese Mental Health Working Plan (2002–2010), which put forward the following principle and priorities. The principle was 'prevention first, integrating prevention with control, primary intervention, extensive coverage, administering according to the law'. The priorities of the first 10 years of the twenty-first century were 'raising awareness of mental health issues in key populations, improving the treatment of the key diseases and expanding the coverage of rehabilitation'. The 'key populations' were children, elderly women and disaster victims. The 'key diseases' were schizophrenia, major depression and dementia. In 2008, the four ministries mentioned above produced the National Guidelines on the Development of the Mental Health System (2008–2015) (Zhang et al., 2002). These national programs have played important roles in the construction and development of the mental health service system, and guiding social resources participating in mental health services.

Since 2004, the central government has allocated special funds annually to strengthen and perfect the training of psychiatrists, and laid the foundation for the human resources required for both institutional and community mental health services. This '686 Project' is intended to improve both the prevention and control of severe mental disorders, to reduce the social and economic impact of mental disorders (in particular, in relation to 'troublesome' patients), and to promote team building among psychiatrists. It is called the '686 Project' because the government invested RMB 6.86 million Yuan as the startup funds in 2004. The main tasks of the project are: (1) to register and evaluate patients with severe mental disorders, and to follow up patients with risk behavior tendencies; (2) to provide certain kinds of medicines free to patients with risk behavior tendencies; (3) to provide free laboratory tests; (4) to deal with emergency patients; (5) to provide urgent hospitalization; (6) to review and rescue patients restricted by locked chains; and (7) to train medical staff to manage and treat severe mental disorders (Ma et al., 2011). By December 2013, the '686 Project' had received RMB 470 million Yuan in total investment from the central and local governments, and had implemented mental health services theoretically covering 1.12 billion people over the whole country.

Generally speaking, the mental health service has developed rapidly. However, despite the increasing investment from the Ministry of Health, there are still problems connected with insufficient resources. The investment in psychiatric hospitals is obviously not enough, especially for the primary psychiatric institutions. As of 2011, there were 690 psychiatric hospitals in mainland China, with a total of 225,641 beds (16.75 beds per 100,000 people). The utilization rate of these beds was high, at up to 97.1 percent. The total number of practitioners (including doctors, nurses, pharmacists, technicians, administrators, etc.) in psychiatric hospitals was 100,734, which included 20,914 psychiatrists (only 1.55 per 100,000 people) (The Ministry of Health of the People's Republic of China, 2012). Compared with international averages of 43.6 beds and 3.96 psychiatrists per 100,000, it is obvious that the mental health services are under-resourced, even more so than in some other developing countries. However, although the service resources are undoubtedly insufficient, the utilization of the related services in some regular institutions is not as high as expected, which suggests that there is inefficiency and waste of existing resources within the mental health services in mainland China (Huang, 2011).

Conclusion

In summary, there are many Chinese traditions, values, beliefs and changes over time influencing the prevalence of mental disorders and the management of mental health services in mainland China. The current status in China is both a challenge and an opportunity for mental health professionals, as well as individuals living with mental disorders and their caregivers.

References

Cheng, Z.R., Gao, H., Zhang, X., Tang, Z.R., Lu, Y.W., Yang, W.Q., Cai, D., Hu, C.Y., Li, H., Li, Y.P., Zhang, Y.P. and Huang, X.Z. (1999) 'The epidemiological survey of mental disorders in Shenzhen', *Medical Journal of Chinese Civil Administration* (Beijing) (in Chinese), 11:32–5.

Cooper, J.E. and Sartorius, N. (1996) *Mental Disorders in China: Results of the National Epidemiological Survey in 12 Areas*, London: Gaskell.

Huang, Y.Q. (2011) 'Status quo and challenge of mental health in China', *Chinese Journal of Health Policy*, 4(9):5–9.

Huang, Y.Q. (2013) 'Epidemiological study of mental disorders in Mainland China', *Taiwanese Journal of Psychiatry* (Taipei), 27(2):101–9.

Huang, Y.Q., Liu, Z.L. and Zhang, M.Y. (2008) *Mental Disorders and Service Use in China*, New York: Cambridge University Press.

Kessler, R.C. and Ustun, T.B. (2004) 'The World Mental Health (WMH) Survey Initiative Version of the World Health Organization (WHO) Composite International Diagnostic Interview (CIDI)', *International Journal of Methods of Psychiatry Research*, 13:93–121.

Kleinman, A. (2004) 'Culture and depression', *New England Journal of Medicine*, 351:951–3.

Lee, S. (2002) 'The stigma of schizophrenia: a transcultural problem', *Current Opinion in Psychiatry*, 15:37–41.

Li, K.Q., Cui, Z., Cui, L.J., Jiang, Q.P., Wu, H.R., Zhang, W.W., Huang, J., Jin, J.X., Wang, X.Y., Xu, J.G., Tao, J., Zhang, Y.P., Zhang, B., Zhang, Y.F., Hou, H.S., Geng, J.P., Zhao, E.Y. and Shi, G. (2007) 'Epidemiological survey of mental disorders in people aged 18 or over in Hebei Province', *Chinese Journal of Psychiatry* (Beijing) (in Chinese), 40:36–40.

Liu, Z.R., Huang, Y.Q., Chen, X., Cheng, H. and Luo, X.M. (2013) 'The prevalence of mood disorder, anxiety disorder and substance use disorder in community residents in Beijing: a cross-sectional study', *Chinese Mental Health Journal* (Beijing), 27:102–10.

Ma, H., Liu, J., He, Y.L., Xie, B., Xu, Y.F., Hao, W., Tang, H.Y., Zhang, M.Y. and Yu, X. (2011) 'An important pathway of mental health service reform in China: introduction of 686 Program', *Chinese Mental Health Journal*, 25(10):725–8.

Shen, Y.C., Zhang, M.Y., Huang, Y.Q., He, Y.L., Liu, Z.R., Cheng, H., Tsang, A., Lee, S. and Kessler, R.C. (2006) 'Twelve month prevalence, severity, and unmet need for treatment of mental disorders in metropolitan China', *Psychological Medicine*, 36:257–68.

Shi, Q.C., Zhang, J.M., Xu, F.Z., Philips, R.M., Xu, Y., Fu, Y.L., Gu,W., Zhou, X.J., Wang, S.M., Zhang, Y. and Yu, Min. (2005) 'Epidemiological survey of mental illnesses in the people aged 15 and older in Zhejiang Province, China', *Chinese Journal of Preventive Medicine* (Beijing) (in Chinese), 4:229–36.

The Mental Health Law of the People's Republic of China (2012) [online], available: www.nhfpc. gov.cn/zwgkzt/pfl/201305/e1ca844160924ab1ba49aa6fe7c1cda5.shtml

The Ministry of Health of the People's Republic of China (2012) *The China Health Statistical Yearbook in 2012*, Beijing: Peking Union Medical College Press.

The State Council of the People's Republic of China (2001) *Major Figures on 2000 Population Census of China*, Beijing: China Statistics Press.

The State Council of the People's Republic of China (2012) *Tabulation on the 2010 Population Census of the People's Republic of China*, Beijing: China Statistics Press.

Twelve Collaborating Units of Epidemiological Survey on Mental Disorders (1986a) 'The methodology and data analysis of epidemiological survey on mental disorders in 12 regions in China', *Chinese Journal of Neurology and Psychiatry* (Beijing) (in Chinese), 19:66–7.

Twelve Collaborating Units of Epidemiological Survey on Mental Disorders (1986b) 'The prevalence of mental disorders, drug dependence and personality disorder', *Chinese Journal of Neurology and Psychiatry* (Beijing) (in Chinese), 19:70–2.

Weng, Z., Zhang, J.X., Ma, D.D., Ma, S.P., Li, X.F., Jiang, W.Q., Xu, L.Y., Chen, D.C., Cao, X.Y., Meng, G.Y., He, Y.Y., Sun, L.M., Zhang, S.J., Zhu, B.J., Cui, W.C., Gong, P.J., Hu, B.W., Liu, Z.X., Mu, Z.P. and Li, X.Q. (1998) 'An epidemiological investigation of mental disorders in Shandong province in 1984 and 1994', *Chinese Journal of Psychiatry* (Beijing) (in Chinese), 31:222–4.

Xie, B. (2013) 'Experiences and lessons drawn from the process of mental health legislation in China', *Chinese Mental Health Journal*, 27(4):245–8.

Xu, T.Y. (1995) 'The history of the modern psychiatry of China', *Chinese Journal of Psychiatry*, 28(3):168–76.

Yang, J.Y., Ruan, Y., Huang, Y.Q., Gao, C.Q., Lu, J., Yao, J., Dang, W.M. and Luo, C. (2009) 'A study on mental disorder prevalence and utilization of health resources in Kunming', *Chinese Health Resources* (Beijing) (in Chinese), 6:277–80.

Zhang, H.Y., Hu, J.Z., Hu, C.Y., Gao, H., Zhang, X., Tang, Z.R., Lu, Y.W., Wu, H.A., Zhang, F.X., Li, H. and Duan, W.D. (2006) 'Epidemiological survey on neurosis in Shenzhen City', *Chinese Journal of Public Health* (Beijing) (in Chinese), 22:866–7.

Zhang, M.Y., Zhu, Z.Q. and He, Y.L.(2002) 'The strategies of the mental health service in China', *Shanghai Archives of Psychiatry*, 14(Supplement):50–2.

Zhang, W.X., Shen, Y.C., Li, S.R., Huang, Y.Q., Wang, J.R., Wang, D.P., Tu, J., Ning, Z.X., Fu, L.M., Ji, L.P., Liu, G.Z., Wu, H.M., Luo, K.L., Zhai, S.T., Yan, H. and Meng, G.R. (1998) 'Epidemiological investigation on mental disorders in 7 areas of China', *Chinese Journal of Psychiatry* (Beijing) (in Chinese), 31:69–71.

Zhao, Z.H., Huang, Y.Q., Li, J., Deng, H.H., Huang, X.M., Su, J.H., Dang, W.M., Yang, Y., Huang, J.K., Zhang, W.M., Deng, Y., Zhou, W.C., Qiu, C., Lu, W.C., Chen, Y.W., Zhong, S.J., Chen, B.Y., Zeng. X.M. and Mei, F. (2009) 'An epidemiological survey of mental disorders in Guangzhou area', *Chinese Journal of Nervous and Mental Disease* (Beijing), 35: 530–4.

13

The care of the mentally ill in Taiwan

Kai-Da Cheng, Yu-Chen Lin, Cheng-Chung Chen and Winston W. Shen

A brief geography of Taiwan

The name "Taiwan" comes from an aboriginal term. Since the 16th century, Taiwan was renamed "Formosa," meaning IIha Formosa, "Beautiful Island" in Portuguese (Mateo and Eugenio, 2002).Taiwan is located east of China, south of Korea and Japan, and north of the Philippines. The area of Formosa (Mateo and Eugenio, 2002), i.e. Taiwan, is about 36,000 square kilometers (14,400 square miles), and the length of Taiwan from the south to the north is greater than its width (Executive Yuan, 2011). The shape of Taiwan island is like the shape of a sweet potato. The Taiwanese thus identify themselves proudly using the nickname, "we are from sweet potatoes."

The Taiwan Strait, or the "Black Ditch" to the Taiwanese, is a 180-kilometer wide strait separating the island of Taiwan from the Asian mainland. The Luzon Strait (Bashi Channel) is the strait between Taiwan and Luzon Island of the Philippines which is 250-kilometer long and connects the Philippine Sea to the South China Sea in the western Pacific Ocean (Executive Yuan, 2011). Taiwan is separated from the Ryukyu Arc, by a distance of 111 kilometers (69 miles) from Hualien to Yonaguni, where the westernmost point of Japan is (Guide for Japanese Islands, 2004). Taiwan thus is an island on the southeast coast of the Asian continent, on the western edge of the Pacific Ocean, forming an important communication link from Southeast Asia to Northeast Asia in the Asia-Pacific region.

About two-thirds of land area in Taiwan is forested mountains, and the rest is hilly country, platforms, highlands, small plains, and basins. The Central Mountain Range stretching across the entire island makes a natural dividing line for rivers on the eastern and the western sides of the island. The west side of the Central Mountain Range has the Yu-Shan (Jade Mountain) range in the middle of Taiwan with its main peak reaching 3,952 meters (12,365 feet), the highest mountain peak in northeastern Asia.

A brief history of Taiwan

The people and area of Taiwan have been ruled by six foreign invaders – the Dutch, the Spanish, Koxinga, the Qing Dynasty, the Japanese, and Chinese Nationalists (Kumingtan, the KMT). Like in other countries history of the island has been written according to political imperatives. The sudden appearance of an agrarian culture around 3000 BC was noted to indicate the arrival of the ancestors of today's Taiwanese aborigines (Olsen and Miller-Antonio, 1992), confirming human presence for millennia.

A wave of male Han Chinese (including Fujianese and Hakka immigrants from the Fujian and Guangdong provinces of mainland China) migrated to Taiwan. Those Han Chinese males married local female Taiwanese aborigines (Tai, 2007), and decided to settle on the island, leading to a multicultural history and forming an intercultural Taiwanese identity. The Spanish in 1628 started to build Fort San Domino and settled in the northern part of Taiwan. However, they were driven out by the Dutch in 1642. (Mateo and Eugenio, 2002). The Dutch then established a presence at Anping (now a part of Tainan city) in the southwestern part of Taiwan in the seventeenth century. Trade and the production of various goods were managed by the Dutch (Blust, 1999).

In 1662, Koxinga (Cheng-gong Cheng, a son of a loyalist father of the Ming Dynasty in China and a mother from Hirado, Nagasaki, Japan) having lost control of mainland China in 1644 then, defeated the Dutch and established a base in Taiwan (Clements, 2004). Cheng's forces were later defeated by the Qing Dynasty of China in 1683. From then, parts of Taiwan became increasingly linked with the Qing Dynasty before the island, along with Penghu, was ceded to the Empire of Japan in 1895, following the First Sino-Japanese War in Manchuria.

Rice and sugar produced in Taiwan were exported to the Empire of Japan (Takekoshi, 1907). Japanese imperial education was implemented in Taiwan and many Taiwanese also fought for Japan during the Second World War. Taiwan was liberated from Japanese rule at the end of World War II in 1945.

In 1949, the KMT lost the Chinese civil war and were defeated in mainland China by the Chinese Communists. The KMT led by Kai-shek Chiang moved the Republic of China (ROC) to Taiwan together with its Nanjing-based archaistic outdated constitution as well as civil and legal systems. The armed forces of the KMT carried out a large-scale massacre killing 10,000 to 30,000 Taiwanese at the end of February 1947 (Durdin, 1947; Kerr, 1965). Later, the KMT declared martial law to rule Taiwan. Since then, the ROC has maintained jurisdiction over an area including the islands of Taiwan, Penghu, Kinmen, Matsu, Wuchiu and some islands in the Southern China Sea as a sovereign country.

Japan formally renounced all territorial rights to Taiwan in 1952 in the San Francisco Peace Treaty (Jean-Marie, 1996; Price, 2001). The KMT ruled Taiwan as a single party state for 40 years, until democratic reforms were promulgated by Ching-kuo Chiang in the 1980s. There is increasing hope that Taiwan will become more democratic and liberal in the coming years.

Many inhabitants of Taiwan are the descendants of immigrants from the various provinces of mainland China as well as from the Chinese southeastern coastal provinces – Fujian and Guangdong. Various ethnic groups have integrated fairly well. Nowadays, nearly 500,000 identifiable indigenous people, the original inhabitants of Taiwan, still live in Taiwan. They consist of 14 different tribes (Covell, 1998).

A brief history of mental health care in Taiwan

The development of the care for the mentally ill in colonial Taiwan started in 1917 when Nakamura, a Japanese professor in Taipei, began to teach knowledge about psychiatric diseases to Taiwanese medical students and physicians (Aoki, 2009; Chen, 1997). But the service for the mentally ill was limited to custodial care until 1922 when treatment for the mentally ill was given at a designated specialized psychiatric hospital in Taipei. In 1934, the colonial government in Taiwan adopted that specialized hospital, and it was named a "sanatorium," and re-built in the same year. This was the first step in having a public psychiatric hospital in Taiwan (Aoki, 2009; Chen, 1997).

After World War II, Taiwanese psychiatrists started to take responsibility for the development of psychiatric care. The prevention of psychiatric diseases became an important focus of medical care in the 1980s when the economy in Taiwan started to improve remarkably. In the following decades, the improvement of psychiatric care was evidenced by the expansion of psychiatric beds, improvement of buildings and equipment, and the requirement of subspecialty certification for a licensed physician to practice psychiatry (Chen, 1997). The Mental Health Act was passed in 1990, to provide social security and human rights for patients with mental illnesses.

The Taiwan National Health Insurance (NHI) law was implemented in 1995, to provide entirely free medical treatment with some copayments (Liao *et al.*, 2013). In the psychiatric field, the government also provided additional budgets for community programs such as community rehabilitation centers and halfway houses, and for compulsory hospitalization. To be eligible for having copayment waived patients need catastrophic disease registration cards from the NHI Bureau. Those eligible include patients with malignance, type I diabetes mellitus, heart transplants, end-stage renal diseases being treated with renal dialysis, acute stroke, dementia, dementia with psychotic symptoms, organic mental disorders, schizophrenic disorders, affective disorders, and delusional disorders when those diseases become chronic to decrease the economic burdens on patients and their families (Liao *et al.*, 2013). The Mental Health Act was revised in 2008, to provide more human rights protection, to regulate the mass media against sensational reporting of suicide victims, and to implement forced community-based psychiatric treatment. Since then, the central government has started new systems of assessing the compulsory hospitalization and community treatment program (Liu *et al.*, 2010). The number of compulsory inpatient treatments for psychotic patients has been deceased from 4,000 to 1,000 patients per year. But the number of compulsory community treatments is still low, being less than 100 patients per year in Taiwan (Liu *et al.*, 2010). These results may be due to busy clinical work in psychiatry, or the difficulties in completing the substantial paper work. Also, the central government does not give much support to the program to provide the possibility that patients with severe mental illness can be admitted compulsorily to daycare or halfway houses (Hsieh *et al.*, 2013). Central government, local psychiatric institutes, and family support groups work hard to reduce stigma in psychiatric patients, to protect patients' human rights, and to help patients with chronic mental illness get jobs in the community. For example, occupational therapists at Kaohsiung Municipal Kai Suyan Psychiatric Hospital have introduced several different initiatives, including a sheltered workshop, selling teams, bakery, and supported work. They have also successfully helped 40 patients per year to get jobs in the community.

Mental health workforce training in Taiwan

There is multi-disciplinary team working in mental health in Taiwan. Five subspecialties are engaged in the mental health team, and each has well-described mental health workforce training requirements. These five subspecialists include psychiatrists, psychiatric nurses, psychiatric social workers, psychologists, and psychiatric occupational therapists. They compose a mental health team, and the psychiatrist is the team leader. All members of the five subspecialties need to pass government sponsored examinations to obtain a license to practice in their discipline. They also need to obtain continuing education credit hours for license renewal every six years. The programs of mental health workforce training are described below.

Psychiatrists

The psychiatrist is the leader of the mental health team and is responsible for coordination of the team. The training program was set up by the Taiwanese Society of Psychiatry (TSOP) in 1988 and revised in 2012. Before becoming a psychiatrist, the candidate physician needs one year of postgraduate training and then a three-year psychiatric residency training course in an approved psychiatric residency training program. The training program includes clinical and lecture courses. The clinical courses include interview training, psychiatric emergencies, psychiatric consultation, forensic psychiatry, disaster psychiatry, and psychotherapy as well as practicum experience in acute wards and chronic wards, and day-ward practicum experience in the three-year residency training. During the clinical courses, they also need to receive training in psychiatric subspecialties such as geriatric psychiatry and addiction psychiatry, as well as child and adolescent psychiatry. Each psychiatric resident has at least one supervisor in the different courses, and is responsible for 15 patients in the acute ward and 50 patients in the chronic ward and day hospital. The lecture courses include psychopathology, psychopharmacology, and other psychiatry-related fields.

Before being able to sit the subspecialty certification examination, the candidate needs to complete a one-year internship, one-year postgraduate training at an approved hospital, and finish up with a third year of psychiatry residency training at an approved hospital. The TSOP also requires the psychiatrist candidate to have a scientific paper submitted and intended for publication before he/she can sit the examination, but this requirement has been discouraged by the Department of Health (or the Ministry of Welfare and Health). The subspecialty certification examination to practice psychiatry is divided into two parts – the written and oral examinations. The setting of the oral examination consists of a psychiatrist candidate, a patient, and three oral examiners from the TSOP subspecialty certification committee members. The pass rate of the Taiwanese subspecialty board in psychiatry is relatively low compared with those of other medical subspecialty certifications in Taiwan. The pass rate of the written examination is 94.6 percent, and that of oral examination has been kept at around 60 percent (calculated from data kept at the TSOP) in the past 18 years from 1995 to 2013. After passing the TSOP oral examination, the candidate physician is certified to practice in psychiatry by the Ministry of Welfare and Health for six years.

Psychiatric nurses

Nurses are key members of the mental health teams. They spend most time caring for patients and play important roles in the team. Differing from other specialties, they are divided into primary nurses and assistant nurses. A primary nurse provides individual nursing planning for patients, and an assistant nurse takes responsibility while the primary nurse is off duty. They have a promotion and seniority system from grades N0 to N4.

Psychiatric or mental health nurses and psychiatric nurse practitioners also exist in Taiwan. The psychiatric nurse practitioners must first pass the licensure of internal medicine or surgical nurse practitioners. Then, they can take the examination for psychiatric nurse practitioners.

Mental health social workers

Mental health social workers are also key members and play important roles in the mental health team. They provide various social welfare resources for patients and refer patients to appropriate services. Since 2010 social workers in Taiwan have had subspecialties, to take care of medical, mental health, child, adolescent, women and family, as well as elderly and disability problems. The mental health social workers provide continuous care for patients and their family.

Psychologists

Psychologists are divided into clinical psychologists and counselors in Taiwan. The clinical psychologists work primarily in hospital. They provide non-pharmacological interventions such as psychotherapy. In addition, they perform psychological tests to help differentiate psychiatric diagnoses. The 2001 law for psychologists in Taiwan states that qualification for the psychologist examination requires a master's degree. As of January 2013, there were 1,218 licensed clinical psychologists in Taiwan, 992 of whom were in active practice. There were also 2,490 licensed counselors, and 1,606 of them were in active practice. Hospitals have been instructed to employ psychologists and counselors in equal numbers.

Psychiatric occupational therapists

Psychiatric occupational therapists evaluate patients' residual function and provide individual occupational therapy for patients. After graduation, they need to follow a two-year program of advanced training. The training program includes physical, pediatric, and mental health. The mental health occupational therapists provide occupational therapy and recreational therapy in acute wards, chronic wards, day hospitals, and community rehabilitation centers.

Highlights of psychiatric epidemiology in Taiwan

Pre-DIS (DSM-III) studies

Among the Asian countries, Taiwan started psychiatric epidemiological studies early. Lin published the first epidemiologic study in Taiwan in 1953. The investigator carried out a three step census survey from 1946 to 1948 on all households and all 19,931 residents in three communities (an urban area, a township, and a rural area). The prevalence per 1,000 population of schizophrenia was 2.2, manic depressive psychosis 0.6, senile psychosis 0.3, other psychosis 0.7, mental retardation 3.4, psychopathic personality 1.0, psychoneurosis 1.2, and all diagnoses 9.4 (Lin, 1953).

A repeated follow-up psychiatric epidemiologic study using the same method was carried out from 1961 to 1963 in three newly chosen communities with a total of 29,184 inhabitants (Lin *et al.*, 1969). The prevalence per 1,000 population of schizophrenia was 1.4, manic depressive psychosis 0.5, senile psychosis 0.4, other psychosis 0.8, mental retardation 4.9, psychopathic personality 1.4, psychoneurosis 7.8, and all diagnoses 17.5 (Lin *et al.*, 1969). Comparison of these two epidemiologic studies shows that prevalence of schizophrenia was decreased between the periods 1946–48 and 1961–66, but the prevalences of mental retardation, psychoneurosis, and all diagnoses were increased (Yeh, 1994).

DSM-III (DIS) studies

The Taiwan Psychiatric Epidemiological Project (TPEP) was conducted from 1982 to 1986, to determine the prevalence of psychiatric disorders defined by the Chinese Modified Diagnostic Interview Schedule (DIS–CM), based on the DMS-III (Hwu *et al.*, 1989). From metropolitan Taipei, two small towns, and six rural villages, the investigators recruited sample subjects numbering 5,005, 3,004, and 2,995, respectively, using a multi-stage random sampling method. The lifetime and one-year prevalences of specific psychiatric disorders were respectively 27 and 17 per 100 people. The lifetime prevalences of any disorders except tobacco dependence were 16.3 percent, 28.0 percent and 21.5 percent in metropolitan Taipei, the small towns, and the rural villages, respectively. The small town sample seemed to have the most disorders. Furthermore, there was a high prevalence of psychophysiological disorder in the metropolitan Taipei sample and a high prevalence of generalized anxiety disorder in the small town and rural village samples. The investigators (Hwu *et al.*, 1996) published part of the study data in 1996 showing the lifetime prevalence of major depressive disorder (MDD), by the Chinese Diagnostic Interview Schedule, was 1.14 percent in Taiwan.

Post-DIS (DSM-III) studies

There have been some sporadic community surveys of mental illness in Taiwan after the DIS. But the largest-scale survey was carried out by Liao and his investigators (Liao *et al.*, 2012). Using the WHO World Mental Health–Composite International Diagnostic Interview tool (Huang, 2013a), Liao *et al.* conducted another survey from 2003 to 2005 (Liao *et al.*, 2012). They found that the lifetime prevalence of major depressive disorder is 1.2 percent in Taiwan.

Current mental health care in Taiwan

There are two systems for mental health care in Taiwan. They are divided into care at general hospitals and care at mental hospitals. Patients with acute, nonpsychotic disorders and dementia are more likely to be treated at general hospitals. But more patients with chronic illness and psychotic conditions are treated at mental hospitals. Taiwan NHI Bureau, the single medical insurance provider in Taiwan, reimburses all the care services, including the fee for the psychiatrists and the fee for the hospitals. Most psychiatrists are employees of hospitals that own and operate clinics. To be eligible for reimbursement from the NHI, hospitals must have complete accredited mental health teams consisting of psychiatrists, nurses, social workers, psychologists and occupational therapists. When patients have acute episodes of psychiatric disorders, they are admitted to acute psychiatry wards for evaluation and treatment. After their symptoms and signs have improved, they are discharged home for clinic follow-up, or are transferred to a chronic ward, day ward or community rehabilitation center for further rehabilitation treatment (Hsieh, et al., 2013). The multi-disciplinary team evaluates patients' function to decide on an appropriate disposition. Day hospital and community rehabilitation are similar units. Patients go to the different units according to their social and occupational functioning.

Except for some free-standing private psychiatric clinics, most psychiatric clinics in Taiwan are located in the premises of hospitals, either general hospitals or public hospitals. Along with acute inpatient and day hospital services, the hospitals own and operate the clinics. Only public psychiatric hospitals operate extra services, such as chronic psychiatric wards, rehabilitation centers, alcohol or substance abuse inpatient services, or forensic psychiatry.

Psychiatric patients who are criminals who have carried out such offences as homicide, sexual assault, stealing, arson, etc., receive specific treatments. Some public hospitals have forensic wards for specific evaluation and treatment. The treatments include pharmacotherapy, psychotherapy, behavioral therapy, and group therapy. Another issue in forensic psychiatry is psychiatric forensic assessment. The courts ask criminals with psychiatric disorder to receive a psychiatric forensic assessment for the judge. When a criminal is not able to make a declaration of intention, receive a declaration of intention, or lacks the ability to discern the outcome of the declaration of intention due to mental disability, the court may order him or her to receive psychiatric forensic assessment prior to the commencement of guardianship.

There are different strengths and weaknesses of the two hospital systems. Psychiatric residents trained at a general hospitals may take a three-month or six-month rotation at psychiatric hospitals for residency training in child and adolescent psychiatry, alcohol and substance abuse psychiatry, or forensic psychiatry during their residency training. Contrarily, psychiatric residents trained at a mental hospital rotate consultation in psychiatry at general hospitals, to compensate for the service not provided at their mental hospitals.

Characteristics of mental health care in Taiwan

The similarities and differences of mental health care in Taiwan vary according to hospital system used. The following describes some salient characteristics of mental health care in Taiwan.

Mental health care is under Taiwan National Health Institutes (NIH) Insurance

The life expectancy in Taiwan in 2012 was averaged at 79.4 years with 76.0 years for males and 82.7 years for females. In 1995, the Taiwan NHI Bureau was established to become a national single medical insurance payer for all medical services, rendered at accredited hospitals in Taiwan. NHI is mainly financed through premiums, which are based on a payroll tax, and is supplemented with out-of-pocket payments and direct government funding (Liao et al., 2013). As a branch of the medicine service, all of the psychiatric service is included in the Taiwan NHI program.

To be eligible for service reimbursement from the Taiwan NHI, hospitals or clinics need to be accredited by the Taiwan Joint Commission on Hospital Accreditation (TJCHA). Established in 1999, TJCHA is a quasi-governmental not-for-profit organization that receives financial support from accreditation fees from participating hospitals and governmental grants. The role of TJCHA is to establish and reform the hospital accreditation system, to introduce international quality indicator systems, to hold the quality improvement contests, to promote annual National Patient Safety Goals, to establish a Taiwan patient-safety reporting system, to promote health professionals' education, and to enhance community healthcare quality (www. tjcha.org.tw/FrontStage/aboutus_en.html). In the past decade, TJCHA stressed the minimal requirements of manpower as well as the adequacy of facilities and equipment of hospitals. TJCHA currently emphasizes on the issue of patients' safety. Of general hospitals in Taiwan, the top 19 hospitals are accredited as medical centers. The number of published papers has also been counted as one of the criteria for being accredited as a teaching facility. For example, the authors' hospitals, Kaohsiung Municipal Kai Suan Psychiatric Hospital and Taipei Medical University-Wan Fang Medical Center are accredited as "teaching" facilities, qualified to teach medical students and train psychiatric residents.

The diagnoses of the DSM system are used by psychiatrists in Taiwan

The nosology of the Diagnostic and Statistical Manual of Mental Disorders is taught to medical students and psychiatry residents in Taiwan. Therefore, all psychiatrists are trained in the DSM concepts. Most senior psychiatrists have been through the diagnostic changes from DSM-III to DSM-IV. In the oral certification examination, candidates are expected to present patients according to the thinking process of the five-axis diagnostic system of DSM-IV. Effective in 2015, DSM-5 (American Psychiatric Association, 2013) will be used in the oral certification examination.

Since the beginning of 2012, the Taiwanese Society of Psychiatry (TSOP) has set up task forces to study and to educate TSOP members with the content of DSM-5. In the past two years, a task force has met regularly to study DSM-5. Some important highlights of changes from DSM-IV to DSM-5 have been presented at TSOP meetings, and short articles published in Taiwanese Newsletter of DSM-5. Because DSM-5 was released by the American Psychiatric Association in May 2013, the November 2013 scientific program at the annual TSOP meeting contained a series of DSM-5 symposia and lectures, presented by the task force members through-out the two-day program. Each of the TSOP members received a free copy of the glossary of Terminology Translation of DSM-5, DSM-IV-TR, ICD-10 and ICD-9 from English to Chinese. For the first time in DSM history, TSOP is planning to publish a Mandarin translation of DSM–5, authorized by the American Psychiatric Association, prepared by TSOP. In November 2014, copies of classic Chinese–translated version of Desk Reference to the Diagnostic Criteria from DSM–5 (American Psychiatric Association 2014) were distributed to all TSOP members. A full–length text classic Chinese–translated version of DSM–5 (American Psychiatric Association 2013) is still under preparation by TSOP. At the same time, some Mandarin names of psychiatric diagnoses are simplified and changed as a destigmatizing effort of TSOP. For example, the new name "the disorder of thought disturbances" in Chinese is to replace for schizophrenia without any connotation of mind–splitting.

The TSOP non-DSM-5 task force members have also published DSM-5-related commentaries in Chinese in the regularly TSOP Newsletter, and in English in the *Taiwanese Journal of Psychiatry* (TJP) owned by the TSOP (Shen 2013a, b). Effective from the June 2013 issue of the TJP, all authors are encouraged to discuss all published clinical cases (currently in the letter-to-the-editor column) according to the concepts of DSM-5 (Wang and Yu, 2013).

The number of new psychiatrists per year is restricted

In 2008, one full year of postgraduate year one (PGY-1) of training at an approved hospital became mandatory in Taiwan before a licensed physician can start any subspecialty residency training. In the case of psychiatry residency training, a physician must finish the PGY-1 training before his/her psychiatric residency. As of October 2013, the total number of psychiatrists in Taiwan was about 1,500. A total of 1,099 psychiatrists has been certified to practice psychiatry in the past 18 years (records kept at TSOP). In the past six years, only 357 psychiatrists (47 in 2008, 36 in 2009, 61 in 2010, 72 in 2011, 69 in 2012, and 72 in 2013) have passed the certification examination to practice in psychiatry. The number of new psychiatrists per year (59.5 psychiatrists per year) compared with that in the past 18 years (61.0 psychiatrists per year), has been roughly unchanged.

Psychiatrists in Taiwan have started to pay attention to psychosocial issues in patients with psychiatric disorders

In the era from the mid-1950s to the mid-1990s, most, if not all, psychiatric research activity in Taiwan was limited to epidemiologic surveys of psychiatric disorders (Lin, 1953; Lin *et al.*, 1969; Hwu *et al.*, 1989; Yeh, 1994). Since the 1990s, the most common published articles from Taiwan have been on topics of biological psychiatry. In each September issue of *TJP*, the titles of papers published by TSOP members in the previous year (about 250–300 papers a year) are compiled. The published topics are mostly in the area of biological psychiatry. For example, 359 articles on second-generation (atypical) antipsychotic drugs have been published from Taiwan from 1993 to 2011 (López-Muñoz *et al.*, 2012). In this bibliometric study, the papers from Taiwan were found to be published in 90 different journals, and eight of the ten journals in which Taiwanese papers were most often published have an impact factor greater than two.

We have noted that papers on psychosocial issues are appearing in the published articles from Taiwan. Examples of topics of those articles include the use of alternative medicine in psychiatry care (Pan *et al.*, 2005), the Yuli model for rehabilitation of psychiatric inpatients (Lin et al., 2009), quality of life among immigrants in Taiwan (Chou *et al.*, 2010), posttraumatic symptoms among disaster victims in Taiwan (Lo *et al.*, 2011), and needs and quality of care of patients with schizophrenia in halfway houses (Hsieh *et al.*, 2013).

Conclusion

In this chapter, the authors have given an overview of mental health care in Taiwan. Readers who are interested in this topic should consult the references cited at the end of the chapter. About 1,500 psychiatrists in Taiwan are busy and working hard treating their psychiatric patients and writing scientific papers at a rate of about 250–300 papers per year.

As shown in the epidemiologic studies, the lifetime prevalence of depression in Taiwan has been found to be 1.14 percent (Hwu *et al.*, 1996) and 1.2 percent (Liao *et al.*, 2012). This finding is similar to the 0.31 percent for lifetime depression reported from China (Huang, 2013b). But the finding from the USA is 4.5 percent. Therefore, the sensitivity of diagnosing depression deserves special attention to cultural differences or the instruments used in epidemiologic studies.

Currently, Taiwan has 1,500 certified psychiatrists for a population of 23 million, giving a ratio of psychiatrists per 100,000 population of 6.5. Among other Asian countries, ratios of psychiatrists are 14.10 in Japan (written personal communication by N. Shinfuku and W. W. Shen in December 2013), 5.12 in South Korea (Fujimoto 2009), 2.3 in Singapore, 0.6 in Thailand, 0.6 in Malaysia, 0.4 in the Philippines, and 0.21 in Indonesia (Yoshida 2009). The authors of the current chapter are afraid that the psychiatrist manpower advantage of Taiwan may be lost to other Asian countries in a few years because psychiatrist manpower in those countries is increasing rapidly. At present, the number of psychiatrist residency training positions in a hospital is decided by the TSOP. Currently TSOP council members are disproportionately represented by private practitioners because the election of the 15 council members is still by outdated by-law systems brought in by the KMT government in the 1940s. Every TSOP member can vote for seven candidates in one ballot instead of only one candidate in one ballot as in the case of the American Psychiatric Association. Even worse, a TSOP member can vote for other TSOP members in their absence. The private practitioners effectively exchange the seven candidates' votes among themselves through pre-voting "horse-trading." The TSOP president is indirectly chosen from among the elected council members. Some years ago, a proposed by-law amendment to vote for a "president-elect" who would have the opportunity to familiarize himself or herself with the business of the TSOP was rejected at general membership meeting because it conflicted with a KMT by-law regulating all professional societies in Taiwan. Thus, the TSOP president is still appointed by indirect elections every two years. The restriction on numbers of residency trainees has been imposed by an interest group looking for a near-sighted reimbursement "pie" from the NHI Bureau. The private psychiatric practitioners on the TSOP council are afraid that more private psychiatrists will compete for patients if more psychiatrists are trained and certified. This situation is somewhat similar to that in Japan when the Japanese Society of Psychiatry Neurology and Psychiatry (JSPN) was "hijacked" by private psychiatrist practitioners from 1970 to 2000 (Shinfuku, 2012). But, after the system at the JSPN was reorganized in the 2000s, the number of new psychiatric residents has remarkably improved in recent years. Now the increased percentage of psychiatrists compared to other medical subspecialties in Japan takes it among the top three medical subspecialties (anesthesiology, psychiatry, and dermatology), and the number of psychiatrists in Japan has been increased 1.5 times in the past 16 years (unpublished data of M. Takeda).

References

American Psychiatric Association (2013) *Diagnostic and Statistical Manual of Mental Disorders, Fifth Edition (DSM–5)*. Arlington, Virginia, USA: American Psychiatric Association, 2013.

American Psychiatric Association with translation into classic Chinese by Taiwanese Society of Psychiatry. *Desk Reference to the Diagnostic Criteria from DSM–5*. Taipei: Ho–Chi Publishing Company, 2014 (in Chinese).

Aoki T. (2009) 'Taiwan', In: Shinfuku N. and Asai K. eds. *World Mental Health Care: Current Status and Future Perspective*, Revised Edition, Tokyo: Herusu Publishing Company, 2009, pp. 147–57 (in Japanese).

Blust R. (1999) Subgrouping, circularity and extinction: some issues in Austronesian comparative linguistics, in E. Zeitoun E. and Li P. J. K. (editors). *Selected Papers from the Eighth International Conference on Austronesian Linguistics*, Taipei: Academia Sinica.

Chen Y. H. (1997) *Developmental History of Medical Care in Taiwan*, Taipei: New Natural Principle, pp. 173–206 (in Chinese).

Chou F. H. C., Chen P. C., Liu R. Y., Ho C. K., Tsai K. Y., Ho W.W., Chao S. S., Lin K. S., Shen S. P., and Chen C. C. (2010) A comparison of quality of life and depression between female married immigrants and native married women in Taiwan. *Social Psychiatry and Psychiatric Epidemiology*, 45, 921–30.

Clements J. (2004), *Pirate King: Coxinga and the Fall of the Ming Dynasty*, London, United Kingdom: Muramasa Industries Limited.

Covell, R.R. (1998) *Pentecost of the Hills in Taiwan: The Christian Faith among the Original Inhabitants (Illustrated Edition)*. Taipei: Hope Publishing House.

Durdin T. (1947) Formosa killings are put at 10,000: foreigners say the Chinese slaughtered demonstrators without provocation. *New York Times,* March 29.

Executive Yuan (2011) *The Republic of China Yearbook* (in Chinese). Government Information Office, Republic of China (Taiwan).

Fujimoto M. (2009) 'Korea', In: Shinfuku N. and Asai K. eds. *World Mental Health Care: Current Status and Future Perspective*, Revised Edition, Tokyo: Herusu Publishing Company, 2009, pp. 138–46 (in Japanese).

Guide for Japanese Islands (in Japanese) (2004) Tokyo: Foundation of Japanese Outlying Islands, Inc.

Hsieh C. J., Chang C., Chen S. C., and Shih Y. W. (2013) Needs and quality of life of patients with schizophrenia living in halfway houses. *Taiwanese Journal of Psychiatry* (Taipei), 27: 283–94.

Huang Y. (2013a) Development of the World Health Organization (WHO) Composite International Diagnostic Interview (CIDI). *Taiwanese Journal of Psychiatry* (Taipei), 27, 334–5.

Huang Y. (2013b) Epidemiological study of mental disorders in China. *Taiwanese Journal of Psychiatry* (Taipei), 27: 101–9.

Hwu H. G., Yeh E. K., and Chang L.Y. (1989) Prevalence of psychiatric disorders in Taiwan defined by the Chinese diagnostic interview schedule. *Acta Psychiatrica Scandinavia*, 79, 136–47.

Hwu H. G., Chang I. H., Yeh E. K., Chang C. J, and Yeh L. L. (1996) Major depressive disorder in Taiwan defined by the Chinese Diagnostic Interview Schedule. *Journal of Nervous and Mental Diseases*, 184, 497–502.

Jean–Marie H. (1996) *The International Status of Taiwan in the New World Order: Legal and Political Considerations*. The Netherlands: Kluwer Law International.

Kerr G. H. (1965) *Formosa Betrayed*, Boston, USA: Houghton Mifflin. Liao C. C., Shen W. W., Chang C. C., Chang H., and Chen T. L. (2013) Surgical adverse outcomes in patients with schizophrenia: a population-based study. *Annals of Surgery*, 2013, 257, 433–8.

Liao S. C., Chen W. J., Lee M. B., Lung F. W., Lai T. J., Liu C. Y., Yang M. J., and Chen C. C. (2012) Low prevalence of major depressive disorder in Taiwanese adults: possible explanations and implications. *Psychological Medicine*, 42, 1227–37.

Liao C. C., Shen W. W., Chang C. C., Chang H., and Chen T. L. (2013) Surgical adverse outcomes in patients with schizophrenia: a population-based study, *Annals of Surgery*, 2013, 257, 433–8.

Lin T. Y. (1953) A study of incidence of mental disorders in Chinese and other cultures. *Psychiatry*, 16, 315–35.

Lin T. Y., Rin H., Yeh E. K., Hsu C. C., and Chu H. M. (1969) 'Mental disorders in Taiwan: fifteen years later: a preliminary report' , In: Caudill W. and Lin T. Y. eds. *Mental Health in Asia and Pacific*, Honolulu: East West Center Press, pp. 66–91.

Liu R. Y., Tsai K. Y., Chou F. H. C., Ho W. W., Chen W. L., and Chen C. C. (2010) The characteristics of severely mental ill patients who need forced hospitalization before and after the amended mental health act in Taiwan. *Taiwanese Journal of Psychiatry* (Taipei), 24: 131–9.

Lo H. W. A, Chen C. C., Chou F. H. C., and Chang H. T. (2011) A comparison of posttraumatic stress symptoms in survivors of the Chi-Chi earthquake and Morakot flood. *Taiwanese Journal of Psychiatry* (Taipei). 25, 167–79.

López–Muñoz F., Shen W. W., Moreno R., Molina J. D., Noriega C., Pérez–Nieto M. A., Rubio G., and Álamo C. (2012) International scientific productivity of second-generation antipsychotic drugs in Taiwan: a bibliometric study. *Taiwanese Journal of Psychiatry* (Taipei), 26: 114–29.

Mateo B. and Eugenio J. (2002) *Spaniards in Taiwan* Vol. II, Taipei: SMC Publishing.

Olsen, J. W. and Miller–Antonio S. (1992) The palaeolithic in Southern China, *Asian Perspectives,* 31: 129–60.

Pan J. J., Chen B. Y., Teng H. W., Lu M. L., and Shen W. W. (2005) The use of alternative medicine among Taiwanese psychiatric outpatients. *Psychiatry and Clinical Neurosciences*, 59, 711–16.

Price J. (2001) *A Just Peace? The 1951 San Francisco Peace Treaty in Historical Perspective*. (A Working Paper, No. 78). Oakland, California, USA: Japanese Policy Research Institute.

Shen W. W. (2013a) Getting used to changes in DSM-5 depressive disorders. *Taiwanese Journal of Psychiatry* (Taipei), 27, 171–3.

Shen W. W. (2013b) The possible changes in the *Fifth Edition of the Diagnostic and Statistical Manual of Mental Disorders*: a summarized exit poll on the eve of the DSM-5 publication. *Taiwanese Journal of Psychiatry* (Taipei), 27, 1: 7–10.

Shinfuku N. (2012) What is happening in the mental health system in Japan: some observations. *Taiwanese Journal of Psychiatry* (Taipei), 26, 70–6.

Tai PT (2007). *The Concise History of Taiwan* (Chinese–English bilingual). Nantou City, Taiwan: Taiwan Historica.

Takekoshi Y. (1907) *Japanese Rule in Formosa*, London: Longmans, Green, and Co.

Wang Y. J. and Yu C. H. (2013) Sleepwalking induced by the extended-release zolpidem under polypharmacy treatment. *Taiwanese Journal of Psychiatry* (Taipei), 2013, 27, 165–6.

Yeh E. K. (1994) Cross-cultural psychiatry of psychiatric disorders: review and future perspective. *Kyushu Psychiatry*, 40, 1–13 (in Japanese).

Yoshida N. (2009) 'Association of South-South Asian Nation (ASEAN)', In: Shinfuku N. and Asai K. eds. *World Mental Health Care: Current Status and Future Perspective*, Revised Edition, Tokyo: Herusu Publishing Company, 2009, pp. 97–106 (in Japanese).

14

Mental health services in Hong Kong

Samson Tse, Roger M. K. Ng and
Linda C. W. Lam

Basic facts about Hong Kong

Hong Kong is a small island with an area of 1,104 km². It is located between the Taiwan Straits, the South China Sea and the Pacific Ocean, making it a strategic city for traffic in Asia and across the globe. It covers the island of Hong Kong, Kowloon peninsula, the New Territories and islands such as Lamma Island and Lantau Island where the world famous Chek Lap Kok international airport is situated. In 1842 after the first Opium War, sovereignty over Hong Kong was handed from China to the United Kingdom and it became a British colony through three different treaties: the Treaty of Nanking (1842), the Treaty of Beijing (1860) and the Convention for the Extension of Hong Kong territory (1898). In 1997, Hong Kong was handed back by the British crown to become a Special Administrative Region of the People's Republic of China.

Starting out as a fishing village, salt production site and trading ground, Hong Kong later evolved into a military port of strategic importance and eventually an international financial centre (History of Hong Kong, undated). Hong Kong is a developed capitalist economy, with a gross domestic product of US$301.6 billion (Cheung *et al.*, 2010) which gives it the world's sixth highest GDP per capita. According to the censuses, the total population of Hong Kong was 6.9 million in 2006 (Census and Statistics Department, 2010) and reached 7.2 million, which is about 0.1 per cent of the world population, in early 2014. Approximately 95 per cent of the population consists of persons of Chinese nationality, and the other 5 per cent are from ethnic minorities (Census and Statistics Department, 2007).

Historical development

The first lunatic asylum in Hong Kong was built in 1875 for non-Chinese people with mental illness, and was eventually relocated and renamed the European Lunatic Asylum in 1885 (Medical Department, 1893). To cater for the increasing needs of local Chinese residents with mental illness, a new Chinese Lunatic Asylum was set up next door in 1891. Due to the vast unmet needs of people with mental illness in Hong Kong, these two small establishments rapidly became overcrowded within a few years of being set up. In view of the increasing demand for asylum care among people with mental illness, the Crown Colonial Government established a formal agreement to transfer patients of Chinese descent to the John Kerr Refuge for the Insane in the city of Canton in Mainland China (Medical Department, 1894). Non-Chinese people with mental illness were repatriated to their mother countries. The formal establishment of these pathways led to a change in the function of the local asylums in Hong Kong from long-term custodial houses to short-term residential placements before transfer to Canton or repatriation.

In 1895, the two asylums merged into a single 140-bed establishment (the Victorian Asylum) to improve management. In line with the Western trend of emphasising the treatment component of mental illness, the asylum was also formally renamed a mental hospital. However, the environment remained largely custodial and overcrowded. The Communist takeover of Mainland China in 1949 witnessed an influx of refugees into Hong Kong and disrupted the transfer of patients to the Canton asylum. This led to a sudden surge in demand for psychiatric care in the local mental hospital. To cope with this increasing demand for inpatient psychiatric care, a new public mental hospital with 1,000 beds, the Castle Peak Hospital, was built in a remote region of Hong Kong in 1961. A further population boom then prompted the establishment of another 1,300-bed public mental hospital, Kwai Chung Hospital. Alongside the opening of these facilities, acute psychiatric beds were also introduced in general hospitals, albeit on a much smaller scale. These were used to care for patients who posed a less significant risk of violence. In the late 1980s, the total number of psychiatric beds in Hong Kong reached its zenith of around 5,000, all of which came under the administration and management of the Department of Hospital Services of the British Colonial Government of Hong Kong. In view of the need to enhance the clinical governance of these mental hospitals and ensure the proper regulation of voluntary and compulsory admissions within the British system, a new Mental Health Ordinance was enacted in 1962 to replace the previous legislation (Lo, 1988). The Ordinance has undergone various minor revisions through the years but is currently heavily modelled after the United Kingdom Mental Health Act of 1983. This revision of local mental health laws also coincided with the transfer of responsibility for hospital administration in 1990 from the Department of Hospital Services to the Hospital Authority of Hong Kong (HA), a newly established statutory organisation fully subsidised by the Hong Kong Government.

Mental health services and new initiatives in the twenty-first century

Psychiatric services

As well as opening more psychiatric beds to cater for unmet needs for inpatient care, the Hong Kong Government followed in the footsteps of the British psychiatric care model by providing regional outpatient care for patients who had been discharged from mental hospitals. By the 1960s, these regional psychiatric clinics had been established in the major regions of the Hong Kong territory and had expanded their function to provide psychiatric care for patients with common mental disorders (CMDs). However, the growth in capacity of outpatient care services could not match the exponentially growing numbers of inpatients discharged from mental hospitals and outpatients with CMDs. As mentioned in the previous section, the HA took over the administration of all public hospitals in 1990, at which time it also assumed responsibility for the clinical governance of public mental health services (for a review of the mental health system in Hong Kong see Cheung et al., 2010).

The mental health services development plan published in 2010 states that over 200,000 Hong Kong citizens were then under the care of the HA's mental health services (Hospital

Authority, 2011). The 2008 service figures indicate that the total number of patients receiving mental health care from the HA was 152,844, with approximately 40,000 suffering from severe mental illness, most of whom had been diagnosed with psychosis. Over 60 per cent of service provision was allocated to the care of people suffering from different forms of CMDs. Over the past few years, the number of patients receiving HA psychiatric services has increased, to 186,907 in 2011/12, with a significant proportion of this growth accounted for by patients with CMDs (Hong Kong Government, 2012).

An extrapolation of prevalence estimates from a recent population survey predicts a far greater number of people suffering from different mental health problems (see the section on 'Mental health research in Hong Kong'). The number of people receiving HA mental health services is only the tip of the iceberg. As there is still very limited provision of mental health care by primary care physicians and private psychiatrists, it is likely that a significant proportion of people living with mental illness have not yet received proper assessment or treatment.

The problem of under-provision has been further compounded by the lack of a comprehensive, district-based primary care system of mental health care for people with CMDs. In view of the pressing need to address the mounting pressure on outpatient caseloads in regional psychiatric clinics, new Integrated Mental Health Clinics were set up in each geographical district in 2012 and run by trained family doctors under the auspices of the HA's primary care clinics. In an effort to ensure the quality of care, these doctors are regularly supervised by experienced psychiatrists. However, the scale and extent of this initiative in primary health care is still relatively small and essentially experimental in nature.

With the advent of community mental health care in the West, Hong Kong followed suit by setting up a community psychiatric nursing service in 1982 and launching community psychiatric teams in 1994. Meanwhile, alternative community-based residential services, such as halfway houses and long-stay care homes, are run by non-governmental organisations (NGOs) to provide medium- to long-term residential options for patients with severe mental illness who have been discharged from hospitals (see the subsection on 'Social welfare and social rehabilitation services'). To ensure the appropriate prioritisation of community care and residential services for patients with a propensity towards violence, a priority follow-up (PFU) system was set up in Hong Kong in 1982. In essence, patients with severe mental illness are categorised as one of three types; PFU (subtarget), PFU (target) and non-PFU. Patients labelled as PFU (subtarget) receive the most intensive level of community care, thereby minimising the likelihood of their falling through the safety net (see the subsection, 'Current pitfalls of the PFU system'). This system was launched well before a similar care prioritisation system was available in the United Kingdom and Australia. Such enhanced support for community care has been coupled with a gradual reduction in the number of inpatient psychiatric beds, with the total having dropped to around 3,600 as of 2013. There has also been a concomitant reduction in the median length of inpatient stay over the last decade, from over 90 to around 60 days. In line with the recent development of assertive treatment and home-based crisis intervention in the West, a systematic effort has been made since 2010 to roll out the case management care model (known as the personalised care programme [PCP]) in 12 districts in Hong Kong (Hospital Authority, 2011). Under this programme, a person with severe mental illness is supported and followed up by a designated case manager who fosters a close alliance with them, co-ordinates and delivers appropriate services and develops an individual care plan taking into account the client's needs and risk profile (Hong Kong Government, 2013a). A service pledge has been made to recruit over 250 case managers to provide individualised home-based care for more than 15,000 patients in all geographical regions of Hong Kong by 2015. The effectiveness of case managers in reducing admissions and mortality rates is currently under investigation by an independent academic institution. The preliminary results are reported to be encouraging.

While ensuring proper quality and standards for mental health professionals delivering care is important to the success of any mental health service, an acceptable level of service cannot be realised without appropriate and effective treatment options. Through an injection of extra funding by the HA, the proportion of patients with schizophrenia being prescribed atypical antipsychotics has jumped from only 10 per cent in 2001 to around 60 per cent in 2013. There is an ongoing initiative to lobby for more government funding, with the aim of ensuring that all patients with appropriate clinical indications for atypical antipsychotics will be entitled to receive them without concern for budgetary constraints. Extra funding has also been allocated in the past couple of years to prescribing anti-dementia drugs and new drugs for the treatment of attention deficit hyperactivity disorder (ADHD), so that more patients with these conditions can receive early pharmacological intervention to minimise their disabilities.

Social welfare and social rehabilitation services

The Social Welfare Department (SWD) is responsible for implementing the government's policies on social welfare and for developing and co-ordinating social welfare services including social security, social rehabilitation services for people with psychiatric disabilities and other related services for specific populations such as young people, the elderly, offenders, and children and families (Hong Kong Government, 2013a). The objective of rehabilitation services is to help individuals with disabilities develop their physical, mental and social potential to the fullest extent. The 1995 White Paper on Rehabilitation has provided a long-term blueprint for the development of rehabilitation services and the Disability Discrimination Ordinance (Cap. 487) which has been in place since 1996 provides persons with disabilities with a legal framework to assert equal opportunities for work, housing and education and to reduce the discrimination and harassment associated with severe mental illness (Hong Kong Government, 2013a). The total health care expenditure in Hong Kong accounts for around 5 per cent of Gross Domestic Product (GDP). Total government expenditure on mental health services accounted for about 0.22 per cent of GDP in 2008–2009. In the same year the government spent HK$3.65 billion on mental health services, up from HK$3.14 billion in 2004–2005. Of these budget allocations, 78 per cent was spent on medical treatment and rehabilitation services and 22 per cent on social rehabilitation services, with 98 per cent of the latter allocated to NGOs for service provision (Cheng, 2011).

Residential services

In 2008–2009, NGOs provided about 3,000 residential care places in institutions such as long-stay homes, halfway houses and supported hostels for persons in recovery from mental illness to support their rehabilitation and re-integration into the community (Cheng, 2011). They also offered about 120 places in self-financing hostels for individuals who are more capable of independent living. Those who are able to live independently and have a long-term housing need may also apply for public housing under the Compassionate Rehousing Scheme of the Housing Authority.

Vocational rehabilitation services

The SWD and NGOs provide a variety of vocational rehabilitation services such as vocational training and sheltered workshops to enhance the vocational skills of persons in recovery. Alternatively, such individuals may find jobs in the open labour market through participating in a supported employment scheme where they undergo on-the-job training and placements.

Furthermore, the Labour Department, the Vocational Training Council and the Employees Retraining Board also offer vocational training and employment support services for members of the public, including persons with psychiatric disabilities, who are looking for retraining opportunities or employment.

Community support services

Community support services include general support services such as counselling and parents/relatives resource centres provided by psychiatric medical social workers and other health professionals. Since October 2010, the SWD has established Integrated Community Centres for Mental Wellness (ICCMW) in Hong Kong through 24 service units (Hong Kong Government, 2013a). ICCMW aim to provide one-stop, accessible and integrated community-based mental health support services. They also provide a single entry point of collaboration between NGOs and HA case managers to ensure service users are receiving an optimal level of support in their own familiar neighbourhood. The services offered by ICCMW seek to meet the varying needs of service users and include community education on mental health, day training, occupational therapy assessment and training, outreach visits, group programmes, counselling, social and leisure activities, drop-in sessions, support for caregivers and, where required, direct liaison with HA psychiatric services for urgent psychiatric consultation and assessment (Social Welfare Department, September 2010). Furthermore, in an effort to establish closer links between HA psychiatric services and ICCMW, the community mental health team in each cluster maintains regular and close liaison with ICCMW staff to facilitate cross-service referrals and skill sharing. In view of the close relationship between the psychiatric, social, housing and police services, a regular multi-disciplinary meeting chaired by SWD and HA representatives is held in each cluster to establish and enhance cross-agency cooperation in the management of patients with mental illness in the community.

Prevention and early detection

In 2001, the HA and SWD jointly launched a number of community-based programmes for the prevention and early identification of mental health problems among different target groups. The Early Assessment and Detection of Young persons with psychosis programme (EASY) was established for people aged 15–25 showing early symptoms of psychosis. A preliminary three-year cohort study suggests that patients receiving this intervention had longer periods of full-time employment, fewer days of hospitalisation, less severe positive and negative symptoms, fewer signs of disengagement from mental health care services and fewer suicides than a historical control group (for further details see Chen et al., 2011). An ongoing randomised controlled trial is being conducted to compare the effectiveness of case management for early psychosis and routine care, with the preliminary results suggesting that case management is superior across various outcome domains. After the 2010–2011 Chief Executive's Policy Address, the EASY target population was expanded to include adults aged 26 to 65 with psychotic symptoms. The Elderly Suicide Prevention Programme (ESPP) was also established to target adults aged 65 or above with suicidal tendencies or depression. A cohort study comparing the two-year completed suicide and suicide re-attempt rates between a historical control group receiving pre-intervention standard care and a group enrolled in the ESPP shows that the latter had a significantly reduced rate of completed suicide but a similar re-attempt rate (Chan et al., 2011). Further studies are now underway to assess the long-term outcomes of patients involved in the ESPP. Last but not least, the Child and Adolescent Mental Health Community Support and Community Mental Health Intervention Projects have also been launched to strengthen support for children and adolescents with emotional or mental health problems.

Recovery-orientated services as emergent practice

There is some indication that mental health services in Hong Kong are gradually embracing the concept of recovery. Most notably, the Mental Health Service Plan for Adults states that '[t]he vision of the future is of a person-centred service based on effective treatment and the recovery of the individual' (Hospital Authority, 2011: 5). Such language might sound familiar to Western professionals, but is seen as a great leap forward and is still a relatively foreign concept to mental health professionals (and trainees) and service users in Hong Kong (Ng *et al.* 2010, 2008; Slade *et al.*, 2014). Even though formal adoption or advocacy of the recovery approach in Hong Kong has only emerged in the last decade, some establishments adopted its principles, such as promoting service user empowerment, in the early 1980s (Tsoi *et al.*, 2014). Most notably, the Richmond Fellowship was the first agency to adopt the Therapeutic Community model in 1984 and remains the only one to have done so (Poon and Lo, undated). The Amity Mutual Support Society, established in 1996 by a group of people recovering from mental illness, was the first formal self-help group to be founded in Hong Kong (Amity Mutual Support Society, 2013). Moreover, the Phoenix Clubhouse, a community adult psychiatric rehabilitation centre established jointly by the Queen Mary Hospital and the University of Hong Kong, was the first to implement the Clubhouse Model in Hong Kong (www.phoenixclubhouse.org/). The Clubhouse is run and managed primarily by its members, all of whom are people recovering from mental illness. Through working and participating in the Clubhouse activities, members are able to use and develop their strengths and abilities, as well as acquiring job-related skills that will help them to return to the open labour market (Raeburn *et al.*, 2013).

Although acute, hospital-based psychiatric care is largely based on the medical model, such as symptomatic and syndromal recovery (Tohen *et al.*, 2000; Judd *et al.*, 2003), there are some exceptions (Tse *et al.*, 2012). For example, in the regional psychiatric unit in Kowloon Hospital, service users have served as representatives on the management committee of the psychiatric rehabilitation team and as peer specialists within the mental health team workforce since 2012. Castle Peak Hospital, the oldest psychiatric institution in Hong Kong, has successfully sought funding to recruit peer specialists as part of its growing user-involved clinical services programme. Within the social services sector, service users play an active role in self-help groups, most of which are sponsored and operated by individual NGOs. These are normally quite informal, bringing together people with various diagnoses or at different stages of recovery. The groups are facilitated by a professional working with individuals in recovery in order to help members to learn how to cope and live with the experience of mental illness. Some self-help groups have a very strong expressive component, using a variety of media (such as painting, sculpture, photography and songwriting) to describe members' recovery experiences. With the gradual development of service user participation in Hong Kong, some of these groups are now evolving to include users as role models or trained facilitators. Some users also work as trainers of caregivers and professionals, or provide input to the design of surveys or other research. Another exciting development is the successful launch of the first multi-agency peer support training course in Hong Kong, run by four NGOs. This three-year pilot project has been funded by MINDSET since August 2012 and aims to train people who have recovered from a mental illness to help others who are still on their recovery journey (for a review of peer support services in mental health, see Davidson and Guy, 2012). All of these developments are welcome. However, a formal, territory-wide and sustained strategy for incorporating service user and caregiver feedback into the design, implementation and evaluation of recovery-oriented services is yet to be established.

Mental health research in Hong Kong

As one of the most prosperous cities in Asia, Hong Kong enjoys free trade and international exchange. Like in most developed cities worldwide, the stress of urban life is the rule rather than the exception. The Hong Kong Special Administration Region is a developed city located at the southern tip of China which was a British colony for a hundred years. Since the change of sovereignty to China in 1997, there has been an exponential increase in cross-border exchange, leading to significant changes in the demographic characteristics of the city's population. Many of those changes are likely to have an impact on mental health care needs.

How common are mental disorders in Hong Kong?

Despite being a major cosmopolitan city, statistics for mental health problems in Hong Kong are far from comprehensive, with few population-based surveys of prevalence. The first such survey was conducted in the 1984 in Shatin, then a satellite town of Hong Kong. The two-phase design involved interviewing over 7,000 community-dwelling adults using the Diagnostic Interview Schedule-III (DIS-III). The prevalence of generalised anxiety and depressive disorders was 7.8 per cent/11.1 per cent and 1.29 per cent/2.44 per cent in men/women respectively, and the overall prevalence of any psychiatric disorder was 19.5 per cent/18.3 per cent in men/women (Chen *et al.*, 1993). Although these findings indicate that mental disorders were widely prevalent, limited community-based research was conducted to further evaluate the mental health care needs of the Hong Kong population. Until the end of the last century, no systematic door-to-door survey of population mental health had been conducted. However, it was recognised that the prevalence estimates of mental disorders needed reconsideration and updating.

Over the past decade, estimates of the prevalence of mood disorders have been based on a few large-scale telephone surveys conducted in the 2000s. A telephone survey of 5,004 participants using the *Diagnostic and Statistical Manual of Mental Disorders*, 4th edition, Diagnostic Interviews, revealed a 12-month prevalence of major depressive episodes of 8.4 per cent. Being a woman and being unemployed were both associated with increased risk, and a significant proportion of respondents also reported frequent thoughts of suicide (Lee *et al.*, 2007). In another telephone survey of 2,005 respondents aged 15–65, the 12-month prevalence of generalised anxiety disorder was 3.4 per cent (Lee *et al.*, 2009).

From these studies, it has been recognised that mood disorders are prevalent conditions in Hong Kong. The impact on psychosocial functioning should not be underestimated. However, despite an increasing public recognition of the significance of mood disorders, there remain major barriers to help seeking and early service utilisation.

The Hong Kong Mental Morbidity Survey

The Hong Kong Mental Morbidity Survey (HKMMS), the first territory-wide door-to-door survey on the community prevalence of mental disorders, was commissioned by the Food and Health Bureau of the Government of the Hong Kong Special Administrative Region in 2010. This survey aimed to provide comprehensive mental health information about Hong Kong citizens and address any significant factors that may provide insights for mental health service planning.

In the second quarter of 2013, interviews were conducted with 5,719 ethnic Chinese adult Hong Kong residents aged 16–75. The study set out to ascertain the community prevalence of common mood disorders, psychosis-related symptoms, at-risk mental states, suicidal ideations, and alcohol and psychotropic substance misuse. The interview schedule comprised an assessment of mental health symptoms using the revised Clinical Interview Schedule adopting the diagnostic algorithm of the *International Classification of Diseases*, 10th edition, for mood disorders. It also studied the major moderating factors that may adversely influence mental health, as well as potentially protective factors that may enhance resilience.

At the time of writing, the final report of the HKMMS is still being prepared. From the interim analysis of the first 4,000 participants, the age- and gender-adjusted one-week overall prevalence rate of CMDs was 14.4 per cent, with the majority being depressive, generalised anxiety, mixed anxiety and depressive disorders. The findings also suggest that being female, being in poorer physical health and having limited social support are associated with a higher risk of developing CMDs. Fewer than 30 per cent of the participants in the HKMMS with diagnosable CMDs had sought professional (medical or non-medical) help for their subjective mental distress over the previous year, indicating the presence of substantial barriers to the pathway of care (Lam and the Hong Kong Mental Morbidity Team, 2013).

Barriers to care

There is now generally increased community awareness of the symptoms of mood disorders, and people are generally more ready to accept that they are common conditions that affect one's health. However, this does not translate into earlier health-seeking behaviours. In a recent study commissioned by the Food and Health Bureau of the Hong Kong government on pathways to psychiatric care, the median duration from symptom onset to first psychiatric consultation was 42 weeks. People presenting with suicidal ideation and agitated behaviour may seek attention earlier, whereas women with depressive symptoms may delay longer in seeking proper psychiatric help (Chan *et al.*, 2012).

Furthermore, a questionnaire survey of attitudes towards mental illness involving 1,035 Hong Kong Chinese respondents found that general acceptance was low. Regular contact with such patients was associated with better knowledge ($p<0.01$) and better acceptance ($p<0.01$) of mental illness. Younger participants, aged 15–19, had less knowledge about mental health problems than other age groups ($p<0.001$) (Siu *et al.*, 2012). A lack of community acceptance of mental illness may make people reluctant to seek help early. Further public education targeting the destigmatisation of mental illness is of primary importance in encouraging early intervention when a problem arises. Apart from the reluctance to seek help, it is also important that there is sufficient provision to allow service users to receive proper care. At present, there are many pressured areas that require attention.

Challenges ahead in the twenty-first century

The need for psychiatric care has been rising significantly over the past few years. Despite an increase in the public resources allocated to mental health services from HK$3.39 billion in 2007/08 to HK$4.42 billion in 2011/12 (Hong Kong Government, 2013b), care provision is still considered grossly insufficient. This is reflected in the very long waiting time for a first assessment appointment in the HA's psychiatric clinics. The complex and diverse service needs of people with serious mental illness (SMI) also require continued attention and innovative approaches. More extensive use of case managers to support recovery from both first episodes and early relapses is of particular importance to long-term functional recovery and prognosis.

Lack of an adequate mental health workforce

The inadequacy of the workforce in the Hong Kong mental health sector is a long-standing problem. The workforce shortage in medical, nursing and allied health professionals can be dated back to the year 2003, when the Hong Kong government drastically cut the amount of subsidies to the universities in the training of doctors, nurses and allied health professionals due to budget constraints. The shortage of doctors and nurses has become apparent in the past five years when senior doctors have retired from the public health service and other experienced doctors have left the public service for the lucrative private medical health market. The private medical market has been booming in the past ten years, partly related to the gradual economic recovery in Hong Kong and partly related to the growth of medical tourism as a result of the relaxation of border controls for visitors from Mainland China. In an effort to increase the number of medical students in the two medical schools in Hong Kong, the government has injected more resources in the past five years. In 2009–2011, a total of 320 medical students were recruited each year into the two medical schools. In 2012–2014, the number of medical students has further increased so that a total of 420 medical students are recruited into the two medical schools each year.

According to the latest WHO *Mental Health Atlas*, Hong Kong has 4.39 psychiatrists per 100,000 population. This is much lower than other developed countries such as England (17.65/100,000) and Japan (10.1/100,000). The nursing workforce is also relatively small. While there are 29.15 mental health nurses per 100,000 population in Hong Kong, the corresponding figures in England and Japan are 83.23 and 102.55, respectively (Chan *et al.*, in press). Since the handover of the sovereignty of Hong Kong to the People's Republic of China in 1997, the training and education of specialist psychiatrists has been overseen by the Hong Kong College of Psychiatrists, a constituent college of the Hong Kong Academy of Medicine. The training of psychiatrists in Hong Kong involves a six-year training curriculum, in which at least three years of full-time clinical training in psychiatry must be spent in one of the accredited training centres in Hong Kong as a junior trainee, before taking the Part 1 and Part 2 clinical examinations of the Fellowship of Hong Kong College of Psychiatrists. Upon successful completion of the two parts of the examinations, eligible trainees are allowed to enrol into at least three more years of clinical training in psychiatry as senior trainees. During the three-year period of higher training, each senior trainee is required to complete a research project and submit a dissertation in preparation for the Part 3 examination. The Part 3 examination comprises an oral viva voce in which three examiners examine and discuss with the trainees the relevant aspects of their submitted dissertations. As of March 2014, the Hong Kong College of Psychiatrists has a register of 48 junior trainees and 71 senior trainees. The number will be expected to increase in the next couple of years as the number of medical graduates will increase. So far, there is no major recruitment problem of medical students into the field of psychiatry in Hong Kong.

The College has also played a pivotal role in raising awareness of the shortage of psychiatrists in Hong Kong since the handover. As of 2013, Hong Kong has around 320 specialist psychiatrists, translating into a ratio of one psychiatrist for 22,000 members of the community. Although this still lags far behind the target of 800 psychiatrists to cover the whole population, there has been a substantial increase over the last 15 years. Similar efforts have been made to recruit, retain and train mental health nurses. As well as offering higher degrees in nursing in local universities, the establishment in 2012 of the Hong Kong Academy of Nursing has served to promote the professional image of the nursing profession. To address the multi-disciplinary nature of the role of case manager in the PCP, the HA has also developed a systematic training programme for all new staff taking up this role. Nevertheless, given the rising demand for mental health services in Hong Kong, there is a pressing need to establish closer links between professional bodies, the HA and universities to develop and increase the mental health workforce. There is also a growing need to develop innovative approaches to recruiting and retaining existing mental health professionals, given the increasing competition from the private sector and other medical specialties.

Limitations of mental health services in the primary care sector

Unlike most developed cities in the West, Hong Kong does not have a comprehensive, region-based primary care service, with the majority of psychiatric services being run by the HA. There is a lack of family physicians and general practitioners with the skills and training required to provide long-term psychiatric care in the community. Although some effort has been made to enhance the knowledge and skills of primary care doctors in terms of the detection and management of CMDs, such as offering postgraduate courses in psychological medicine in local universities, the number of doctors with adequate training remains limited. The lack of any incentive for primary care doctors in the private sector to accept patients with CMDs is another important issue. At present, only about 100 psychiatrists work in the private sector, and so this area can provide only very limited services which are insufficient to cater for the level of demand. The primary care sector should play a more important role in the management of CMDs in the near future, thus reducing the service loads of HA mental health services.

Insufficient provision of medical, vocational and social rehabilitation services and poor coordination among the sectors

Social and mental health needs frequently coexist, and the management of mental health problems demands that due attention be paid to social needs as well. In Hong Kong, the SWD and the HA come under different administrative structures, so the allocation of resources is at best unco-ordinated and at worst competitive. It is of paramount importance that a strategic work group involving representatives from both sectors be established to ensure the co-ordination and formulation of long-term joint mental health strategies. One important area that still lacks co-ordination is the planning of psychiatric rehabilitation services. With the aim of optimising the use of HA psychiatric beds, a number of long-stay patients with complex needs have been discharged into the community for residential care. However, there has not been a concomitant increase in the number of supervised residential beds in the voluntary sector. In catering for such unmet demand in the community, numerous private hostels of dubious quality have sprung up over the past ten years. Although there is a registration system in place for such hostels, run by the SWD, this is a voluntary process and there is a real risk that those operating at suboptimal standards will not apply.

Although paid employment or engagement in a meaningful social programme is seen as critical to successful re-integration for individuals with mental illness, there is a lack of community vocational and social services for persons in recovery (Tsang et al., 2011; Tsoi et al., 2014). Research shows that unemployment, or problems finding meaningful work that is commensurate with one's qualifications, is associated not only with psychological distress, depression and anxiety, lowered self-esteem and the risk of alcohol and drug abuse, but also impacts negatively on social inclusion or a sense of belonging (Tsang et al., 2010; Tse et al., 2014). When establishing such services, it is important to bear in mind how they can be blended seamlessly with the existing day hospital, occupational therapy and physical therapy services offered on an outpatient basis by the HA. Without a good interface and bridging process, patients may either fall through the cracks or be included within particular services for an unnecessarily long time, impeding their re-integration into the community.

Inadequate support for families and carers and self-help organisations

Based on a territory-wide survey of persons with disabilities and chronic diseases conducted by the Census and Statistics Department in 2006–2007, there were 86,600 persons with mental illness living in Hong Kong and 56,300 (65 per cent) were responsible for the day-to-day care of someone else (Hong Kong Government, 2008). The majority of studies of families or caregivers have been conducted from the perspective of the individual adult. Given that most individuals live within the context of a family and the wider society, it is somewhat surprising that the examination of caregiving from a family perspective has so far been minimal by comparison. Even less is known about Hong Kong families in this context (Li *et al.*, 2013; Lam *et al.*, 2013). Much has been written about the challenges and problems faced by family members and caregivers when supporting a person with mental illness. Such research tends to focus on the individual and to take a deficit- rather than strengths-based approach. Strengths-based approaches build on families' capacity to maximise the protective factors in their lives and thereby minimise the impact of risk factors, such as abusive behaviours towards family members with mental illness or clinical depression in caregivers. Given that Hong Kong is a society made up of predominantly ethnic Chinese people with a strong family orientation, future support for work involving caregivers and family members will be both relevant and meaningful.

Lack of sustained efforts to enhance public understanding and acceptance of mental illness

Countering a lack of understanding of mental illness, and the subsequent stigma and discrimination, is an ongoing battle in Hong Kong and beyond (Fung *et al.*, 2010). Over the years the SWD, the HA and the Department of Health have organised various community and education activities jointly with other government departments and NGOs. Such activities have aimed at increasing mental health literacy and acceptance of persons with mental illness, but have been piecemeal in nature, without any clear overarching vision. Systematic anti-stigma and mental health literacy programmes, under the direction of a designated work group on mental health education, would be a more effective and consistent approach to enhancing public awareness of these important issues. Furthermore, the outcomes of such media and education campaigns need to be systematically evaluated and monitored through relevant performance indicators (Mak and Cheung, 2012). Such outcome-based evaluations would generate important information about their effectiveness and inform the planning of subsequent mental health education campaigns.

Current pitfalls with the PFU system

The PFU system was established in 1983 to enable patients with a history of severe mental illness who had a documented history of, or propensity towards, violence to be registered and closely followed up. However, the current definition of violence is a narrow one and focuses on violence towards others, rather than self-harm or self-neglect. Furthermore, due to concerns about personal privacy, access to the PFU register is restricted to HA mental health professionals and the information is not shared with other agencies such as the SWD, Housing Authority, police or other care providers. This is an issue that demands careful discussion and collaboration between sectors so as to achieve the fine balance between personal freedom and protection of the public. To compound matters further, each psychiatric institution maintains a separate registry, resulting in inconsistencies in the definition and subsequent registration of patients with the PFU system: 'as such, some people may be over- or under-evaluated, resulting in inappropriate labelling or discharge. There is a need to standardize the system to deliver fair and proper standards of care and services' (Expert Panel for Better Community Care of Psychiatric Patients in Hong Kong, 2010: 4).

Upcoming challenges and moving forward

Increasing attention to childhood psychiatric conditions

Not only does the public display increasing awareness of adult psychiatric problems, but attention to childhood psychiatric conditions has also been increasing dramatically of late. In recent years, there has been intense demand from parents for an earlier and more comprehensive service for children suffering from developmental neuropsychiatric conditions. The newly established Child and Adolescent Psychiatric Clinics for children with autistic spectrum disorders and ADHD have growing waiting lists, reflecting an immense amount of unmet need. Furthermore, the services currently offered by the HA focus mainly on the management of autistic spectrum disorders and ADHD, with other common childhood psychiatric conditions such as emotional disorders receiving less attention. There is still a long way to go before an adequate workforce offering a comprehensive model of care can be made widely available to children in need of psychiatric services.

Substance abuse

The changing social demographics of Hong Kong have also had an impact on the pattern of substance abuse. In the last century, the conventional psychiatric drugs of abuse were heroin and related narcotics. Over the last decade, this pattern has changed and the use of psychotropic medication such as ketamine, amphetamine and other stimulants now dominates. The age of onset of substance abuse has also fallen dramatically, making this a real problem in the primary or early secondary school years. As psychiatric complications and co-morbidity are commonly associated with psychotropic substance abuse, the burden of care for this group of young people is also expected to increase. Apart from psychiatric treatment, public education and early detection are extremely important measures required to prevent such problems from emerging in the early phases of life.

Ageing community

The triumph of good medical care has increased the life expectancy of Hong Kong citizens. In 2012, they were expected to enjoy the second longest lifetimes in the world (Ng, 2012). Rapid ageing has also led to a change in the pattern of mental health care needs. Advanced age is associated with a higher prevalence of major neurocognitive disorders (such as dementia) with high psychiatric morbidity. People with progressive cognitive decline and psychiatric disturbances require special attention and skilled intervention due to their complex medical and psychiatric needs. Apart from late onset conditions, an increasing number of people with SMIs and CMDs are also reaching old age. The usual psychiatric care they are offered may require adjustment as medical comorbidity may emerge, affecting the safety profiles and efficacies of maintenance therapy.

The way forward

This chapter has provided a brief review of the development of services to respond to the emerging challenges of mental illness in the unique context and setting of the Hong Kong Special Administrative Region of Mainland China. Over the years, there have been various modes of intervention available for people with mental health problems in Hong Kong, ranging from inpatient care and pharmacological treatments through to personalised care programmes or community-based interventions offered jointly by service users. It is recognised that mental health service delivery has become more community- and strengths-based and recovery-oriented over the past decade. However, the burden of care has not reduced. The stresses of living, better public understanding of mental health needs and changing socio-demographic patterns also demand careful forward planning from the government. To deal with these changes, there is also a need for a carefully planned research programme within the mental health area to guide policy development and foster cultural and community responsiveness. The challenge for the future is to determine whether the overall improvements in psychiatric and social welfare services achieved so far can be sustained over time, and whether an adequate and effective workforce can be developed in order to address the rapidly growing mental health needs of the population.

References

Amity Mutual Support Society (2013) available: www.amss1996.org.hk/index.php/about-us

Census and Statistics Department (2007). *Women and men in Hong Kong: Key statistics* (2006 edition). Hong Kong Special Administrative Region, China.

Census and Statistics Department (2010). Mid-year population for 2010. Retrieved November 25, 2010 from www.censtatd.gov.hk/press_release/press_releases_on_statistics/index.jsp?sID=2594&sSUBID =16625&displayMode=D

Chan, S. S., Leung, V. P., Tsoh, J., Li, S., Yu, C.-S., Gabriel, K., Poon, T., Pan, P. C., Chan, W. and Conwell, Y. (2011) 'Outcomes of a two-tiered multifaceted elderly suicide prevention program in a Hong Kong Chinese community', *American Journal of Geriatric Psychiatry*, 19(2), 185–96.

Chan, W. C., Chow, P. P., Lam, L. C., Hung, S. F., Cheung, E. F., Dunn, E., Ng, R. M. and Fu, J. (2012) *Mental health problems in community: A study of the pathway to care in Hong Kong. Final report*, Hong Kong Food and Health Bureau, Hong Kong Government.

Chan, W. C., Lam, L. C. and Chen, E. Y. (in press) 'Letter from Hong Kong: Recent development of mental health services', *Advances in Psychiatric Care*.

Chen, C.-N., Wong, J., Lee, N., Chan-Ho, M.-W., Lau, J. T.-F. and Fung, M. (1993) 'The Shatin community mental health survey in Hong Kong: II. Major findings', *Archives of General Psychiatry*, 50(2), 125–33.

Chen, E. Y., Tang, J. Y., Hui, C. L., Chiu, C. P., Lam, M. M., Law, C. W., Yew, C. W., Wong, G. H., Chung, D. W. and Tso, S. (2011) 'Three-year outcome of phase-specific early intervention for first-episode psychosis: A cohort study in Hong Kong', *Early Intervention in Psychiatry*, 5(4), 315–23.

Cheng, I. (2011) *Mental health services in selected places*, Hong Kong: Legislative Council Secretariat: Research Division.

Cheung, E. F. C., Lam, L. C. W. and Hung, S.-F. (2010) 'Mental health in Hong Kong: Transition from hospital-based service to personalised care', *International Psychiatry*, 7(3), 62–4.

Davidson, L. and Guy, K. (2012) 'Peer support among persons with severe mental illnesses: A review of evidence and experience', *World Psychiatry*, 11(2), 123–8.

Expert Panel for Better Community Care of Psychiatric Patients in Hong Kong (2010) *Recommendations on improving the mental health policy in Hong Kong*, Hong Kong: Hong Kong Association for the Promotion of Mental Health.

Fung, K. M., Tsang, H. W. and Chan, F. (2010) 'Self-stigma, stages of change and psychosocial treatment adherence among Chinese people with schizophrenia: A path analysis', *Social Psychiatry and Psychiatric Epidemiology*, 45(5), 561–8.

History of Hong Kong (undated). Retrieved April 22, 2014 from http://en.wikipedia.org/wiki/History_of_Hong_Kong

Hong Kong Government (2008) *Social data collected via the General Household Survey: Special Topics Report No.48: Persons with disabilities and chronic diseases*, Hong Kong: The Census and Statistics Department.

Hong Kong Government (2012) *Legislative Council Q4: Number of persons receiving psychiatric services provided by the Hospital Authority (HA)*, Hong Kong Information Centre, http://gia.info.gov.hk/general/201205/30/P201205300297_0297_94676.pdf

Hong Kong Government (2013a) *Fact sheet – Rehabilitation*, Hong Kong: Information Services Department.

Hong Kong Government (2013b) *Hong Kong 2012. Hong Kong Government Yearbook*, Hong Kong: Information Services Department.

Hospital Authority (2011) *Mental health service plan for adults 2010–2015*, Hong Kong.

Judd, L. L., Hagap, S. A., Schettler, P. J., Coryell, W., Endicott, J., Maser, J. D., Solomon, D. A., Leon, A. C. and Keller, M. B. (2003) 'A prospective investigation of the natural history of the long-term weekly symptomatic status of bipolar II disorder', *Archives of General Psychiatry*, 60(3), 261–9.

Lam, C. W. and the Hong Kong Mental Morbidity Team (2013) *Modulating factors of common mental disorders – preliminary results of Hong Kong Mental Morbidity Survey*, Poster presentation at the World Psychiatric Association International Congress 2013, Vienna, Austria.

Lam, P. C., Ng, P. and Tori, C. (2013) 'Burdens and psychological health of family caregivers of people with schizophrenia in two Chinese metropolitan cities: Hong Kong and Guangzhou', *Community Mental Health Journal*, December, 1–6.

Lee, S., Tsang, A. and Kwok, K. (2007) 'Twelve-month prevalence, correlates, and treatment preference of adults with DSM-IV major depressive episode in Hong Kong', *Journal of Affective Disorders*, 98(1), 129–36.

Lee, S., Ma, Y. L., Tsang, A. and Kwok, K. (2009) 'Generalized anxiety disorder with and without excessive worry in Hong Kong', *Depression and Anxiety*, 26(10), 956–61.

Li, D., Li, S. M., Tsang, H. W., Wong, A. H., Fung, K. M., Tsui, M. C., Chung, R. C., Yiu, M. G., Tam, K. and Lee, G. T.-h. (2013) 'Development and validation of perceived rehabilitation require questionnaires for caregivers of people with schizophrenia', *International Journal of Psychiatry in Clinical Practice*, 17(4), 1–9.

Lo, W. H. (1988) 'Development of legislation for the mentally ill in Hong Kong', *Journal of Hong Kong Psychiatric Association*, 8, 6–9.

Mak, W. W. and Cheung, R. Y. (2012) 'Psychological distress and subjective burden of caregivers of people with mental illness: The role of affiliate stigma and face concern', *Community Mental Health Journal*, 48(3), 270–4.

Medical Department (1893) *Annual report of the Medical Department*, Hong Kong.

Medical Department (1894) *Annual report of the Medical Department*, Hong Kong.

Ng, K.-C. (2012) 'Hong Kong women live the longest', *South China Morning Post*, Hong Kong, 27 July, www.scmp.com/article/1007812/hong-kong-women-live-longest

Ng, R. M., Pearson, V., Lam, M., Law, C. W., Chiu, C. P. and Chen, E. Y. (2008) 'What does recovery from schizophrenia mean? Perceptions of long-term patients', *International Journal of Social Psychiatry*, 54(2), 118–30.

Ng, R. M., Pearson, V., Chen, E. E. and Law, C. W. (2010) 'What does recovery from schizophrenia mean? Perceptions of medical students and trainee psychiatrists', *International Journal of Social Psychiatry*, 57(3), 248–62.

Poon, A. and Lo, K. (undated) 'Can the therapeutic community empower the residents in the halfway house: A practical experience in the Richmond Fellowship of Hong Kong', available: www.richmond.org.hk/aspac2004/aspac2004notes/abstract/P_abs.pdf

Raeburn, T., Halcomb, E., Walter, G. and Cleary, M. (2013) 'An overview of the clubhouse model of psychiatric rehabilitation', *Australasian Psychiatry*, 21(4), 376–8.

Siu, B., Chow, K., Lam, L., Chan, W., Tang, V. and Chui, W. (2012) 'A questionnaire survey on attitudes and understanding towards mental disorders', *East Asian Archives of Psychiatry*, 22(1), 18–24.

Slade, M., Amering, M., Farkas, M., Hamilton, R., O'Hagan, M., Panther, G., Perkins, R., Shepherd, G., Tse, S. and Whitley, R. (2014) 'Uses and abuses of recovery: Implementing recovery-oriented practices in mental health systems', *World Psychiatry*, 13, 12–20.

Social Welfare Department (September, 2010) *Collaboration guidelines among integrated community centres for mental wellness, psychiatric service and personalised care programmes of the Hospital Authority, Medical Social Services Units and other welfare services units*, Hong Kong: Rehabilitation and Medical Social Services Branch.

Tohen, M., Hennen, J., Zarate, C. M., Baldessarini, R. J., Strakowski, S. M., Stoll, A. L., Faedda, G. L., Suppes, T., Gebre-Medhin, P. and Cohen, B. M. (2000) 'Two-year syndromal and functional recovery in 219 cases of first-episode major affective disorder with psychotic features', *American Journal of Psychiatry*, 157(2), 220–8.

Tsang, H. W., Leung, A. Y., Chung, R. C., Bell, M. and Cheung, W.-M. (2010) 'Review on vocational predictors: A systematic review of predictors of vocational outcomes among individuals with schizophrenia: An update since 1998', *Australian and New Zealand Journal of Psychiatry*, 44(6), 495–504.

Tse, S., Cheung, E. F. C., Kan, A., Ng, R. M. and Yau, S. (2012) 'Recovery in Hong Kong: Service user participation in mental health services', *International Review of Psychiatry*, 24(1), 40–7.

Tse, S., Chan, S., Ng, K. L. and Yatham, L. N. (2014) 'Meta-analysis of predictors of favorable employment outcomes among individuals with bipolar disorder', *Bipolar Disorders*, 16(3), 217–29.

Tsoi, E., Lo, I., Chan, C., Siu, K. and Tse, S. (2014) 'How recovery-oriented are mental health services in Hong Kong? Snapshots of service users' perspectives', *Asia Pacific Journal of Social Work & Development*, 24(1–2), 82–93.

Section 4

Far East

Overview

Nori Takei

This section deals with three Far East countries: North Korea, South Korea and Japan. As the three countries are geographically close to each other, population and cultural exchange among them has a long history. In fact, the people share some attributes related to religion, such as Buddhism and Confucianism, and culture including the use of ideographs (Chinese characters). However, the three countries have their own histories and thus unique characteristics in a number of respects. One of clear difference is in political principles; North Korea is a socialistic (totalitarian) country whereas the South Korea and Japan are democratic countries. North Korea has taken a stance of isolation from the world and, as a result, no diplomatic relations exist between North Korea and the neighbouring democratic countries.

This has a bearing on the current status of psychiatry in these countries. In the chapter by Kim, it is surprising to learn that North Korea may be using rather old-fashioned medicine in psychiatric practice, since it says that 'coma therapy had been used until recently' in North Korea. As, there are no diplomatic relations, the chapter relies chiefly upon reports from defecting North Korean physicians, and the high prevalence of mental health problems that has been frequently reported in defectors cannot per se be extended to the resident North Korean population, it is difficult to understand precisely what psychiatric practice is like and the prevailing mental health problems in contemporary North Korea. However, Dr Kim's chapter presents a picture suggesting that the people in North Korea may be receiving poor mental health care, especially those who have minor psychiatric conditions such as depression and anxiety and stress-related disorders. As documented, the recession after the economic crisis in North Korea in the 1990s may have affected vulnerable populations in that country. Although the information gathered in this book is not intended to influence (mental) health care systems practised in particular countries, health policy-makers and professionals would benefit from referring to the approaches and health programmes that have been found to be effective and successful in other nations.

It becomes clear from chapters by Lee, Park and Park (South Korea), and Suda, Sugihara and Takei (Japan) that the two nations have followed similar patterns in giving weight to biological psychiatry after the 1980s. The differences are in the influence and introduction of new approaches from modern world psychiatry in their practices. In South Korea, young doctors are reported to have been educated in the USA during the Korean War that broke out in the

1950s and were further influenced by the USA after the war. In contrast, Japanese psychiatry has long been influenced by German psychiatry, namely psychopathology. Psychodynamic theories were introduced after World War II, but psychopathological tenets remained dominant in Japan. Japan has experienced a rather slow process of transition from 'classical' (traditional) psychiatry to modern psychiatry (i.e. biologically orientated and evidence-based practices).

In developed counties, there is a shift towards emphasising community mental health care provision and improving the quality of primary mental health care, through which preventive medicine can be delivered. It is of interest to note that clinical practices in the two countries, both belonging to the OECD, still rely heavily on hospital-based medicine, i.e. long-stay hospitalisation. This may need reform, since more appropriate allocation of expenditures for caring for a wide range of mentally afflicted populations would be sensible when we cannot be sure that the economic growth that supports the social security and health care systems will continue in these countries. Both countries have faced an economic downturn.

Even under strong influences from Western psychiatry, unique characterstics originating from traditions in these countries also exist. For instance, *Tao psychotherapy* (South Korea) and Morita therapy (Japan) are described in this section. These therapeutic approaches may be linked to a culture-bound reasoning process, which Buddhism may underlie.

Stigma attached to mental disorders is a global issue. Kim presents a shocking report on this problem in North Korea: 'Since psychiatric disorders should not exist in the ideal society, the presence of mental illness would be regarded as socially undesirable even by the government'. Rectifying and eradicating stigmatisation is challenging but has to be tackled by working together to provide optimal care for sufferers beyond single nations.

15

History and perspective on psychiatry in Japan

Shiro Suda, Genichi Sugihara and Nori Takei

Geography

Japan is an island nation in East Asia. According to the Government, Japan's population was estimated to be around 128 million as of 2010 (www.e-stat.go.jp/SG1/estat/List.do?bid= 000001034991), the world's tenth most populous country. The land area is 377,923 km^2 in total, which is roughly equal to that of Germany. The Gross Domestic Product (GDP) was US$5,960 billion in 2012, the third largest in the world. Japan has one of the highest life expectancies in the world at 86.4 and 79.6 years of age for females and males, respectively (www.mhlw.go.jp/toukei/saikin/hw/life/life09/01.html). However, Japan has experienced net population loss due to a decrease in birth rate, making it face the concerns of a growing ageing population combined with a low birth rate.

History of psychiatry in Japan

In the Middle Ages

The earliest record of psychiatric disorders in Japan appears in '*Syoku Nihon Gi*', published in 797 AD. The Empress gave birth to Prince Syomu in 701. After childbirth, she developed stupor and was bedridden for a long time. However, after 36 years, she achieved remission at the first contact with a priest. This episode was thought to be a case of the catatonic subtype of schizophrenia with spontaneous remission after persistent stupor (Okada, 2002). This is the first documented case of psychiatric disorder in Japan and the existence of such an old reference is mostly attributable to the Tenno system, which is the Japanese Imperial system that has lasted at least 1,500 years, and in which the Imperial family's genealogy has been documented and kept extraordinarily well.

Around the same era, epilepsy and insanity became recognised as diseases. In 984 AD, the '*Ishinbou*', the oldest medical textbook extant in Japan, was published. The '*Ishinbou*' included details about epilepsy and insanity, which were thought to be caused by the infiltration of bad feelings. In general, these mental abnormalities were considered to be due to possession by a fox spirit, and shamans engaged in treatment. Notably, the concept of 'possession by evil spirit' was generally accepted as an aetiology of psychiatric disorders in Japan, which is coincidentally identical to Western traditional culture.

Based on Buddhism-linked compassion, individuals who suffered from epilepsy and insanity were given special care. In 723 AD, the first relief facility (*Hiden In*) was built to take care of the afflicted on the premises of the 'Kohuku-ji' temple in the city of Nara, which is located 25 miles south of Kyoto. Torture and any types of abuse against such individuals were prohibited in an ordinance at that time, which was modelled after that of China (*T'ang*); however, it is doubtful whether this regulation was adhered to in real life (Okada, 2002). Indeed, children who could not walk by the age of three were made victims and released into the sea or rivers from ships.

In the late fourteenth century, moxibustion (*kyu*) and herbal medicine, which were techniques of traditional Chinese medicine, were first introduced for the treatment of epilepsy and insanity (Okada, 2002). From the early seventeenth century to the mid nineteenth century (i.e. the Edo era), trading and cultural exchange with foreign countries were strictly restricted under the national seclusion policy of Japan, which promoted the independent development of medicine within the country. Most treatment facilities were built in the precincts of temples or shrines, where various original treatments had been practised for mentally ill patients. Aside from moxibustion and herbal medicine, these treatments included cold-water ablutions under a waterfall, hot springs recuperation, locking up in a small box (to restrict movement of excited patients), sleep therapy using alcohol and persuasion therapy (Okada, 2002). It can be pointed out that these treatments were relatively gentle and humane, when compared with those practised in Western countries in these times, such as trephining and phlebotomy (Foerschner, 2010).

Before the early nineteenth century, a prototype psychiatric confinement system had been established. Under the system, individuals with psychiatric disorders were kept in confinement houses in temple premises or placed under house arrest (Okada, 2002; Hashimoto, 2011). However, a doctor's certificate was required for confinement to avoid illegal abuse. It is of note that there was no systemic persecution and violence against patients with mental problems in Japan up to the mid nineteenth century. In addition, in the law of that time, such individuals received reduced sentences for any crime; instead, allied responsibilities were imposed on their family members as supervisors in a form of collective punishment. The principle of 'allied responsibilities of family' is grounded in the Japanese societal system, in which the household head represents authority and responsibility for all family members. This tradition still remains in Japan, influencing Japanese ways of living and thinking as well as the judicial system.

In the modern era

In the mid nineteenth century, the feudal system that had been run by the Samurai hierarchy ended and Japan opened the door to outside cultures. After 250 years of national seclusion, the restrictions on trade and cultural exchange were totally dismantled and various Western cultures began to rapidly percolate into Japan. Medicine also encountered such a cultural influx. Because of the strong impact of Western medical practices, Japanese traditional medicine fell into decline. Japan introduced German systems of medicine, and 'modernised' medicine prevailed across the nation. After 1874, psychiatric wards had begun to be accommodated in military hospitals around Japan. In 1875, the first public psychiatric hospital was founded in the precincts of the 'Nanzen-ji' temple in Kyoto. Following this, new psychiatric hospitals were opened one after the another (e.g. Kato Fu-ten Hospital in 1878, the first private psychiatric hospital in Japan, and Tokyo Tenkyoin in 1879, the predecessor of Tokyo Metropolitan Matsuzawa Hospital). The first department of psychiatry was established in the University of Tokyo, School of Medicine, in 1886. The total number of psychiatric facilities rose to 24 with over 2,000 beds (0.45 beds per 10,000 population) in 1901 and to 137 with over 20,000 beds (2.9 beds per 10,000 population) in 1935 (Okada, 2002).

The development of the legal systems related to persons with mental disorders was deeply affected by the Japanese family system described above. The first act in relation to mental health was issued in 1872, in which a statement that unaccompanied mentally ill persons should be restrained by the police was incorporated (Okada, 2002). Subsequently, in 1874, the police officially stated that mentally ill persons should always be looked after by supervisors, appointed from their families, and who should be committed to take *all* responsibilities for their behavioural problems (Okada, 2002). Furthermore, the Japanese criminal code in 1882 imposed fines of between fifty sen and one yen fifty sen (approximately US$100 and US$300 in today's currency) on those families who failed to comply with their legal obligation to monitor family members with mental problems and let them wander on the streets (Suzuki 2011). Therefore, to circumvent punishment under the criminal law, persons with mental illness were placed under house arrest, or even jailed if they had no family members or relatives, and no one could take familial responsibility. This fundamental principle, i.e. the responsibility of the family for care provision and management of individuals with psychiatric problems, constituted a cornerstone of later mental health policy and is still in operation.

In 1900, the government of Japan established the Mental Patients' Custody Act, which was the first national legislation for regulating the confinement of mentally ill persons. This act was intended to uphold social order and security as well as to prevent misuse of confinement and custody for the mentally handicapped. In order to restrict patients in an institution or under house arrest, their families were required to designate one of them to serve as a 'custodian', who took all responsibility for care and confinement of the patient and medical expenses, and for filing an application for confinement with the government office via the police. When an appropriate custodian could not be found, the mayor of the municipality where the patient lived would take over the duties of custodian (Okada, 2002; Suzuki, 2011). Under the act, the place of confinement had to meet 'proper' facility criteria for safe custody of the patient and be licensed by the government. However, the definition of confinement and custody remained unclear. Furthermore, the numbers of psychiatrists and mental hospitals at the time were so limited that most of the confinement facilities were built in the custodian's house, i.e. their home. In reality, however, the act was administered to confine patients at home under the control of the police. Home custody was the second most common way of caring for mental patients in the first half of the twentieth century in Japan (Hashimoto, 2011). Indeed, the number of registered mental patients in 1940 was 81,356 (11.4 per 10,000 population), while the numbers of hospitalised patients and patients under home custody were 12,291 and 6,207, respectively (Okada, 2002).

As with the Western countries, there was no established treatment for mental illnesses at that time in Japan and most inpatients lived in a bubble without any special care or psychiatric examinations. In Japan, shock therapies (i.e. insulin shock therapy, cardiazol convulsive therapy and electroconvulsive therapy) were introduced and carried out in the 1930s and were reported to be effective. However, these methods were not popular treatments, since services using these approaches were not covered by insurance policies. In these circumstances, it is particularly worth noting that Dr Shoma Morita originated a purpose-centred, response-oriented therapy that was later called 'Morita therapy' in the 1930s. This unique therapy is still used in clinical settings and well acknowledged among Japanese psychiatrists as one of the most empirically effective *cognitive* behavioural therapies for anxiety disorders ('anxiety neurosis' in the old-fashioned terminology). Although cognitive behavioural therapy (CBT) may be now very popular all over the world, including Asian countries, and has become an established treatment for various types of mental problems, it may be surprising for readers in the West to note that one of the CBTs was initiated in the early twentieth century in the Far East. Morita therapy was influenced by the Zen principles of Buddhism. The basic concept is that neurotic symptoms are understood as the expression of the total process constituting the inner conflicts, or the sufferings arising from them, and the unsuccessful efforts of patients to stop rumination or worry, or deny or eliminate their conflicts, and that all of these processes are linked with anxiety. The specific approach (guidance) of Morita therapy is to instruct sufferers to accept the emotion of anxiety as it is, not to eagerly seek a cure, to conquer or suppress anxiety. Successful patients can leave behind their mindset that is fixated on their anxiety and start using their energy more effectively and realistically (Kondo, 1953; Morita *et al.*, 1998). However, despite such a seemingly effective therapeutic approach and a long history attached to it, no practitioners who have been involved with this technique have succeeded in in proving its effectiveness in a rigorous manner using scientific research methods (i.e. randomised controlled trials, RCTs). Consequently, Morita therapy has been less used and is becoming obsolete. This is regrettable.

Perspectives on psychiatry in Japan

Mental health policy

As mentioned above, the first national legislation covering the mentally ill in Japan was the Mental Patients' Custody Act, enacted in 1900, which legalised home custody (Ito and Sederer, 1999). Home custody was a common way to look after patients with mental illness until the end of World War II. The practice of home custody was ended after the enactment of the Mental Hygiene Act in 1950, which required medical treatment in hospitals for people with mental disorders. Then, the Law on Mental Health and Welfare of Persons with Mental Disorders (Mental Health and Welfare Law), was introduced in 1995; it acknowledged for the first time that mental illness is a disability and incorporated strict criteria for involuntary hospitalisation. It was hoped that this law would help reduce stigma, as it states that people with mental disorders should be treated equally to those with physical disabilities (Ito and Sederer, 1999).

Japan's Mental Health and Welfare Law established four legal conditions for admission to psychiatric hospital: (1) voluntary admission with the consent of the patient, (2) involuntary admission by order of the prefectural governor for a patient who is likely to hurt himself/herself or others because of mental disorder, (3) involuntary admission to protect patients from a medical perspective, and (4) emergency temporary admission by order of a certified psychiatrist. All involuntary admissions are reviewed in terms of patient rights by a Psychiatric Review Board composed of two or more certified psychiatrists, one or more lawyers, and one or more additional mental health or welfare professionals in each prefecture.

Despite the enactment of these laws on mental health and welfare, Japan had no specific legal regulations for offenders with mental disorders (Nakatani *et al.*, 2010). In response to the demand for a comprehensive forensic mental health system, Japan enacted the Act on Medical Care and Treatment for Persons Who Have Caused Serious Cases under the Condition of Insanity (the Medical Treatment and Supervision Act) in 2005. This Act provides a hybrid solution straddling the judicial and medical system, with a District Court, composed of a judge and a specially qualified psychiatrist, serving as a gatekeeper (Haraguchi *et al.*, 2011). The Act aims to improve conditions for the mentally ill, to prevent associated violent behaviours, and to promote the social rehabilitation of persons who have caused serious forensic cases to others while they were under the condition of insanity, through ensuring continuous and appropriate medical care as well as providing necessary treatment and instruction.

Mental health system and psychiatric epidemiology

Mental health care is naturally part of the whole health care system in Japan. The health care system in Japan is unique in several aspects. Although the system has gained a reputation as guaranteeing the nation's people equal chances of receiving good-quality medical care, a number of problems have emerged as Japan has been suffering from persistent recession. Annually increasing medical costs have become the nation's burden. The cost of personal medical care is covered in a universal health care insurance system. Health insurance is mandatory for residents of Japan. In general, individuals are required to assume responsibility for 30 per cent of the costs, while the government takes care of the remaining 70 per cent. With a few exceptions, the medical fee for every medical service is set by a government committee. This system of provision of the universal health care across the nation ('the system of the public health insurance for the whole nation') that was established in the 1960s is considered to be positive and maybe even admirable practice.

One of the negative aspects of the health care system in Japan is the fact that there are no general practitioners (GPs) in the nation. Any individual can access any doctor without referral, i.e. they can directly see even specialists at a university hospital at their own discretion. This has posed problems of a shortage of medical resources and a convergence of patients to specific medical facilities. The same holds true for mental health care services.

The Ministry of Health, Labour and Welfare in Japan has reported that the number of persons who visit medical facilities due to mental problems is on the increase. The number of patients was approximately 2.2 million in 1996, while it was 3.2 million in 2011. The social cost of mental disorders in Japan in 2008 was estimated to be over US$110 billion. In parallel with the increase in the number of patients with mental disorders, the number of psychiatric clinics (private mental clinics) in Japan appears to have increased; 3,198 psychiatric clinics were in operation in 1996, but the number rose to 5,629 in 2008.

Japan is encountering several issues regarding care for inpatients in psychiatric hospitals. It has been highlighted that, in comparison with the trend in the West, the number of psychiatric beds in Japan is remarkably large. The introduction of the Mental Hygiene Act in 1950 led to a four-decade-long increase in the total number of psychiatric beds. A socially influential incident also contributed to the argument for necessity of mental care in hospital. In 1964, US Ambassador Edwin Reischauer was stabbed by a young Japanese boy with a diagnosis of schizophrenia. Such events, albeit unusual and infrequent occurrences, associated with the social stigma that persons with mental illness are dangerous gave momentum towards the increase in psychiatric beds. Consequently, the number of psychiatric beds, which was 10.1 per 10,000 population in 1960, reached 24.9 per 10,000 population in 1975, and peaked at 29.0 per 10,000 population in 1990 (Tsuchiya and Takei, 2004). The total number of psychiatric beds in Japan was 342,194 in 2012 for a total population of approximately 128 million, resulting in 26.7 per 10,000 population. Although the number of psychiatric beds in Japan is in decline, the number of psychiatric beds per 10,000 population in Japan is conspicuously high compared with the figure in any other G7 countries, for example the USA (3.4 per 10,000) and the UK (5.0 per 10,000) (www.who.int/gho/publications/world_health_statistics/2013/).

Another problem with the mental care system in Japan is the long-term hospitalisation of the mentally ill population. According to the Ministry of Health, Labour and Welfare in Japan, a breakdown of all inpatients in psychiatric hospitals (n = 304,394) by length of stay as of the year of 2011 is as follows: the number of patients with a period of admission of 1–5, 5–10, 10–20 and over 20 years are, respectively, 87,976 (28.9 per cent), 42,489 (14.0 per cent), 34,549 (11.4 per cent) and 34,799 (11.4 per cent). As a result, nearly 40 per cent of patients (37 per cent with a period of admission longer than five years) are viewed as the long-stay. It is no surprise that 48 per cent of the inpatients were elderly (over 65 years old). One of the reasons why the number of inpatients has grown in Japan is certainly problems on patients' and their families' side; elderly individuals with mental disorder, mainly schizophrenia, have difficulties in living in the local community due to a lack of daily skills and/or social support, and families may feel it is easier to rely on hospitals for provision of care. The bureaucracy may also be blamed for lack of leadership, since the Ministry of Health, Labour and Welfare, as a policy-maker, is in a powerful position to modify the system of mental health care. The Ministry, at last, started a 'discharge facilitation programme for individuals with mental illness' in 2004. Although the number of inpatients with mental disorder who can be discharged from hospital was estimated, by the government, to be approximately 70,000, this may be an understatement. This figure corresponds to a fraction of the total numbers of the inpatient population in Japan.

In modern medicine, patients have a right to purse quality of life (QOL) while they tend to have difficulties in enjoying life because of the handicap caused by having an illness. QOL is a major issue for individuals with mental disorders as well (Lehman, 1983). In these circumstances, at international level, the quality of care especially in psychiatric hospitals in Japan may face criticism as it ranks low compared with the care provided in general hospitals. This is because the minimum requirements for staff (i.e. the number of physicians) in psychiatric hospitals are set to lower than those for general hospitals by the Medical Law. The Law permits a lower minimum number of psychiatrists for hospitals with psychiatric beds (48 beds per psychiatrist) than in general hospitals (16 beds per physician).

Psychiatric training and practice

Maintaining the quality of medicine is naturally linked with the system of educational training. The medical/psychiatric training system in Japan has been delineated in an article by Tsuchiya and Takei (2004). Briefly, for medical students, a minimum six-year period of education and training at medical school is required. Postgraduate medical students are then qualified to take the National Examination for Physicians (NEP). Those who pass the NEP are eligible to take a two-year postgraduate training course offered by teaching hospitals. After the training course, any physician can claim that he or she is a psychiatrist. From a practical and an ethical point of view, the Mental Health and Welfare Law authorises some psychiatrists ('designated psychiatrists') to conduct psychiatric assessments in relation to legal procedures such as involuntary admission and restrictions on patients' freedom. To obtain such a designation, a psychiatrist must have at least five years of clinical experience, including at least three years of training in psychiatry (at psychiatric hospitals, or sections of psychiatry in general hospitals or university hospitals). In addition, he or she must attend a three-day course run by experienced psychiatrists that covers legal, ethical, clinical and forensic issues. Then, applicants are required to submit eight case reports to the Ministry of Health, Labour and Welfare. Qualification is judged merely on the quality of the report.

There has, thus far, been no other systematic training for psychiatrists available across the nation. However, there is a welcome movement, in Japan, that paves the way for developing specialists who can contribute to enhancement of the quality of mental health care provision; that is, a training programme for cognitive behavioural therapy (CBT). On the other hand, the

Japanese Society of Psychiatry and Neurology, the largest association of psychiatrists in Japan, has lately started to authorise psychiatrists who succeed in passing an examination to designate themselves as a psychiatry specialist. In addition, given awareness of the necessity for well-prepared and systematised training programmes that are applied across the nation in an identical fashion to provide highly qualified psychiatrists (i.e. specialists) (Takei 1995), the Japanese Society of Psychiatry and Neurology has set up educational programmes in which physicians can learn and achieve international standards of psychiatry. However, the impacts of such non-governmental authorisation (e.g. whether psychiatry specialists would have better clinical practices, leading to better outcomes and higher satisfaction in patients and families, than non-specialists) have not been evaluated or reported. Similar issues have been raised regarding designation by the non-governmental associations in the field of paediatrics and forensic psychiatry.

Psychopharmacological treatments in Japan do not differ from those practised in Western countries; patients can receive newly developed medications, although there may be a drug lag (i.e. a delay in the approval of new drugs). Although Morita therapy, which can be classified as one of the CBTs as described above, is still in use in practice, CBT is, in general, not yet widely available. Because of the problems arising from ill-integrated health care systems in Japan as discussed above (e.g. no catchment area system for health care provision) and lack of strong regulation by the government, individuals who seek psychiatric care receive restricted services. A relevant and visible example of this is the following fact: the average amount of time a psychiatrist spends with a patient is about 5–10 minutes.

Social/explanatory models of mental illness

Traditionally, progress in psychiatry in Japan had been strongly influenced by practices in Germany and France. Thus, some psychiatrists' views are influenced by German and/or French traditional *psychopathology*. In addition, psychoanalytic/psychodynamic perspectives still prevail in the general population, including some psychiatrists and psychologists. Such a trend or fashion has been attributable to directions and dogmata advocated by a few leading professionals in the field. However, many psychiatrists, especially those who began practice after the late 1980s, have become accustomed to and use standard nomenclatures and classification systems, such as ICD and DSM. Furthermore, new understanding and knowledge derived from recent progress in biological psychiatry research have been introduced to not only clinical psychiatrists but also the general population via the mass media. Although there are still discrepancies and misunderstandings between a 'science-based' discipline and other perspectives or views, the former should soon establish itself in the field of psychiatry.

Topics of interest specific to Japan

On 11 March 2011, 9.0 magnitude earthquakes occurred in the east part of Japan. The earthquake and subsequent tsunami killed over 15,000 people. In addition to the earthquake and tsunami, because of the radiation leaks caused by the Fukushima nuclear power plant accidents, about 347,000 people had to be evacuated. The evacuees are considered to be at risk of mental disorders, including post-traumatic stress disorder, depression and anxiety disorder. Although many sufferers, including vulnerable children, are assumed to exist, nation-led prospective studies have not been initiated (Takei, 2011; Sugihara and Suda, 2011). Natural disasters are not rare and a large-scale flood or hurricane disaster may happen in any country at any time. The nation has lost an opportunity to contribute to world research outputs, especially a detailed probe into the psychological aftermath and process of recovering from disasters in a defined population. Reliable data on mental breakdown or exacerbation of pre-existing psychiatric problems among the victims are not available in relation to the 11 March disasters. Nevertheless, many mental health professionals have participated as volunteers in the disaster areas, as national guidelines for post-disaster mental health were issued in 2001 by the National Centre of Neurology and Psychiatry, which was based on valuable lessons about post-disaster mental health from two previous major disasters at Kobe in 1995 and Niigata in 2006 (Kim and Akiyama, 2011). As of 2014, three years after the disaster, people in the disaster areas are still facing hardship even in living a normal life, with the majority of the victims residing in temporary housing. Two of the authors (SS, GS) themselves have participated in volunteer work; a wide range of disaster-related mental health problems were evident among the evacuees, which included depression, post-traumatic stress disorder, alcohol misuse, insomnia and worsening of pre-existing psychiatric illness; and psychological problems, such as irritability, hypersensitivity, hyperactivity (especially in children at school), and 'burnout' among support staff and officials. To clarify and quantify the psychological problems and to provide optimal care for the victims, special attention continues to be paid to this population. This is the nation's duty, and reporting on how they progress in terms of health is the duty of professionals who are involved in assisting the victims at risk.

References

Foerschner, A. (2010) 'The history of mental illness: From "skull drills" to "happy pills"', *Student Pulse*, 9, 1–4.

Haraguchi, T., Fujisaki, M., Shiina, A., Igarashi, Y., Okamura, N., Fukami, G., Shiraishi, T., Nakazato, M. and Iyo, M. (2011) 'Attitudes of Japanese psychiatrists toward forensic mental health as revealed by a national survey', *Psychiatry and Clinical Neuroscience*, 65(2), 150–7.

Hashimoto, A. (2011) *Seishinbyousya to Shitaku-kanchi*. Tokyo: Rikka Shuppan.

Ito, H. and Sederer, L. I. (1999) 'Mental health services reform in Japan', *Harvard Review of Psychiatry*, 7(4), 208–15.

Kim, Y. and Akiyama, T. (2011) 'Post-disaster mental health care in Japan', *The Lancet*, 378(9788), 317–18.

Kondo, A. (1953) 'Morita therapy: A Japanese therapy for neurosis', *The American Journal of Psychoanalysis*, 13, 31–7.

Lehman, A. F. (1983) 'The well-being of chronic mental patients', *Archives of General Psychiatry*, 40(4), 369–73.

Morita, S., Kondo, A. and LeVine, P. (1998) *Morita Therapy and the True Nature of Anxiety-Based Disorders (Shinkeishitsu)*. Albany: State University of New York Press.

Nakatani, Y., Kojimoto, M., Matsubara, S. and Takayanagi, I. (2010) 'New legislation for offenders with mental disorders in Japan', *International Journal of Law and Psychiatry*, 33(1), 7–12.

Okada, Y. (2002) *Nihon Seishinka Iryoushi*. Tokyo: Igakusyoin.

Sugihara, G. and Suda, S. (2011) 'Need for close watch on children's health after Fukushima disaster', *The Lancet*, 378(9790), 485–6.

Suzuki, A. (2011) 'The state, family, and the insane in Japan, 1900–45' in Porter, R. and Wright, D., (eds.), *The Confinement of the Insane: International Perspectives, 1800–1965*. Cambridge, UK: Cambridge University Press, pp. 193–225.

Takei, N. (1995) 'Postgraduate psychiatric training in Japan', *The Lancet*, 345(8954), 926.

Takei, N. (2011) '*hisaiji no kenkou kanri daikibo na tuisekitchousa hitsuyou*' (Health management for children who encountered the disasters: need of large scale national prospective studies). Watashi no_shiten_(My view), *Asahi Newspaper* (August 5 issue).

Tsuchiya, K. J. and Takei, N. (2004) 'Focus on psychiatry in Japan', *British Journal of Psychiatry*, 184, 88–92.

16

South Korea

Min-Soo Lee, Yong Chon Park and
Seon-Cheol Park

Introduction

South Korea is a country in the southern portion of the Korean Peninsula in East Asia and its official name is the Republic of Korea. It has a border with North Korea (the Democratic People's Republic of Korea) to the north and borders across the seas with China to the west and Japan to the east. The history of Korea is about 5,000 years old. Several dynasties governed the Korean Peninsula, and the government of the Republic of Korea was established after the elections limited to South Korea in 1948. The Korean War began in 1950 when the armed forces of North Korea attacked South Korea and the war lasted for three years. The division of South and North Korea has continued since then. Rapid and vigorous social, economic, and political changes during the past several decades have occurred in South Korea. The South Korean agrarian society of the 1960s and 1970s was converted into an industrial society in the 1980s, and into an information society in the 1990s. The total population of South Korea stands at about 51 million as of July 2011.

Brief history of modern psychiatry in South Korea

Since an old history book of Korea described how one man's anxiety was cured by bitter but good advice in 630 AD (Han, 1967), the Korean traditional culture could have an abundant background in psychiatric care or treatment. However, the history of modern psychiatry in Korea has been quite short (Chang and Kim, 1973). Its impact was not significant in Korea in the eighteenth century, although Galen's neuroanatomical and neurophysiological theory, which had been introduced and quoted by a scholar of *Silhak* (the Realist School of Confucianism), could make the scholars of the Conservative School of Confucianism question the mind–body theory of Korean folk medicine (Lee and Rhi, 1999; Rhi, 1999). The dawn of modern psychiatry in Korea began in the late nineteenth century (Lee, 2004). There are several milestones in the introduction of modern Western psychiatry into Korea. In 1886, Jaejungwon (the first Western medical institution in Korea) first published an annual report of clinical practice patterns for diseases of the nervous system including diagnoses of chorea, delirium tremens, hysteria, globus hystericus, idiocy, insanity, mania, dementia, melancholy, and insomnia

(Park and Yeo, 1999). In around 1910, the first lecture on "mental diseases" in Korea was given at Daehan Hospital, which was a modern hospital founded by the order of the emperor of the Korean Empire in 1907 (Chung *et al.*, 2006). In 1913, the first psychiatric ward and department of psychiatry in a modern hospital of Korea were established during the forced Japanese annexation of Korea (Rhi, 1994). In 1913, Dr Charles Inglis McLaren (1882–1957), a medical missionary from the Australian Presbyterian Church, started giving lectures about psychiatry and neurology at Severance Union Medical School, and, until 1938, he continued to deliver lectures about psychiatry and neurology and treating psychiatric and neurological patients (Yeo, 2008; Min, 2011). Meanwhile, mentally ill patients were regarded as violent, dangerous, and eugenically inferior beings by Koreans who were influenced by newspapers and educated by regulatory authorities under the Japanese rule. However, the Korean people, who had had superstitious beliefs about the mentally ill, began to accept the relatively modern approach to treating patients (Lee, 2013). In other words, modern Western psychiatry was introduced into Korea by Japanese psychiatrists who had accepted German psychiatry and moved to Korea during the forced Japanese annexation of Korea, and also by Western Christian missionaries who had a humanitarian approach (Rhi, 1999).

In September 1945, the Korean Neuropsychiatric Association (under the name of the Chosun Neuropsychiatric Association) was first founded among a number of academic meetings of clinical specialties in Korea, and it was composed of about 20 members limited to the internists and psychiatrists of the time. In 1950, the outbreak of the Korean War resulted not only in devastating consequences but also offered an opportunity to advance psychiatry in South Korea. Many young psychiatrists, who were recruited to become military medical officers, visited military hospitals in the United States during the war. The first returning group of Korean civilian psychiatrists, who had gone to the United States for residency training and further study after their military service, became the forerunners of contemporary Korean psychiatry (Lee, 2004). Hence, education and training in psychiatry in South Korea was changed from the German-psychiatry-based system to an American-psychiatry-based system (Rhi, 1999). In 1953, the first psychoanalytic psychotherapy in South Korea was conducted by Dr Rhee Dong-Shick (1920–) for a patient with a psychogenic headache (Huh, 2009). In 1955, antipsychotics including reserpin and chlorpromazine were introduced into psychiatric practice in South Korea (Kim and Rhi, 1996).

Psychiatry in South Korea has progressed via Westernization and modernization to catch up with and assimilate the psychiatry of the developed countries. Due to the influence of psychoanalytic psychiatry taught in the United States at the end of World War II, the first-generation psychiatrists in South Korea principally studied psychodynamic psychiatry (Lee, 2004). In the 1970s, psychotherapy and cultural psychiatry in South Korea contributed to establishing related academic meetings including the Korean Academy of Psychotherapists (1974), the Korean Society for Analytical Psychology (1978), and the Korean Association of Psychoanalysis (1980). In the 1980s, progress in biological psychiatry was initiated in South Korea, under the influence of biology-based research in psychiatry in the United States (Lee, 2004; Rhi, 1999). In the 1990s, biological psychiatry grew with the evolution of basic science including molecular biology, genetics, electrophysiology, and neuroimaging, and the introduction of various diagnostic and treatment skills into South Korea. Hence, neuroimaging, genetic, and other biological disciplines in psychiatry have been actively investigated.

Bridging the gap between developed countries and South Korea in the research fields of biological psychiatry contributed to attaining a world-class level of biological research in South Korea (Chung and Lee, 2008). Moreover, because of the consistent increase in the number of psychiatric hospitals and clinics, 84 university-affiliated and training hospitals, 253 general hospitals, 129 mental hospitals, 861 private psychiatric clinics, and 1,327 psychiatric clinics and hospitals had been established by 2011 (Park *et al.*, 2013).

Culture, society, and psychiatry in South Korea

The relationship between cultural context and psychiatry should be discussed in the diagnosis of psychiatric disorders. The mode of symptom presentation of psychiatric disorders is often influenced by cultural contexts (Kleinman *et al.*, 1978). Hence, culture-related specific disorders and the epidemiology of mental disorders in South Korea need to be discussed because they are mainly shaped by the pathogenetic or psychoplastic effects of sociocultural influences (Tseng, 2007). First, a culture-bound syndrome manifests as an esoteric clinical presentation limited to cultures in traditional society (Bhugra *et al.*, 2007). *Hwabyung* (火病 in Chinese characters) and *shinbyung* (神病), which are included in the culture-bound syndromes of the *Diagnostic and Statistical Manual*, Fourth Edition (DSM-IV) (American Psychiatric Association, 1994), is well-known as a culture-bound syndrome in South Korea. *Hwabyung* has a literal meaning of anger disorder or fire disorder. While *hwabyung* had not been listed as a single disease entity in any medical literature of Korea and other Sinosphere countries, it had been used as a popular name indicating a disease caused by *hwa* (火, anger or emotional disturbance) by Korean people. To identify its distinctive symptomatology or presentation, *hwabyung* had been regarded as a unique emotional illness in Korea. The sufferers of *hwabyung* were predominantly Korean middle-aged women, suffering repressed or suppressed anger of long duration, and typical manifestations included insomnia, dysphoria, indigestion, anorexia, dyspepsia, palpitations, generalized aches and pains, and a feeling of a mass in the epigastrium (Lin, 1983; Min, 2008a; Min *et al.*, 2009).

When studying *hwabyung*, there are two perspectives. One view is that *hwabyung* is not a disease entity, but an anger-related comprehensive process which results in emotional discomfort, multiple somatic complaints, and death (Lee, 1978). Meanwhile, *hwabyung* has also been suggested to be a distinctive disease entity differentiated from depressive disorder, generalized anxiety disorder, and somatic symptom disorder (Lee, J. *et al.*, 2012). The Korean culture-specific pathogenesis of *hwabyung* has been speculated to be as follows (Chung and Cho, 2006): *Jeong* (情) is an emotional and psychological bond which is considered a distinct and unique phenomenon of the collective nature of Korean society. *Haan* (恨) is another Korean culturally unique phenomenon, and an intense repressed or suppressed anger which results from broken *jeong*. Finally, *haan* can incur *hwabyung* with multiple and complex emotional and somatic symptoms.

In addition there is *shinbyung*, which literally means divine disorder. *Shinbyung* is one of the possession syndromes evolved in an attempt to project traumatic suffering on the shamanistic world. *Shinbyung* has been suggested as a Korean culture-related syndrome because its pathogenesis is related to Korean shamanism, and its symptomatology and clinical progress do not correspond to dissociative disorder under Western psychiatric nosology and taxonomy (Kim, 1972; Yongmi, 2000). However, because of the impacts of globalization, urbanization, and industrialization, the geographical localization of culture-bound syndromes has increasingly slid into oblivion, and abandonment of the definition has been suggested (Bhugra *et al.*, 2007). *Shinbyung* and other possession syndromes are present across the world beyond Korea and Siberia. In addition, *hwabyung* and *shinbyung* were excluded from the culture-bound syndromes of the DSM-5 (American Psychiatric Association, 2013). *Hwabyung* and *shinbyung,* as cultural-bound syndromes, commonly have diagnostic vagueness and arbitrariness. However, the terms indicate characteristic symptom presentations of psychiatric patients and help psychiatrists to communicate the patients' distress and life history more deeply and immediately in South Korea, because they are popular words representing their own cause and symptomatology among Korean people (Kim, K., 1994; Suh, 2013).

Second, delusional and hallucinatory contents, which are sensitively influenced by cultural or political underpinnings in South Korea, can partly present the cultural characteristics and etiologies of symptomatological contexts. A series of transcultural studies on the psychopathology of patients with schizophrenia demonstrated that Korean patients with schizophrenia tend to present with delusions regarding love/sex, dysmorphobia, and religious or supernatural matters as compared with Korean–Chinese, Chinese, and Taiwanese patients with schizophrenia (Kim et al., 1993; Kim et al., 2001a; Kim et al., 2001b; Kim, 2006). Moreover, in the 1990s and 2000s a study on the chronological changes in delusional themes of Korean patients with schizophrenia revealed that a significant increase in rejection as a persecutory behavior was not observed in men but was in women (Oh et al., 2012). These findings suggest that a rapid and vigorous process of acculturation in South Korea is reflected by the social and cultural shaping of schizophrenic symptomatology.

Third, a specific clinical group, related to social and historical contexts in South Korea, also needs to be discussed. North Korean defectors in South Korea are special clinical patients who have been generated by the division of South and North Korea for the last 60 years. The communication block and cultural and socio-political differences between South and North Korea have resulted in and exacerbated adaptation problems of North Korean defectors in South Korean society. North Korean defectors are often diagnosed with depression and post-traumatic stress disorder, and are encumbered with comprehensive adaptation problems of a broken family, conflict in the family due to role conversion, attitudes of the mass media to refugees, problems of education for living, and difficulties in establishing a support system. Thus, South Korean psychiatrists need to understand the characteristics of North Korean defectors and develop adequate interview skills and treatment plans (Jeon, 1997; Lee, Y.H. et al., 2012; Min, 2008b). In addition, all the survivors of the Korean forced comfort women (sexual slaves) of the Japanese army during World War II have suffered from lifetime post-traumatic stress disorder (Min et al., 2004).

Furthermore, the cultural influences on psychiatry in South Korea can be present in the treatment modes for psychiatric disorders. Despite the introduction of Western psychiatry into South Korea, the practitioners of traditional medicine, shamanistic rituals, faith healing, and other folk remedies have been asked to help psychiatric patients (Kim, 1999; Kim, 2005). In other words, shamanism, Buddhism, and folk medicine has been regarded as a cultural mechanism that could have preventive and curative effects on psychic conflicts or distresses in traditional Korean society (Chang and Kim, 1973). The illness behavior patterns of Koreans with psychiatric disorders, which are influenced by the ancestral curative mechanism of traditional Korean society, are characterized by the following features: (a) multiple help-seeking behaviors, (b) non-compliance with modern psychiatry, (c) preference for medical facilities that treat physical disease rather than psychiatric disorders, (d) preference for magico-religious therapies, (e) preference for dietary supplements, and (f) preference for advice from non-professional lay persons. Because of the crucial hindrance of these illness behavior patterns on psychiatric practice, culture-relevant psychiatric approaches are needed in South Korea. Hence, the cultural background of patients should be considered in a therapeutic process that transcends the cultural hindrances in South Korea (Kim, 1998; Rhi et al., 1995). A humanistic approach based on the personality of the psychiatrist (Park and Kim, 1998), application of some folk medicine treatment methods including herbal medications (Song, 1998), and comprehension of archaic languages of shamanic culture and translation into medical concepts of modern psychiatry (Rhi, 1998) are considered culture-relevant psychiatric approaches.

The influences of cultural factors on psychotherapeutic practice have concerned many psychiatric scholars. In particular, *Tao psychotherapy* has been presented as a solution to the issue as founded by Dr Rhee Dong-Shick in South Korea, and defined by the converged form of the Eastern *Tao* (道) and the essence of Western psychotherapy (Kang, 2006). *Tao* has been presented as the ideal human nature of Korea, and aims at strengthening the ego, which is insightful of its own inner and outer worlds, and to be free of ego from emotional or psychic conflicts. Hence, *Tao* corresponds to the archetype of Western psychotherapy, including existential psychotherapy and dasein analysis (Cho, 2008; Craig, 2008). *Tao* is regarded as the ultimate in humanism by Dr Rhee, and *Tao psychotherapy* is metaphorically defined by the following description (Rhee, 2008): "The therapist with his personality brings spring to the patient who is shivering in a frozen land." *Tao psychotherapy* has significance in that theoretical backgrounds of psychotherapy for Koreans have been extracted from the Korean traditional culture. However, *Tao psychotherapy* does not correspond to the culture-specific psycho-therapeutic methods like the Morita and Naukan therapies of Japanese psychiatry (Kim, K., 1994).

Mental health system in South Korea

The mental health system in South Korea has progressed tremendously within the past few decades, despite its institutional and practical limitations (Lee, 1999). Due to rapid and progressive industrialization and urbanization of an agrarian-centered society in South Korea in the 1970s and 1980s, patients with severe mental illness were separated from the family and community and many of them were institutionalized in religious establishments and affiliated unauthorized facilities. As a result, the institutionalized patients were placed in non-therapeutic and inhuman situations (Ryu, 1982). Given this situation, the Korean Neuropsychiatric Association suggested definite proposals for the Korean Mental Health Act of 1988 (Kim, E., 1994). The Ministry of Health and Social Affairs collected the opinions of the Korean Neuropsychiatric Association and other organizations and submitted the 1992 government draft proposals to the National Assembly. In 1995, the first version of the Korean Mental Health Act was passed by parliament. The first version of the Korean Mental Health Act was formed with the underpinnings of an industrial society model from the cautious viewpoint that mentally ill people had been recognized as dangerous and refractory. Moreover, the shift from traditional hospitalization-oriented services to community-based rehabilitation-oriented services was emphasized. Specifically, procedures for involuntary admission of mentally ill patients were introduced, and strict criteria for mental health professionals and facilities were defined. In other words, the mental health policies of the Korean government intended to suppress hospitalization of the mentally ill for a lengthy period and were directed toward community mental health. Although community-based rehabilitation programs were developed in 1995, and the WHO collaborating center for psychiatric rehabilitation and community mental health in 2003 by Yong-In Mental Hospital (Lee, 2004), the support plans for public community mental health services were poor. Thus, the community mental health directed ideas of the first version of the Korean Mental Health Act were limited to a declarative level at the time (Suh, 2010).

Since the enactment of the Mental Health Act in 1995, medical treatment for severe mental illness including schizophrenia in South Korea has been mainly conducted using inpatient-oriented treatment, long periods of hospitalization, and poor psychosocial treatment, as compared with the United States and European countries (Chang *et al.*, 2008). Furthermore, as of 2005, only 138 social rehabilitation centers and 28 alcohol rehabilitation centers had been established in South Korea, compared to 1,048 psychiatric medical facilities. The future tasks in developing a mental health system in South Korea are that community-based rehabilitation services should be promoted and absorb the unnecessarily institutionalized chronic psychiatric patients (Kahng and Kim, 2010). In addition, community-based services should be comprehensively grown and strengthened in the realms of mental health promotion, prevention of mental illness, psychiatric rehabilitation, case management, residential facilities, and crisis intervention (Suh, 1999). Hence, as of 2013, the Korean Mental Health Act has been revised several times and is supposed to be renamed the Korean Mental Health Promotion Act, with the intention of decreasing the socioeconomic costs of chronic mentally ill people through early detection and treatment of psychiatric patients and to strengthen the human rights of individuals in South Korea.

Psychiatric epidemiology in South Korea

There have been two nationwide epidemiological studies in South Korea. In 1984, a psychiatric epidemiological study was carried out using the DSM-III (American Psychiatric Association, 1980) and Diagnostic Interview Schedule III (Robins *et al.*, 1981). The findings were characterized by a higher prevalence of alcohol abuse among men in Seoul compared with that in the United States. In addition, the prevalence of psychiatric disorders tended to increase with increasing age. Overall, the findings were characterized by a lower rate of psychiatric illness including schizophrenia, mood disorders, and alcohol use disorder in South Korea compared with that in the United States and could have been influenced by the cultural factors of the Korean agrarian society at the time (Lee *et al.*, 1990a; Lee *et al.*, 1990b). In 2001, the Korean Epidemiological Catchment Area (KECA) study was carried out using the DSM-IV (American Psychiatric Association, 1994) and the Composite International Diagnostic Interview (World Health Organization, 1990). That study was aimed at revealing the changes in epidemiological

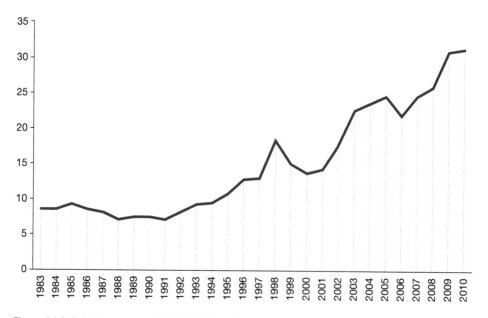

Figure 16.1 Suicide rates per 100,000 in South Korea, from 1983 to 2010

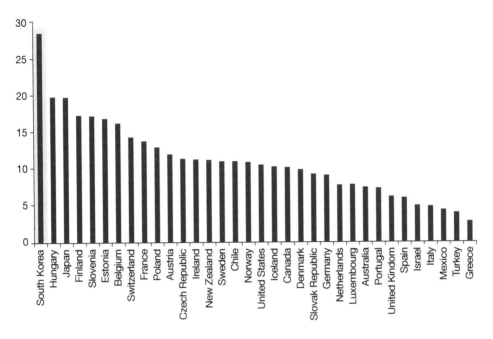

Figure 16.2 Suicide rates in South Korea and other OECD countries

findings from Westernization and industrialization in South Korea. Compared with the findings of Lee *et al.*'s study (1990a), the lifetime prevalence of alcohol use disorder decreased and the prevalence of other psychiatric disorders did not change. The prevalence of psychiatric disorders in South Korea was higher than in other East-Asian countries and most European countries, but lower than in the United States (Cho *et al.*, 2007). In 2006, the Korean Epidemiological Catchment Area Study Replication showed that the lifetime prevalence of substance use disorder had decreased markedly and that the prevalence of psychiatric disorders had decreased slightly compared to the findings of previous studies (Lee *et al.*, 1990a; Cho *et al.*, 2007; Cho *et al.*, 2010). The three epidemiological studies all demonstrated that alcohol use disorder was highly prevalent in South Korea.

Notably, completed suicides have been increasing rapidly and vigorously in South Korea since the early 1990s as shown in Figure 16.1. A total of 15,566 South Koreans committed suicide in 2010. The suicide rate of 2010 per 100,000 was 31.2 and increased 130.2 percent from that of 2000. In addition, suicide was the most common cause of death for South Koreans aged 10–40 years old. Moreover, the suicide mortality rate in South Korea was high compared with those in other OECD countries, as shown in Figure 16.2, and its rate of increase is the highest (Hong *et al.*, 2006; Jeon, 2011; Jeon, 2012). In addition, the rate of suicide attempts in South Korea was 3.2 percent and it is much higher than in China (1.0 percent), Japan (1.9 percent) and 17 other countries including Africa, the Americas, Europe, and Asian countries (2.7 percent; Lee *et al.*, 2009; Nock *et al.*, 2008; Ono *et al.*, 2008). Because of these rapid increases in suicide deaths, depression has become a fundamental public health issue in South Korea (Park and Park, 2012). The lifetime prevalence of major depressive disorder was 6.7 percent (4.8 percent in men and 9.1 percent in women), and has increased by 0.2 percent annually for the last decade (Jeon, 2012). The economic cost of depression in Korea was estimated to be US$4,049 million, which included US$152.6 million for direct healthcare costs, US$3,880.5 million for indirect costs and US$2,958.9 million for morbidity costs (Chang *et al.*, 2012). Despite the impacts of depression on the mental health of the Korean population, most research in this realm has been limited to biological psychiatry. The Clinical Research Center for Depression (CRESCEND) study, as the first large, prospective, observational and clinical study of a nationwide sample of Korean depressed patients, has provided epidemiological data using psychometric scales to measure a number of clinical variables and reported diverse epidemiological findings for clinical features and progress of Koreans with depressive disorders (Kim *et al.*, 2011).

A rapid increase in the elderly population in South Korea is one of most important issues in psychiatric epidemiology. Since the number and proportion of the elderly population in South Korea have increased very dramatically, the doubling times of the elderly population are just about two decades (11.0 percent increase in 2010). By 2040, the proportion of the elderly population is expected to be one-third of the national population in South Korea. According to the cumulative findings of psychiatric epidemiological surveys, about 10 percent of the elderly population suffers dementia. In addition, ranges in the prevalence of clinically significant depressive symptoms, alcohol use disorder, and sleep difficulties were 9.1–33.0 percent, 13.6 percent, and 22–58 percent, respectively. Thus, the socioeconomic burden from the elderly population expected in the near future should be attended to and mitigated via the establishment of a preventive policy for elderly psychiatric disorders (Cho *et al.*, 2011).

Special issues for psychiatry in South Korea

The social stigma, prejudice, and discrimination against patients with psychiatric disorders may be the most difficult problem faced in the clinical practice of psychiatrists in South Korea. To overcome the current problems and to strengthen the preventive approach, reforms were carried out in the clinical psychiatry of South Korea. First, in 2010, the Korean term for the department of psychiatry was changed to a new name representing the medicine of mental health promotion and wellbeing (精神建康醫學科). The aims of changing the Korean term for the department of psychiatry were to: (a) alleviate the metaphorically negative image of the Korean term for spirit or mind (*jungshin*, 精神), (b) expand the areas for therapeutic intervention from symptomatic treatment to mental health promotion, and (c) establish psychiatry's reputation for medical expertise in South Korea (Ahn, 2011; Park, 2012). Second, in 2011, the Korean name for schizophrenia was also changed from *jungshinbunyeolbyung* (精神分裂病) to *johyeonbyung* (調絃病). *Jungshinbunyeolbyung* has a literal meaning of mind-splitting disorder and is a Korean pronunciation of *seishin-bunretsu-byo*, which has been approved as the Japanese translation for schizophrenia (Sugihara and Takei, 2013). The literal meaning of *johyeon* is to tune a string instrument, which is derived from a passage in a Buddhist text from sixteenth-century Korea: "Studying is similar to tuning the strings of a Korean string instrument in which tightness and looseness should be befitting." Hence, *johyeonbyung* literally means attunement disorder and metaphorically presents as a neuroimaging-study-suggested theory that schizophrenia can be a disease of brain connectivity, and phenomenologically denotes the actual Gestalt during schizo-phrenic experiences (Lee *et al.*, 2013, 2014). In addition, the Korean terms for schizophrenia-spectrum disorders including schizophreniform, schizoaffective disorder, schizotypal disorder, schizoid personality disorder, and schizotypal personality disorder were also renamed by using *johyeon* in 2012 (Park *et al.*, 2011). Third, Bipolar Day has been held by the Korean Society for Depressive and Bipolar Disorders since 2005. Bipolar Day is aimed at educating the public about the clinical features of bipolar disorder, to detect unrecognized bipolar symptoms, and to screen for bipolar disorders (Hwang *et al.*, 2012). Consequently, the changes in the psychiatry of South Korea, including changing the Korean terms for department of psychiatry and schizophrenia and holding Bipolar Day, are expected to overcome the social stigma of psychiatric disorders and heighten the accessibility of psychiatric interventions in South Korea.

Finally, innovative diagnostic and therapeutic practices in psychiatry are also being carried out in South Korea. Subjects with early psychosis (attenuated psychosis syndrome in the DSM-5) have been detected with psychometric tools including the Structured Interview for Positive Symptoms and managed with the preventive interventions including pharmacotherapy and cognitive-behavioral therapy in several special clinics in South Korea (Yoo *et al.*, 2007). In addition, Seoul Early Management and Improvement Services, which is a community-based detection, assessment, and allocation service for early psychosis, has been also established (Lee and Ahn, 2013). Furthermore, since 2001, the Korean Medication Algorithm Projects for Major Psychiatric Disorder have developed evidence-based guidelines, relevant to South Korean medical environments, for schizophrenia, bipolar disorders, depressive disorders and obsessive compulsive disorder (Ahn *et al.*, 2006). Meanwhile, evidence-based, pharmacological and non-pharmacological treatment guidelines for depression in Korea have been developed by CRESCEND (Park *et al.*, 2014; Won *et al.*, 2014). More specifically, the non-pharmacological treatment guideline for depression is characterized by recommendations for exercise therapy, bibliotherapy, cognitive-behavioral therapy, interpersonal psychotherapy, and short-term psychodynamic supportive psychotherapy. These evidence-based, clinical practice guidelines for major psychiatric disorders in Korea are expected to be essential in organizing and improving treatment and management.

Conclusions

Psychiatry in South Korea has developed quickly with its modernization and Westernization, in accordance with the vigorous and rapid industrialization and economic growth of South Korea in the several decades since the extremely difficult historical events of the Japanese annexation, the Korean War and the division of North and South Korea. Outstanding progress in biological psychiatry has been made because the proactive efforts of researchers have resulted in excellent academic products since 1980. Despite its excellent growth, psychiatry in South Korea for the twenty-first century has an unresolved identity problem. The identity of psychiatry in South Korea can shed light on *Tao psychotherapy*, the theoretical underpinnings of which are based on *Tao*, as the essence of Korean traditional culture. Moreover, changing the Korean term for schizophrenia, which was conducted with reference to the phrase *johyeon* of a Korean Buddhist text should be re-emphasized as an endeavor to establish the identity of psychiatry in South Korea. Meanwhile, despite their exclusion from the DSM-5, *hwabyung* and *shinbyung* represent the specific clinical manifestations of psychiatric problems in South Korean. Because of the political instability in North Korea, psychiatric care for North Korean refugees in South Korean society and adjacent countries is an important issue. Social problems, including the rapid increase in the proportion and number of elderly people, is a future challenge for psychiatry in South Korea. Despite several limitations and hindrances, an emphasis on transition from long-term hospitalization to community-based rehabilitation services in South Korea should also be noted. As the rapid development and economic growth of South Korea have been regarded as a role model for developing countries, the successful and significant modernization and identity establishment of psychiatry in South Korea is expected to provide an excellent role model for the quantitative and qualitative growth of psychiatry and mental health systems in developing countries.

References

Ahn, D.H. (2010) 'Special Issue', *Journal of Korean Neuropsychiatric Association*, 49: 533–7 (in Korean).

Ahn, Y.M., Kwon, J.S., Bahk, W.M., Kim, C.E., Park, J.I., Lee, S.Y., Yi, J.S., Lee, C.H., Jang, H.S., Jun, D.I., Chung, S.K., Chung, I.W., Cho, H.S., Joo, Y.H., Choi, Y.S., Kim, Y.S., Lee, H.S. and Feasibility of Korean Medication Algorithm for Schizophrenia Project Group (2006) 'The feasibility of the Korean Medication Algorithm for the treatment with schizophrenic patients (II): the problem of applying the algorithm to the real clinical situation and opinion of revision', *Korean Journal of Psychopharmacology*, 17: 35–49 (in Korean).

American Psychiatric Association (1980) *Diagnostic and Statistical Manual of Mental Disorders* (3rd ed). Washington (DC): American Psychiatric Press.

American Psychiatric Association (1994) *Diagnostic and Statistical Manual of Mental Disorders* (4th ed). Washington (DC): American Psychiatric Press.

American Psychiatric Association (2013) *Diagnostic and Statistical Manual of Mental Disorders* (5th ed). Washington (DC): American Psychiatric Press.

Bhugra, D., Sumathipala, A. and Sribaddana, S. (2007) 'Culture-bound syndromes: a re-evaluation', in Bhugra, D. and Bhui, K. (eds) *Textbook of Cultural Psychiatry,* Cambridge: Cambridge University Press.

Chang, S.C. and Kim, K. (1973) 'Psychiatry in South Korea', *American Journal of Psychiatry*, 130: 667–9.

Chang, S.M., Cho, S.J., Jeon, H.J., Hahm, B.J., Lee, H.J., Park, J.I. and Cho, M.J. (2008) 'Economic burden of schizophrenia in South Korea', *Journal of Korean Medical Sciences,* 23: 167–75.

Chang, S.M., Hong, J.P. and Cho, M.J. (2012) 'Economic burden of depression in South Korea', *Social Psychiatry and Psychiatric Epidemiology*, 47: 683–9.

Cho, M.J., Kim, J.K., Jeon, H.J., Suh, T., Chung, I.W., Hong, J.P., Bae, J.N., Lee, D.W., Park, J.I, Cho, S.J., Lee, C.K. and Hahm, B.J. (2007) 'Lifetime and 12-month prevalence of DSM-IV psychiatric disorders among Korean adults', *The Journal of Nervous and Mental Disease*, 195: 203–10.

Cho, M.J., Chang, S.M., Lee, Y.M., Bae, A., Ahn, J.H., Son, J., Hong, J.P., Bae, J.N., Lee, D.W., Cho, S.J., Park, J.I., Lee, J.Y., Kim, J.Y., Jeon, H.J., Sohn, J.H. and Kim, B.S. (2010) 'Prevalence of DSM-IV major mental disorders among Korean adults: a 2006 national epidemiological survey (KECA-R)', *Asian Journal of Psychiatry*, 3: 26–30.

Cho, M.J., Lee, J.Y., Kim, B.S., Lee, H.W. and Sohn, J.H. (2011) 'Prevalence of the major mental disorders among the Korean elderly', *Journal of Korean Medical Science*, 26: 1–10.

Cho, S.C. (2008) 'The significance of Taopsychotherapy', *The Korean Journal of Psychotherapy*, 22: 26–31 (in Korean).

Chung, C.K and Cho, S. (2006) 'Conceptualization of jeong and dynamics of hwabyung', *Psychiatry Investigation*, 3: 46–54.

Chung, W., Lee, N. and Rhi, B.Y. (2006) 'The introduction of the Western psychiatry into Korea (II): psychiatric education in Korea during the forced Japanese annexation of Korea (1910–1945)', *Korean Journal of Medical History*, 15: 157–87 (in Korean).

Chung, Y.C. and Lee, S.H (2008) 'Biological psychiatry in Korea', *International Review of Psychiatry*, 2008; 20: 419–24.

Craig, E. (2008) 'In honor of Rhee Dongshick's 88th birthday: Taopsychotherapy in the horizon of Western psychotherapy', *The Korean Journal of Psychotherapy*, 22: 43–50 (in Korean).

Han, D.S. (1967) 'A reference to the first authentic case of mental illness in Korea', *The Seoul Journal of Medicine*, 1: 9–11 (in Korean).

Hong, J.P., Bae, M.J. and Suh, T. (2006) 'Epidemiology of suicide in Korea', *Psychiatry Investigation*, 3: 7–14.

Huh, C.H. (2009) 'Examining Korea's first case of psychoanalytic psychotherapy: a brief psychotherapeutic treatment for a patient with psychogenic headache', *The Korean Journal of Psychotherapy*, 23: 60–4 (in Korean).

Hwang, T.Y., Youn, B.Y., Woo, Y.S. and Bahk, W.M. (2012) 'Report on 2011 Bipolar Day', *Journal of Korean Society for Depressive and Bipolar Disorders*, 10: 43–7 (in Korean).

Jeon, H.J. (2011) 'Depression and suicide', *Journal of Korean Medical Association*, 54: 370–5 (in Korean).

Jeon, H.J. (2012) 'Epidemiologic studies on depression and suicide', *Journal of Korean Medical Association*, 55: 322–8 (in Korean).

Jeon, W.T. (1997) 'Review of adaptation and mental health of refugees and perspectives and counter-plots in the Korean reunification process', *Journal of Korean Neuropsychiatric Association*, 36: 3–18 (in Korean).

Kahng, S.K. and Kim, H. (2010) 'A developmental model overview of mental health system in Korea', *Social Work in Public Health*, 25: 158–75.

Kang, S.H. (2006) 'Tao psychotherapy and assimilation of Western psychotherapy in Asia', *The Korean Journal of Psychotherapy*, 20: 17–22 (in Korean).

Kim, E. (1994) 'Analysis of recent proposals of the Korean Mental Health Act', *Mental Health Research*, 13: 139–54 (in Korean).

Kim, J.K. and Rhi, B.Y. (1996) 'Psychiatric care in Korea between 1945–1955', *Journal of Korean Neuropsychiatric Association*, 35: 342–55 (in Korean).

Kim, K. (1972) 'Psychoanalytic consideration of Korean shamanism', *Journal of Korean Neuropsychiatric Association*, 11: 121–9 (in Korean).

Kim, K. (1994) 'Cultural psychiatry in Korea', *Journal of Korean Neuropsychiatric Association*, 33: 939–52 (in Korean).

Kim, K. (1998) 'Illness behavior and psychiatric practice in Korea', *Mental Health Research*, 17: 1–3 (in Korean).

Kim, K. (1999) 'Psychiatry in Korea 21 century – quo vadis?', *Journal of Korean Neuropsychiatric Association*, 38: 5–11 (in Korean).

Kim, K. (2005) 'Culture-relevant psychotherapy in Korea: clinical insight', in Tseng, W.S., Chang S.C. and Nishizino, M. (eds) *Asian Culture and Psychotherapy: Implication for East and West*, Honolulu: University of Hawai'i Press.

Kim, K. (2006) 'Delusions and hallucinations in East Asians with schizophrenia', *World Cultural Psychiatry Research Review*, 1: 37–42.

Kim, K., Li, D., Jiang, Z., Cui, X., Lin, L., Kang, J.J., Park, K.K., Chung, E.K. and Kim, C.K. (1993) 'Schizophrenic delusions among Korean-Chinese and Chinese: a transcultural study', *The International Journal of Social Psychiatry*, 3: 190–9.

Kim, K., Hwu, H., Zhang, L.D., Lu, M.K., Park, K.K., Hwang, T.Z., Kim, D. and Park, Y.C. (2001a) 'Schizophrenic delusions in Seoul, Shanghai and Taipei: a transcultural study', *Korean Journal of Medical Science*, 16: 88–94.

Kim, K., Zhang, L.D., Lu, M.G., Park, K.K., Park, Y.C. and Kim, D. (2001b) 'Schizophrenic hallucinations in Shanghai and Seoul: a transcultural study ', *Journal of Korean Neuropsychiatric Association*, 40: 767–76 (in Korean).

Kim, T.S., Jeong, S.H., Kim, J.B., Lee, M.S., Kim, J.M., Yim, H.W. and Jun, T.Y. (2011) 'The clinical research center for depression study: baseline characteristics of a Korean long-term hospital-based observational collaborative prospective cohort study', *Psychiatry Investigation*, 8: 1–8.

Kleinman, A., Eisenberg, L. and Good, B. (1978) 'Culture, illness and care: clinical lessons from anthropological and cross-cultural research', *Annals of Internal Medicine*, 88: 251–8.

Lee, B.H. (2013) 'Modern approach to treating mental patients in colonial Chosun', *Korean Journal of Medical History*, 22: 29–78 (in Korean).

Lee, C.K., Kwak, Y.S., Yamamoto, J., Rhee, H., Kim, Y.S., Han, J.H., Choi, J.O. and Lee, H.Y. (1990a) 'Psychiatric epidemiology in Korea. Part I: gender and age differences in Seoul', *The Journal of Nervous and Mental Disease*, 4: 242–6.

Lee, C.K., Kwak, Y.S., Yamamoto, J., Rhee, H., Kim, Y.S., Han, J.H., Choi, J.O. and Lee, H.Y. (1990b) 'Psychiatric epidemiology in Korea. Part II: urban and rural differences', *The Journal of Nervous and Mental Disease*, 4: 247–52.

Lee, H.Y. (2004) 'Past, present and future of Korean psychiatry', *Psychiatry Investigation*, 1: 13–19.

Lee, J., Min, S.K., Kim, K.H., Kim, B., Cho, S.J., Lee, S.H., Choi, T.K. and Suh, S.Y. (2012) 'Differences in temperament and character dimensions of personality between patients with Hwa-byung, an anger syndrome, and patients with major depressive disorder', *Journal of Affective Disorder*, 138: 110–16.

Lee, M.S. and Ahn, S.R. (2013) 'The analysis of community-based identification, assessment and allocation system for early psychosis', *Korean Journal of Schizophrenia Research*, 16: 32–7 (in Korean).

Lee, N. and Rhi, B.Y. (1999) 'The introduction of Western psychiatry into Korea (I): from the mid seventeenth century to 1911, the time of Japanese forced annexation of Korea', *Korean Journal of Medical History*, 8: 233–68 (in Korean).

Lee, S., Tsang, A., Huang, Y.Q., He, Y.L., Liu, Z.R., Zhang, M.Y., Shen, Y.C. and Kessler, R.C. (2009) 'The epidemiology of depression in metropolitan China', *Psychological Medicine*, 39: 735–47.

Lee, S.H. (1978) 'The diagnosis of hwabyung', *Psychiatry Bulletin*, 1: 1–10.

Lee, Y.H., Lee, W.J., Kim, Y.J., Cho, M.J., Kim, J.H., Lee, Y.J., Kim, H.Y., Choi, D.S., Kim, S.G. and Robinson C. (2012) 'North Korean refugee health in South Korea (NORNS) study: study design and methods', *BMC Public Health*, 12: 172.

Lee, Y.M. (1999) 'Development of the National Mental Health System through delegation to primary sector', *Mental Health Research*, 18: 12–22 (in Korean).

Lee, Y.S. and Kwon, J.S. (2011) 'Special Issue', *Journal of Korean Neuropsychiatric Association*, 50: 16–19.

Lee, Y.S., Kim, J.J. and Kwon, J.S. (2013) 'Renaming schizophrenia in South Korea', *The Lancet*, 382: 683–4.

Lee, Y.S., Park, I.H., Park, S.C., Kim, J.J. and Kwon, J.S. (2014) 'Johyeonbyung (attunement disorder): renaming mind splitting disorder as a way to reduce stigma of patients with schizophrenia in Korea', *Asian Journal of Psychiatry*, 8: 118–20.

Lin, K.M. (1983) 'Hwa-byung: a Korean culture-bound syndrome?', *American Journal of Psychiatry*, 140: 105–7.

Min, S.K. (2008a) 'Clinical correlates of hwa-byung and proposal for a new anger disorder', *Psychiatry Investigation*, 5: 125–41.

Min, S.K. (2008b) 'Divided countries, divided mind 1: psycho-social issues in adaptation problems of North Korean defectors', *Psychiatry Investigation*, 5: 1–13.

Min, S.K. (2011) 'Professor Charles I. McLaren, MD (1): his life and medical philosophy', *Journal of Korean Neuropsychiatric Association*, 50: 172–86 (in Korean).

Min, S.K., Lee, C.H., Kim, J.Y. and Shim, E.J. (2004). 'Posttraumatic stress disorder of former comfort women for the Japanese army during World War II', *Journal of Korean Neuropsychiatric Association*, 43: 740–8 (in Korean).

Min, S.K., Suh, S.Y. and Song, K.J. (2009) 'Symptoms to use for diagnostic criteria of hwa-byung, an anger syndrome', *Psychiatry Investigation*, 6: 7–12.

Nock, M.K., Borges, G., Bormet, E.J., Alonso, J., Angermeyer, M., Beautrais, A., Bruffaerts, R., Chiu, W.T., de Girolamo, G., Gluzman, S., de Graaf, R., Gureje, O., Haro, J.M., Huang, Y., Karam, E., Kessler, R.C., Leipine, J.P., Levinson, D., Medina-Mora, M.E., Ono, Y., Posada-Villa, J. and Williams, D. (2008) 'Cross-national prevalence and risk factors for suicidal ideation, plan and attempts', *British Journal of Psychiatry*, 192: 98–105.

Oh, H.Y., Kim, D. and Park, Y.C. (2012) 'Nature of persecutors and their behaviors in the delusions of schizophrenia: change between the 1990s and the 2000s', *Psychiatry Investigation*, 9: 319–24.

Ono, Y., Kawakami, N., Nakane, Y., Nakamura, Y., Tachimori, H., Iwata, N., Uda, H., Nakane, H., Watanabe, M., Naganuma, Y., Furukawa, T.A., Hata, Y., Kobayashi, M., Miyake, Y., Tajima, M., Takeshima, T. and Kikkawa, T. (2008) 'Prevalence of and risk factors for suicide-related outcomes in the World Health Organization World Mental Health Surveys in Japan', *Psychiatry and Clinical Neuroscience*, 62: 442–9.

Park, H.W. and Yeo, I.S. (1999) 'The first annual report of the Korean Government Hospital', *Yonsei Journal of Medical History*, 3: 1–44.

Park, J.I., Oh, K.Y. and Chung, Y.C. (2013) 'Psychiatry in Korea', *Asian Journal of Psychiatry*, 6: 186–90.

Park, S.C., Lee, Y.S. and Kwon, J.S. (2011) 'Special Issue', *Journal of Korean Neuropsychiatric Association*, 49: 533–7 (in Korean).

Park, S.C., Oh, H.S., Oh, D.H., Jung, S.A., Na, K.S., Lee, H.Y., Kang, R.H., Choi, Y.K., Lee, M.S. and Park, Y.C. (2014) 'Evidence-based, non-pharmacological treatment guideline for depression in Korea', *Journal of Korean Medical Science*, 29: 12–22.

Park, Y.C. and Kim, K.I. (1998) 'The psychiatric practice relevant to the Korean culture', *Mental Health Research*, 17: 4–13 (in Korean).

Park, Y.C. and Park, S.C. (2012) 'Why do suicide and depression occur?', *Journal of Korean Medical Association*, 55: 329–34 (in Korean).

Park, Y.N. (2012) 'New challenge for psychiatry: from symptomatic treatment to mental health promotion', *Journal of Korean Neuropsychiatric Association*, 51: 101–6 (in Korean).

Rhee, D.S. (2008) *Introduction to Taopsychotherapy: Beyond Freud and Jung*, Seoul: Hangangsoo (in Korean).

Rhi, B.Y. (1994) 'Psychiatric care and its change under the Japanese government in Korea with special reference to the clinical activities at the colonial governmental hospital: "Chosun-Chong-Dok-Bu Ui-Won" (1913–1927)', *Korean Journal of Medical History*, 3; 147–69 (in Korean).

Rhi, B.Y. (1998) 'Patients with shamanistic background and psychiatric care', *Mental Health Research*, 17: 14–24 (in Korean).

Rhi, B.Y. (1999) 'Hundred years' psychiatry in Korea (1899–1999)', *Korean Journal of Medical History*, 8: 157–68 (in Korean).

Rhi, B.Y., Ha, K.S., Kim, Y.S., Saskai, Y., Young, D., Woon, Tai-Hwang, Laraya, L.T. and Yanchun, Y. (1995) 'The health care seeking behavior of schizophrenic patients in 6 East Asian areas', *International Journal of Social Psychiatry*, 41: 190–209.

Robins, L.N., Helzer, J.E., Croughan, J. and Ratcliff, K.S. (1981) 'National Institute of Mental Health Diagnostic Interview Schedule: its history, characteristics and validity', *Archive of General Psychiatry*, 38: 381–9.

Ryu, S.J. (1982) 'Direction of the Korean Mental Health Act', *Soonchunhyang University Papers*, 5: 309–17 (in Korean).

Song, J.Y. (1998) 'Psychiatric management of patients who are familiar with traditional medicine', *Mental Health Research*, 17: 25–36 (in Korean).

Sugihara, G. and Takei, N. (2013) 'Renaming schizophrenia with proper public education is an optimal way to overcome stigma', *Psychological Medicine*, 43: 1557–8.

Suh, S. (2013) 'Stories to be told: Korean doctors between hwa-byung (fire-illness) and depression, 1970–2011', *Culture, Medicine and Psychiatry*, 37: 81–104.

Suh, T. (1999) 'Models of mental health delivery system in Korea', *Mental Health Research*, 18: 1–11 (in Korean).

Suh, T. (2010) 'History of the Korean Mental Health Act', *Journal of Korean Neuropsychiatric Association*, 49: 144–8 (in Korean).

Tseng, W.S. (2007) 'Culture and psychopathology: general view', in Bhugra, D. and Bhui, K. (eds) *Textbook of Cultural Psychiatry*, Cambridge: Cambridge University Press.

Won, E., Park, S.C., Han, K.M., Sung, S.H., Lee, H.Y., Paik, J.W., Jeon, H.J., Lee, M.S., Shim, S.H., Ko, Y.H., Lee, K.J., Han, C., Ham, B.J., Choi, J., Lee, H., Hwang, T.Y., Oh, K.S., Hahn, S.W., Park, Y.C. and Lee, M.S. (2014) 'Evidence-based pharmacological treatment guideline for depression in Korea, revised edition', *Journal of Korean Medical Science*, 29: 468–84.

World Health Organization (1990) *Composite International Diagnostic Interview (CIDI)*, Geneva: World Health Organization.

Yeo, I. (2008) 'The establishment of SUMC (Severance Union Medical College) psychiatry department and the formation of the humanistic tradition', *Korean Journal of Medical History*, 17: 57–74 (in Korean).

Yongmi, Y.K. (2000) 'Shin-byung (divine illness) in a Korean woman', *Culture, Medicine and Psychiatry*, 24: 471–86.

Yoo, S.Y., Lee, K.J., Kang, D.H., Lee, S.J., Ha, T.H., Wee, W., Lee, A.R., Song, J.Y., Kim, S.N. and Kwon, J.S. (2007) 'Characteristics of subjects at clinical high risk for schizophrenia: natural follow up study in "Seoul Youth Clinic": pilot study', *Journal of Korean Neuropsychiatric Association*, 46: 19–28 (in Korean).

17

North Korea

Seog Ju Kim

Country location and geography

North Korea is located in East Asia in the northern part of the Korean Peninsula (Palka and Galgano, 2003). North Korea shares its northern border with the People's Republic of China along the Amrok river and the Duman river, and with Russia along the Duman river. North Korea was separated from South Korea along the Demilitarized Zone on its southern border after the 1953 Korean War ceasefire. Its west coast is on the Yellow Sea, while its east coast is on the East Sea of Korea. The capital of North Korea is Pyŏng'yang. Its Gross Domestic Product per capita is estimated to be US$1,800 in 2011 (Central Intelligence Agency, nd).

During the Cold War era, health care was at the forefront of ideological battles between the two Koreas. North Korea boasted of constructing one of the top-ranked public health systems in the 1970s. However, the North Korean health care system virtually collapsed after the prolonged economic hardships during the 'Arduous March' in the late 1990s. According to a survey conducted in 1999, 89 percent of North Korean refugees reported the experience of 'illness without access to medical care' (Lee *et al.*, 2001). The current status of mental health in North Korea should be understood in the light of this historical context.

According to the country profile of the World Health Organization (nd), the estimated total population of North Korea was 24,763,000 in 2012 (World Health Organization, 2010). Life expectancy at birth was 65 years for males, and 72 years for females in 2009. The probability of dying under five years old was 29 per 1,000 live births in 2009. The proportion of the population under 15 years old was 21.98 percent, whereas the proportion over 60 was 12.74 percent in 2009. Government expenditure on health was US$4.2 per capita in 2008.

Mental health policy

In 2003, the Ministry of Public Health in North Korea presented mental health as one of the top ten national health priorities for the next five years (2004–2008): to be more specific, mental health was the eighth priority on the list (World Health Organization, 2003). However, there is very little information regarding the mental health policy of the North Korean government. The lack of the information has been regarded as inevitable due to the closed and exclusive social system of North Korea.

Psychiatric hospitals in North Korea are called '49th hospitals (*sashipguho*)'. In terms of consent to hospitalization in a mental hospital, some former North Korean doctors, who have defected to South Korea, have reported that the opinions of doctors were much more decisive than the consent of family members in North Korea (Kim *et al.*, 2012). However, one former North Korean doctor mentioned that the consent of family members was necessary for admission to psychiatric wards. Furthermore, as the patients in mental hospitals in North Korea were usually considered to be severely psychotic or mentally retarded, the opinions of patients themselves were reported to be less important than those of family members or doctors in deciding admission.

According to the report of one former North Korean doctor (Kim *et al.*, 2012), there were certain guidelines for seclusion or restraint during the hospitalization in the 49th hospitals. However, other former North Korean doctors did not know even of the existence of such guidelines. Although there is a report that some patients experienced violence or harassment during their hospitalization in the 49th hospitals, former North Korean doctors did not witness violence to or harassment of patients.

Although political issues are very important in North Korean medical education (Park and Park, 1998), there is no evidence of systematic abuse of psychiatry for political purposes in North Korea. This is unlike other former socialist countries, in which political dissidents were admitted to mental hospital with psychiatric diagnoses. This difference may be due to the presence of concentration camps for political dissidents in North Korea. Reactionaries and political dissidents were not classed as psychiatric patients because most of them could not avoid arrest and harsher punishments. It also may be due to the intentional confinement of psychiatry to biological issues segregated from political issues.

Psychiatric epidemiology

The data for psychiatric epidemiology in North Korea are largely unknown. Even for vulnerable populations such as prisoners in the political prisoner camps or victims of the long-term starvation in the 1990s, no data are available for psychiatric epidemiology. Some researchers have investigated the prevalence of psychiatric disorders or psychiatric symptoms in North Korean defectors in South Korea and China. The prevalence of psychiatric disorders in North Korean defectors has been reported to be very high in a number of previous research reports. However, since the psychiatric status of North Korean defectors has been significantly affected by their migration trajectories and their adjustment to a new society (Min 2008), this cannot directly represent the psychiatric epidemiology of inhabitants of North Korea.

According to former North Korean doctors' reports (Kim *et al.*, 2012), only those with full-blown psychotic symptoms or those with vividly bizarre behaviors are regarded as psychiatric patients even by doctors in North Korea. The sphere of psychiatry is thus mainly confined to schizophrenia and bipolar disorders with psychotic features. Most inpatients in mental hospitals, so-called '49th hospitals' in North Korea, were diagnosed with schizophrenia and a few with manic episodes of bipolar disorders. Other neurotic disorders, such as non-psychotic mood disorders, anxiety disorders or somatoform disorders do not get much attention from North Korean psychiatry and are rarely diagnosed. The focus on psychosis in North Korean psychiatry could be influenced by the predominance of biological etiologies rather than psychosocial etiologies for mental illness in the former communist countries. Moreover, due to the economic difficulties and the spread of infectious disease, governmental priority would have been given to life-threatening and urgent medical problems such as infectious diarrhea or tuberculosis rather than mental illness. Among psychiatric disorders, only psychosis has been a major concern in North Korea, as it has been considered a disease that could hinder social safety.

Former North Korean doctors reported that depressive disorders or anxiety disorders were rarely treated in mental hospitals (Kim *et al.*, 2012). However, the possibility of a high prevalence of depression or anxiety disorders in North Korea cannot be excluded given the stressful situations such as economic poverty, political surveillance, violence or imprisonment. A panel study reported that North Korean defectors had commonly experienced traumatic or stressful events when they had lived in North Korea (Kim and Oh, 2010). The traumatic or stressful events in North Korea include the starvation to death of family/relatives/close neighbors (68.1 percent), life-threatening coldness or shortage of food (58.2 percent), being eyewitness to the public execution of acquaintances (42.8 percent), severe beating (29.9 percent), imprisonment (24.4 percent) and torture (18.9 percent).

Among North Korean defectors, depression or posttraumatic stress disorder (PTSD) was reported to be very common. Among North Korean defectors in the border region between China and North Korea, 56 percent of respondents were suspected to have PTSD (Lee *et al.*, 2001). In the above-mentioned study, the vast majority of North Korean defectors reported clinically significant levels of anxiety (90 percent) and depression (81 percent). According to a study conducted using the Structured Clinical Interview of the DSM-III-R (SCID), the prevalence of PTSD among North Korean resettlers in South Korea was 29.5 percent (Jeon *et al.*, 2005). A follow-up study of this population showed that 88.8 percent of patients diagnosed with PTSD recovered after three years (Hong *et al.*, 2006). Based on a survey using the Center for Epidemiologic Studies Depression Scale (CES-D), 29 percent of North Korean refugees in *Hanawon* (see Glossary) showed depressive symptoms (Han, 2001). Among North Korean defectors who stayed in South Korea for more than six months, 51.5 percent of respondents demonstrated clinically significant symptoms of depression on the CES-D scale (Eom and Lee, 2004).

Therefore, non-psychotic depression or anxiety disorders are likely to be under-diagnosed in North Korea. The epidemiology of non-psychotic psychiatric disorders in North Korea may be affected by the fact that the diagnostic classification system of North Korean medicine is different from that of other countries. Diseases without delusion, hallucination or impaired reality testing are usually not diagnosed as psychiatric disease in North Korea. In the textbook of family medicine in North Korea, somatic symptoms of anxiety or depression were described in the internal medicine or the neurology section of the disease classification system (Choi, 2004). North Koreans with mood or anxiety disorders tend to express their symptoms as somatic ones rather than psychological ones. Somatic symptoms may be culturally and politically acceptable in North Korea, while psychological symptoms may not. These somatic symptoms are often diagnosed as 'cardiac neurosis (*Simjang Sin'gyŏngjŏng*)' and 'neurasthenia (*Sin'gyŏng Soeyak*)', rather than mood or anxiety disorders. These diseases are treated by general physicians or neurologists rather than psychiatrists in North Korea (Kim *et al.*, 2012). The textbook of family medicine in North Korea stated that cardiac neurosis could progress to neurasthenia (Choi, 2004). Neurasthenia is considered to be caused by the imbalance of the autonomic nervous system, which can also progress into 'dysautonomia (*Jayulsin'gyŏng Siljojŏng*)'. The clinical manifestations of cardiac neurosis are palpitation, chest discomfort, dyspneic sensation, dizziness, nausea and agitation. Symptoms of cardiac neurosis resemble symptoms of anxiety disorders such as panic disorders. Clinical symptoms of dysautonomia also include depressive mood, anxiety, fatigue, insomnia, nightmare and palpitations, which are quite similar to those of major depressive disorders. The chief complaint of neurasthenia patients is usually somatic anxiety symptoms or insomnia. Neurasthenia patients usually experience excessive dreaming or worry, nervousness and loss of concentration. These symptoms are interpreted as the signs of abnormal body status in North Korea rather than as signs of psychological or psychosocial distress. Usually physicians other than psychiatrists issue the medical certificate for neurasthenia, which sometimes can be used for exemption from labor. However, former North Korean doctors reported that they knew by their clinical experiences that these disorders (cardiac neurosis, neurasthenia and dysautonomia) were more common among those who experienced stressful situations and that they would be associated with emotional problems.

According to a World Health Organization (WHO) report, the rate of excessive alcohol consumption (i.e. drinking more than one bottle per person, per sitting) was 26.3 percent among North Korean males (World Health Organization, 2010). Before the economic devastation, alcohol had been strictly controlled by the government and alcohol abuse was not so common. However, during the economic devastation, alcohol use increased through illegal bootlegging in North Korea. Alcohol-related problems have been reported to be common in North Korean defectors in South Korea (Jeon et al., 2008). However, according to former North Korean doctors' reports (Kim et al., 2012), alcohol abuse or dependence were rarely diagnosed in North Korea. Only acute and vivid alcohol intoxication was treated in hospitals. There is also a possibility of under-diagnosis of alcohol dependence in North Korea. Although it remains unclear, plausible reasons for the under-diagnosis of alcohol-related problems in North Korea may be: the shortage of alcoholic beverages due to the economic crisis, the permissive culture for alcohol drinking or ignorance of alcohol-related disorders.

Opium has been cultivated in North Korea for medical purposes for treating diarrhea or pain because of the shortage of drugs during the economic devastation in the 1990s. According to North Korean defectors, the opioid can also be purchased in the private market, and this illegal use is not as well-controlled as before the 1980s. Therefore, there is a risk of high prevalence of opioid abuse. In addition, some North Korean defectors have reported that illegal use of methamphetamine is not rare in North Korea. Although there are no exact data for prevalence of methamphetamine- or opioid-related disorders in North Korea, there is a possibility of a high prevalence of these substance-related disorders.

In North Korea, there is no internship or resident training for any medical specialty including psychiatry. The government or Party officials decide the workplace of all medical graduates. After that decision, those who work in a 49th hospital or 49th department become psychiatrists without additional training in psychiatry. Doctors must follow the Party's decision on the medical specialty assigned to them. According to the former North Korean doctors' reports, psychiatry is not a popular discipline among medical graduates in North Korea. Other core medical specialties (gibon'gwa) such as internal medicine, surgery, obstetrics and gynecology, and pediatrics are more helpful for becoming a high-ranking official in medical society in North Korea. Moreover, psychiatric hospitals (49th hospitals) are located in geographically isolated rural areas, which makes being a psychiatrist even more unattractive. In addition, the former North Korean doctors reported that psychiatrists have less informal sources of income than other physicians or surgeons. According to the former North Korean doctors' reports, to solve the problem of the unpopularity of psychiatry, the Party introduced a few social benefits such as exemption from both the one-month mobilization for collecting medicinal herbs and agricultural labor, as well as special vacations twice a year.

Mental health systems

North Korean psychiatry is influenced by psychiatry in former communist countries. As in other former communist countries, biological therapy has been regarded as the mainstay of North

Korean psychiatry. However, pharmacological or other biological treatments in North Korea have been outdated due to the closed social system and the distressed economy. Old typical antipsychotics such as chlorpromazine have been prescribed to psychotic patients in the 49th hospitals. Former North Korean doctors have reported that insulin coma therapy had been used until recently (Kim *et al.*, 2012). Sedatives such as benzodiazepine and barbiturate are also prescribed in psychiatric wards in North Korea. After the economic devastation and the destruction of the public health system in the 1990s, North Koreans can easily buy sedatives from the private market, though it is illegal. Parenteral administration or high-dose abuse of these sedatives by self-administration in North Korea are suspected nowadays. The pharmaco-therapy for neurasthenia or cardiac neurosis is usually conducted by general physicians in North Korea. For neurasthenia or cardiac neurosis, which shows symptoms similar to anxiety disorders or depression, benzodiazepines are commonly prescribed (Kim *et al.*, 2012). Former North Korean doctors did not know about atypical antipsychotics or antidepressants.

Usually, psychodynamic or cognitive psychotherapy has not been conducted in psychiatric clinics in North Korea. The only occupational therapy practiced for inpatients in 49th hospitals was subsistence farming. However, former North Korean doctors reported that their emotional support or reassurance could influence the symptoms of cardiac neurosis or neurasthenia (Kim *et al.*, 2012). Therefore, some forms of supportive psychotherapeutic approach may be provided empirically for neurotic patients.

Inpatient rather than outpatient treatment is the norm in North Korean psychiatry. Psychiatric practices are separated from other medical specialties or primary health services in North Korea. Physicians should transfer full-blown psychotic patients to the 49th ward with the approval of the vice president of the hospital. The North Korean mental health delivery system is composed of the 49th Prevention Center (49th ward) or the department of psychiatry in provincial hospitals. Each province had one 49th hospital in the past. There are unverified reports by former North Korean doctors that the number of 49th hospitals has been reduced. If it is true that the North Korean government has reduced the number of the 49th hospitals, the reason for this strategy remains unclear. It may be related to governmental efforts to deinstitutionalize mental patients, the concealment of negative social images from people or the economic difficulty in the govern-mental health sector. In addition to 49th hospitals, there were 49th wards for hospitalization of 49th patients in military hospitals or upper-level hospitals. In these hospitals, there was usually one doctor in charge of 49th patients, i.e. psychiatric patients. If there was no one in charge of psychiatry, doctors in charge of internal medicine usually covered the clinical role for psychiatric outpatients and inpatients.

According to the former North Korean doctors' reports, more than 100 patients were hospitalized in each 49th hospital (Kim *et al.*, 2012). Doctors in the 49th hospital each took care of about ten hospitalized patients. Discharge from the 49th hospital was determined by the doctor's assessment of the patients' recovery. According to the former North Korean doctors' reports (Kim *et al.*, 2012), some patients were discharged early in spite of significant remaining psychotic symptoms, because their family members had to provide food for them due to the famine during the economic devastation. Most patients visiting the outpatient clinics were former patients discharged from the 49th hospitals.

No data are available for a community health system or rehabilitation program for patients with mental illness in North Korea. Former North Korean doctors did not know of the existence of community mental health systems. It is possible that most patients with psychosis are admitted to 49th wards long-term or are neglected in their homes without proper management.

Social/explanatory model(s) of mental illness

The explanatory model for the etiology of mental illness in North Korean psychiatry is predominantly shaped by the tradition of biologically oriented psychiatry in former communist countries. Pavlovian theory that every mental process abnormality originates from the pathology of 'superior nervous activity' became the basis of medical education and clinical practices in North Korean psychiatry. However, contrary to the denial of genetic elements in the etiology of mental illness in Soviet psychiatry, former North Korean doctors thought that schizophrenia and other psychotic disorders were clearly affected by genetic effects (Park et al., 2014). There seems to be virtually no discussion of psychosocial and psychodynamic etiology of mental illnesses in North Korean clinics. Former North Korean doctors reported that the concept of unconsciousness was not included in the etiology of mental illness in North Korea (Kim et al., 2012). According to their memory, only familial or other personal problems, which were not directly related to the social system per se, were considered as potential causes of neurasthenia in North Korean medical practice. However, attributing the cause of mental illness to ideological issues such as remnants of capitalism was rare in North Korean clinics. Development of psychiatric disorders was generally considered to be due to biological causes or brain abnormalities. Former North Korean doctors believed that ideological, political or social issues have nothing to do with psychiatry.

Patients with mental illness experience stigmatization in the North Korean community. In North Korea, psychiatric patients are understood to show bizarre and stupid behaviors. Laypersons call a psychiatric patient a '49th'. Sometimes, '49th' is used as a derogatory term to insult another person. However, there is hardly any mention of mental illnesses or psychiatric patients in the mass media, since the mass media in North Korea is permitted to broadcast only about desirable aspects of North Korean society. Since psychiatric disorders should not exist in the ideal society, the presence of mental illness would be regarded as socially undesirable even by the government. Psychiatric patients in North Korea are admitted to hospitals in geographically remote areas. The isolation of psychiatric patients from the social network might be related to the protection of the ideal society from potentially socially undesirable individuals.

Topics of interest specific to North Korea

WHO identified three major challenges for mental health care in North Korea (World Health Organization, 2003, 2010). The first challenge was the need for to shift institutional mental health care to community care. As a model for deinstitutionalization in 2003, WHO proposed initiating a program for the community-based management of psychosis and epilepsy as well as the reduction of hospital beds and cost of care. The second challenge was the availability of psychotropic drugs. The last challenge, which was added in the new 2009–2012 plan, was the integration of mental health services within the entire health care system including primary health care. For this, the training of health care workers in the primary health care centers in the management of psychosis and epilepsy was proposed.

After the economic devastation, the North Korean government encouraged traditional Korean medicine and the prescription of herbal medicine. Emphasis on traditional Korean medicine also represents and symbolizes a politically independent North Korea. Therefore, herbal medicines are also prescribed for patients with neurasthenia or cardiac neurosis because of the shortage of drugs and for political reasons.

According to a North Korean doctor's report, the suicide rate was not reported to be high in North Korea. Suicide is taboo and prohibited in North Korea. Suicide is interpreted as a counterrevolutionary act of rebellion and betrayal against the state. Former North Korean doctors reported that, if a person commits suicide, the social ranks (*seong-bun*) of his/her family members are downgraded (Kim *et al.*, 2012). Social rank affects every aspect of the lives of North Koreans including jobs, social benefits, education and residence. Therefore, suicide is strongly discouraged due to North Koreans' concerns for the wellbeing of their children, siblings and parents. Even if there is a suicide, doctors and family members try to hide the case by giving a different cause of death in the death certificate. On the contrary, WHO estimated very high suicide rates in North Korea (38.5 per 1 million). However, WHO acknowledged that data acquisition was difficult for North Korea. It has been suggested that deaths in state custody might be calculated as suicide in North Korea as in former communist countries. However, the suicide rate had been increased in the post-socialist transition in many former socialist countries (Park *et al.*, 2014). In addition, the current suicide rate of South Korea ranks among the highest in the world. Therefore, although the current suicide rate in North Korea remains unclear, there would be a potential risk of a dramatic increase in suicides in North Korea after Korean reunification.

North Korea is in a state of dynamic coexistence of characteristics from both the former communist society and a society in post-socialist transition. In light of the mental health crisis in transitional societies, enormous challenges for mental health may be waiting for any future unified Korea. There is a need to prepare in advance blueprints of programs for the potential reorganization of education, diagnosis, treatment and a community mental health system in North Korean psychiatry.

Glossary

Hanawon: a government-sponsored educational facility for the settlement of North Korean refugees during their initial phase in South Korea.

Jayulsin'gyŏng Siljojŏng: dysautonomia.

Sashipguho: 49th hospital, mental hospital in North Korea, also a derogatory term for a psychiatric patient.

Simjang Sin'gyŏngjŏng: cardiac neurosis.

Sin'gyŏng Soeyak: neurasthenia.

References

Central Intelligence Agency (nd). *CIA World Factbook: North Korea*. Retrieved 27 October 2013, from www.cia.gov/library/publications/the-world-factbook/geos/kn.html

Choi, T.S. (2004) *Guidebook for Family Medicine*, Kwahak-Bekwasajeon-Chulpansa.

Eom, T., and Lee, K. (2004). The relationship among social problem solving capability, social support and depression of North Korean defectors. *Korean Journal of Family Social Work*, 18, 5–32.

Han, I. (2001). Depressive traits of North Korean defectors. *Korean Journal of Family Social Work*, 11, 78–94.

Hong, C., Yoo, J., Cho, Y., Eom, J., Ku, H., Seo, S., Jeon, W. (2006). A 3-year follow-up study of posttraumatic stress disorder among North Korean defectors. *Journal of Korean Neuropsychiatric Association*, 45(1), 49–56.

Jeon, W., Hong, C., Lee, C., Kim, D., Han, M., and Min, S. (2005). Correlation between traumatic events and posttraumatic stress disorder among North Koreans in South Korea. *Journal of Traumatic Stress*, 18, 147–54.

Jeon, W., Yu, S., Cho, Y., and Eom, J. (2008). Traumatic experiences and mental health of North Korean refugees in South Korea. *Psychiatry Investigation*, 5, 213–20.

Kim, H., and Oh, S. (2010). The MMPI-2 Profile of North Korean female refugees. *Korean Journal of Psychology*, 29(1), 1–20.

Kim, S., Park, Y., Lee, H., and Park, S. (2012). Current situation of psychiatry in North Korea: from the viewpoint of North Korean medical doctors. *Korean Journal of Psychosomatic Medicine*, 20(1), 32–9.

Lee, Y., Lee, M., Chun, K., Lee, Y., and Yoon, S. (2001). Trauma experience of North Korean refugees in China. *American Journal of Public Health*, 20(3), 225–9.

Min, S. (2008). Divided countries, divided mind 1: psycho-social issues in adaptation problems of North Korean defectors. *Psychiatry Investigation*, 5, 1–13.

Palka, E., and Galgano, F. (2003). *North Korea: A Geographical Analysis*. West Point, NY: US Military Academy Press.

Park, Y.J., and Park, H. (1998). A study on medical educational system in North Korea. *Korean Journal of Medical History*, 7, 63–76.

Park, Y.S., Park, S., Jun, J., and Kim, S. (2014). Psychiatry in former socialist countries: implications for North Korean psychiatry. *Psychiatry Investigation*, in press.

World Health Organization (nd) *Country Profile: Democratic People's Republic of Korea*. Retrieved October 27 2013, from www.who.int/countries/prk/en/

World Health Organization (2003). *WHO Country Cooperation Strategy 2004–2008: DPRK*. Geneva: WHO.

World Health Organization (2010). *WHO Country Cooperation Strategy 2009–2013: DPRK*. Geneva: WHO.

Section 5

Southeast Asia: Indonesia, Malaysia and the Philippines

Overview

Thambu Maniam

Four countries are included in this section – Indonesia, Malaysia, the Philippines and Singapore. While they share some historical similarities, there are also experiences unique to each country. These nations were colonies of the Western powers until the second half of the twentieth century. This had a major impact on the development of psychiatric services in these countries. The Philippines was the first country to be colonized, initially by the Spanish, and later by the USA; Indonesia was next, by the Dutch; then Singapore and lastly Malaysia, both by the British. Indonesia is the most populous nation in this region; the city state of Singapore is the most developed.

Malaysia and Singapore share many similarities with respect to psychiatry because of their geographical proximity, shared history and close cultural ties. In all four countries, for the most part, the colonial rulers set up the first formal mental health services, usually based on the form of care available in their home countries. Mental asylums made their debut in Southeast Asia around the end of the nineteenth and the beginning of the twentieth century. So the initial psychiatric services were custodial in nature. Gradually, in keeping with the development of psychiatry in the West, mental health services underwent a change: the size of psychiatric institutions began to shrink, general hospital psychiatric units grew and community services began to develop. This has not always been a smooth process of changeover. Money saved from downsizing psychiatric hospitals has not always been channeled to develop community facilities, something that is not unique to Asia. In tandem with these developments Mental Health laws have begun to change too, to become more liberal, more cognizant of the rights of patients and to promote more humane treatment of the mentally ill. Up to less than two decades ago the mental health law of the east Malaysian state of Sabah was called the Lunatic Ordinance. The telex address for the psychiatric hospital near the state capital of Sarawak used to be 'Alienist'! All these have fortunately changed since 2001.

Psychiatry has struggled to be accepted as part of the mainstream of medicine. The stigma that is attached to psychiatric illness and patients, also sticks to psychiatrists, psychiatric paramedics, psychiatric wards and medications. Little wonder mental health services are underfunded. It appears that only recently psychiatry is emerging from its status as the Cinderella of medicine – though the long-awaited demise of her 'stepmother' is not quite here yet.

This change did not come of its own accord. Change never does. It occurred through the untiring efforts of many leaders in psychiatry in the region who have managed to remove bureaucratic hurdles and initiate changes. Such hurdles may be due to administrative inertia, ignorance or simply a lack of political will. These do not change if they go unchallenged. Psychiatrists are generally seen as amiable people who prefer the non-confrontational approach. In some cases this has produced unfortunate results for patients, who themselves are voiceless. In Southeast Asia patient advocacy groups are not strongly placed to influence policy. Any that exist are very much dependent on professionals for leadership. Happily in some countries there is emerging a nascent movement of non-government organizations to give voice to the needs of the disadvantaged.

Southeast Asian countries to a great extent initially depended on Western countries for the training of psychiatrists, but by the end of the twentieth century, the vast majority of specialists were being trained locally. Taking Malaysia as an example, the official approach is to train specialists within the country, then send them for subspecialty training overseas. This gives psychiatrists basic training in the local context, while giving them exposure to international practices.

Sadly, Southeast Asian countries have faced many disasters in recent years, the most notable being the Indian Ocean tsunami of 2004, earthquakes and volcanic eruptions in the Philippines and Java, and the more recent disappearance of the Malaysian Airlines Flight MH 370 with more than 200 people on board. At the time of writing the disappearance of the aircraft still remains an absorbing mystery. Psychiatrists and other mental health workers have had to attend to the mental health needs of those affected in the aftermath of these tragedies. In the process expertise in responding to disasters has been developed among local mental health personnel. This should open up rich areas of research in coming years.

A particularly interesting aspect of mental health services in this region is the role of cultural beliefs about mental illness and their impact on care-giving. Prevalent beliefs about malevolent spirits causing psychiatric disorders, or no-less malevolent neighbors employing charms and black magic to make one sick, make work in mental health care challenging. Southeast Asians move between modern scientific medicine and traditional shamanic treatments quite smoothly. It is not uncommon to find a person with a PhD from a respectable Western university seeking the help of a *bomoh* for his mental health problems, while at the same time taking his psychiatric medications. Culture bound syndromes such as *Amok* and *Latah* have their origin in this region. The term *Koro* is thought to be of Malaysian origin, as are *Amok* and *Latah*.

In this chapter the authors who are themselves practicing psychiatrists trace the history of the development of mental health services in their respective countries and describe the current state of services. They highlight some unique aspects of mental disorders and societal perceptions towards them. It is hoped that this will contribute to the available literature on this important aspect of health care in developing countries.

18

Indonesia

Hervita Diatri and Albert Maramis

Indonesia (van der Kroef, 1951) is the largest archipelagic country in the world, it consists of 17,508 islands that lie between two continents, Asia and Australia, and between two oceans, the Pacific and Indian. Because of this geographical position, Indonesia is also called 'Nusantara', which literally means 'archipelago in between' (Portal Nasional RI, 2010). The total area of Indonesia is 1,919,440 km², which consists of land 1,826,440 km² and water 93,000 km² (Asian Center for the Progress of Peoples, 2007).

According to Ministry of Internal Affairs Regulation number 18/2013 on Code and Data of Government Administration Territory, in 2013 there were 33 provinces, 497 districts/ municipalities (399 districts and 98 municipals), 6,994 sub-districts *(kecamatan)*, 8,309 urban villages *(kelurahan)* and 72,944 rural villages *(desa)* (Ministry of Internal Affairs, 2013).

The population of Indonesia is 237,556,363 according to the 2010 Census (Statistics Indonesia, 2011); males 119,507,580 and females 118,048,783. The three provinces that have the largest populations are West Java (43,021,826), East Java (37,476,011) and Central Java (32,380,687). In the period 2000–2010, the population growth rate was 1.49 per cent per year. The distribution of the population is concentrated in Java (58 per cent) and Sumatera (21 per cent) Islands. The average population density is 124 per km². DKI Jakarta (the capital city of Indonesia) is the province with the highest population density of 14,440 per km², while the lowest density is in West Papua with eight per km².

Indonesia is categorized as a lower-middle-income country with its US$3,563 gross national income per capita in 2012; a significant rise from US$2,200 in 2000 (The World Bank Group, 2014).

From the 2013 Human Development Report, Indonesia's Human Development Index (HDI) value was 0.629 for 2012; this is the medium human development category at 121th rank among 187 countries and territories (UNDP, 2013). In 2011, Indonesia was ranked 124th out of 187 countries. However, comparison of ranks and values with previous reports cannot be made because of differences in underlying data and methods (UNDP, 2013).

Mental health policy

Indonesia's dedicated law for mental health started in colonial times with *Het Reglement op het Krankzinnigenwezen (Stbl. 1897 No. 54)* or The Regulation on the Institutions for the Insane. Based on that regulation, mental hospitals could not receive patients direct from the community, they only received patients from the attorney's office, the police and government institutions with an indication of severe mental disorder.

Twenty years after its independence, Indonesia developed its own mental health law, Law Number 3/1966 on Mental Health. This mental health law contained only 14 articles within seven chapters, and mostly dealt with treatment and hospitalization of people with mental illness (Indonesian Parliament, n.d.a). This mental health law was repealed when Law Number 23 Year 1992 on Health was passed. In the health law there were four articles on mental health that regulated the scope of mental health and service providers, rehabilitation and compulsory treatment (Indonesian Parliament, n.d.b). Unfortunately, government regulations to make this law operational were never developed.

The 1992 Health Law was amended by Law Number 36 Year 2009 on Health. In Chapter IX there are eight articles on mental health (Articles 144–151) that cover the objectives and scope of the mental health programme: whose is the responsibility and what are the responsibilities for public information and education on mental health, treatment of mental illness, rights of people with mental illness including homeless people, and forensic psychiatric examination (Indonesian Parliament, n.d.c). Currently, a new mental health law is being developed as a legislation initiative by the Parliament.

It is interesting to observe that, with their autonomy and special status, Aceh Province had developed their own provincial regulations (*Peraturan Daerah/Perda*, or *Qanun*) on health (Qanun Aceh Nbr. 4/2010). Regulations on mental health were incorporated in that *Qanun*, Chapter XXII, Articles 148–169. The number of articles on mental health in the health *Qanun* was three times the number in the national health law, covering issues like the scope of the mental health programme, duties and responsibilities of the government of Aceh, principles of the mental health service, hospitalization and discharge, referral, mental health facilities, guardianship, and management of persons with mental disorder (Government of Aceh, n.d.).

The first Mental Health Policy was developed in 2001 and stated that a comprehensive and integrated mental health programme would be needed to accomplish the mission to: (a) enhance the mental health state of the individual, family, and community; (b) promote the quality and coverage of mental health services; (c) enhance the community's capacity to maintain their mental health; and (d) promote the professionalism of mental health workers particularly in science and technology, skills, and ethics (Directorate of Community Mental Health, 2001). A new Mental Health Policy is being developed since the first one expired some years ago. A series of initial meetings have been organized and the policy is scheduled to be finalized in 2014.

Psychiatric epidemiology

In 2007, Indonesia for the first time carried out a national survey on mental health. It was a part of the first Basic Health Research that was implemented by the National Institute for Health Research and Development. The Basic Health Research 2007 was a descriptive cross-sectional survey using a sample of households and household members that were identical to other nationwide surveys and censuses. The sample collected consisted of 258,366 households and 987,205 household members. Non-random errors such as the development of new districts, census blocks that were unreachable, missing households, differences in the time of data collection, estimation at district level could not be done for every indicator, and biomedical data that only represent urban census blocks were limitations of this survey. The survey was carried out in twenty-eight provinces in 2007, while the other five provinces (Papua, Papua Barat, Maluku, Maluku Utara and East Nusa Tenggara) were surveyed in August–September 2008, (National Institute of Health Research and Development, 2008).

The survey had two sets of questions on mental health, the first were on severe mental disorders. The national prevalence of severe mental disorder (psychosis/schizophrenia) was 4.6 per thousand, with the provinces of DKI Jakarta (20.3 per thousand), Nanggroe Aceh Darussalam (18.5 per thousand), Sumatera Barat (16.7 per thousand), Nusa Tenggara Barat (9.9 per thousand) and Sumatera Selatan (9.2 per thousand) being the five highest, and Maluku (0.9 per thousand) the lowest.

The second set of questions used the Self Reporting Questionnaire (World Health Organization, 1994), 20 items, to cover mental emotional disorders (depression and anxiety). National prevalence for a mental emotional disorder in the people 15 years old and older was 11.6 per cent. Nanggroe Aceh Darussalam, Sumatera Barat, Riau, Bangka Belitung, DKI Jakarta, Jawa Barat, Jawa Tengah, Jawa Timur, Nusa Tenggara Barat, Nusa Tenggara Timur, Sulawesi Tengah, Sulawesi Selatan, Gorontalo and Papua Barat were the 14 provinces that had prevalences above the national prevalence.

The ten districts/cities that had the highest prevalence of mental emotional disorders were Luwu Timur (South Sulawesi) (33.7 per cent), Manggarai (East Nusa Tenggara) (32.4 per cent), Aceh Selatan (Aceh) (32.1 per cent), Purwakarta (West Java) (32.0 per cent), Belitung Timur (Bangka and Belitung) (31.0 per cent), Banjarnegara (Central Java) (30.5 per cent), Boalemo (Gorontalo) (29.9 per cent), Cirebon (Central Java) (29.9 per cent), Central Aceh (Aceh) (29.6%) and Kota Malang (East Java) (29.6 per cent), while the ten districts/cities with the lowest prevalence were Yahukimo (West Papua) (1.6 per cent), Pulang Pisau (Central Kalimantan) (1.7 per cent), Karimun (Riau Islands) (1.9 per cent), Jayapura (Papua) (1.9 per cent), Sidoarjo (East Java) (1.9 per cent), Tabalong (South Kalimantan) (2.1 per cent), Maluku Tengah (Maluku) (2.4 per cent), Kota Baru (South Kalimantan) (2.4 per cent), Kudus (Central Java) (2.4 per cent) and Muaro Jambi (Jambi) (2.4 per cent).

From the Basic Health Research 2007, it was shown that mental emotional disorders were more prevalent in women, those with low educational level, the unemployed and those in the first quintile of household expenditures.

Treatment gap

As in other developing countries, Indonesia has the problem of a treatment gap. According to WHO documentation, in 2005 the treatment gap (the percentage of people who need treatment but did not receive it for various reasons) for psychotic disorder in West Java was 96.5 per cent; more or less the same as in several areas in India (Director General of Health Services, Ministry of Health, Republic of Indonesia, 2014).

There has been progress in that the Government of Indonesia is going to include in the National Medium-term Development Plan 2015–2019 the target of decreasing the treatment gap by 10 per cent in 2019. It was decided that to meet the indicator there will be two major programmes: community empowerment and improvement of mental health services in health facilities. Community empowerment aims to develop communities that are concerned about mental health, and public campaigns and mental health information through the media, especially electronic media and the internet (Director General of Health Services, Ministry of Health, Republic of Indonesia, 2014).

To improve mental health services in health facilities, Indonesia is following the World Psychiatric Association survey on three major strategies to decrease treatment gaps (Director General of Health Services, Ministry of Health, Republic of Indonesia, 2014):

1. Increase the number of psychiatrists and other mental health professionals;
2. Increase the involvement of well-trained non-specialist mental health service providers; and
3. Increase the active participation of people with mental illness and their families.

The three strategies show that it is not enough to only develop services in hospitals. It is important to develop a community-based mental health service system through development of mental health services in primary care, involvement of consumers, families and community/religious/women leaders as mental health cadres, and development of Mental Health Alert Villages.

The effectiveness of these major strategies has been proven in Aceh, where there was a decrease in the treatment gap for severe mental disorders. Since 2005, the three strategies have been implemented and become a model for community mental health service development in Indonesia. On average, the decrease in the treatment gap is 29 per cent in Aceh Province, the highest in Indonesia, and in several districts it is more than 45 per cent (Aceh Provincial Health Office, 2013).

The treatment gap for common mental disorders is greater. Data from public health centres that are actively delivering mental health services are still very limited, less than 3 per cent of the estimated number of cases, even though mental and emotional disorders like depression cause great disability and burden (Diatri, 2013). Improvement in many areas, like regulation, financing, inter-sectoral collaboration, advocacy, community empowerment, quality of human resources, service development in health facilities and monitoring–evaluation systems is urgently needed. Further discussion of the situation and future plans can be found in the following section.

Mental health service systems

During the colonial Dutch rule, Indonesia (or the Dutch East Indies) set up its first mental hospital. Based on a recommendation by Drs Bauer and Smit and the Governor General's Decree dated 14 May 1867, the construction of Bogor Mental Hospital was started in 1876 and it was opened officially on 1 July 1882. In 1902, the second mental hospital was opened in Lawang, East Java. Then another two were opened in 1923, Magelang and Sabang Mental Hospitals. These were custodial-type hospitals with large capacities, around 1,000–2,000 beds. Sabang Mental Hospital was destroyed during an attack by the Allied Forces in the World War II (Arsawakoi [Indonesian Mental Hospital and Drug Dependence Hospital Association], n.d.).

There were four types of institution for the care of psychiatric patients at that time: The first was the four mental hospitals *(Kranzinnigengestichten)*. Those hospitals were always full, patients could not be discharged and new patients could not be admitted, therefore annex facilities *(Annex inrichtingen)* of the existing mental hospitals were built, as in Semplak (Bogor) in 1931 and in Pasuruan (near Lawang) in 1932. The second was temporary hospitals for acute psychotic patients *(Doorgangshuizen)*. The patients there could be sent home if they were stabilized but would be sent to the mental hospitals if they needed longer treatment. Third was *Verpleegtehuizen*, which literally means nursing home, which functioned like *Doorgangshuizen* but the head was a registered nurse under supervision of a general practitioner. The last was the Colony, a shelter for stabilized psychiatric patients. They lived in people's houses in the community and did farming work in the area, but under supervision. The receiving families were given a 'living allowance' (Maramis and Maramis, 2009).

After independence, in 1966, prevention, treatment and rehabilitation were accepted as the three principles of mental health care. A comprehensive system of mental health services was envisioned involving the existing public health centres (Pusat Kesehatan Masyarakat/Puskesmas), but mental hospitals were still the major player providing in and outpatient services, consultation to other hospitals and public health education. Twenty-two new mental hospitals were established so there were 26 among 31 provinces at that time (Pols, 2006).

In 2000, after changing to a decentralized system, most of the centrally owned mental hospitals were handed over to sub-national governments. Currently, only four mental hospitals and one drug dependence hospital are owned by central government: Dr Marzoeki Mahdi Mental Hospital in Bogor, Dr Soeharto Heerdjan Mental Hospital in Jakarta, Dr Soeroyo Mental Hospital in Magelang, Dr Radjiman Wediodiningrat Mental Hospital in Lawang and the Drug Dependence Hospital (Rumah Sakit Ketergantungan obat/RSKO) in Cibubur (Arsawakoi [Indonesian Mental Hospital and Drug Dependence Hospital Association], n.d.).

After the focus on mental hospitals for a very long time, the role of primary and secondary care in mental health services was very limited. On the other hand, mental hospitals became giant mental health centres and treated the whole spectrum of cases, from those that actually can be treated in primary and secondary care, to specialized and sub-specialized cases. It is understood that such a situation leads to a low quality of services, as can be seen from (Working Group 2 Indonesia Mental Health System Development Taskforce, 2009):

1. Increasing stigma of mental health that resulted in low acceptance of mental health efforts by the community.
2. Limited accessibility and affordability of mental health services that resulted in a high treatment gap and treatment discontinuation.
3. Budget efficiency was difficult to achieve because treatment costs became too expensive as a result of difficulties of accessibility, treatment discontinuity, relapses and readmissions.
4. Low effectiveness, particularly in relation to the ability of patient and family to manage mental health problems at home.
5. Problems in treatment effectiveness and patient safety during hospitalization were another challenge, since the ratio of health workers to patients was not high enough.
6. Hospital-based comprehensive mental health efforts need huge resources, which could not be met because of their low priority.
7. Low quality of service, which has the potential for mistreatment that will drive the patient and family away from the health service.

Based on an understanding of the above problems, several components of the mental health service system have been developed, i.e. a mental health service integrated into the existing health service from primary to tertiary care level, formal and informal community-based mental health services, and a specialized institutional mental health service (Figure 18.1).

Each component of the mental health service system has its own roles and tasks as can be seen in Figure 18.2.

The number of facilities (Table 18.1) is obviously not sufficient and various efforts are needed to solve the lack of quantity before we talk about quality. From the quality aspect, only 58 per cent of mental hospitals have class A national accreditation; among general hospitals, only 43 per cent have been accredited (Directorate General of Health Services, Ministry of Health,

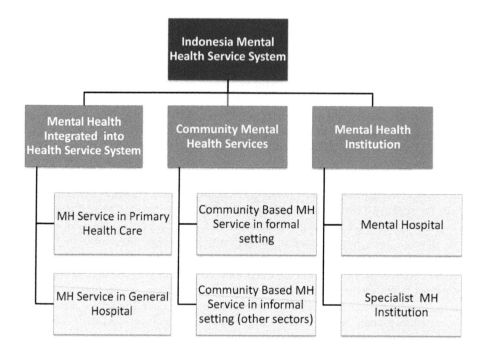

Figure 18.1 Structure of the mental health service system in Indonesia (Directorate of Mental Health, Ministry of Health, Republic of Indonesia, 2008).

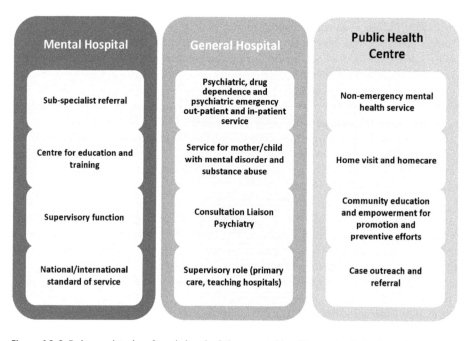

Figure 18.2 Roles and tasks of each level of the mental health service in Indonesia (Mangaweang, 2014).

Table 18.1 Number of mental health facilities in Indonesia (Directorate General of Health Services, Ministry of Health, Republic of Indonesia, 2013; Director General of Health Services, Ministry of Health, Republic of Indonesia, 2014)

Level of service	Number (national)	Number with mental health services	Ratio/ 100,000 population
Public health centre	9,005	2,702 (30%) – 10% are in Aceh	1.13
General hospital (public and private)	1,728	181 (10.5%)	0.08
Specialized hospitals[a]	500	34 (6.8%)	0.01
Mental hospital	47	In 26 of 4 provinces in Indonesia	0.02
Drug dependency hospital	1	In Jakarta (capital city)	

[a] Specialized hospitals provide care for one area or one particular type of disease, based on medical specialties, age groups, organ, or type of disease

Republic of Indonesia, 2013). The effort to integrate services is expected to answer the problems of quantity and quality.

Integration of health services is important in improvement of the quality of the mental health service, because it will be able to (Working Group 2 Indonesia Mental Health System Development Taskforce, 2009):

1. Decrease stigma and increase community acceptance of mental health services.
2. Improve accessibility and affordability.
3. Ensure early detection and prompt intervention and treatment continuity.
4. Overcome the lack of human resources.
5. Increase the chance of a more comprehensive approach in a team including other disciplines.
6. Increase cost effectiveness.

Challenges and obstacles in the process of integration are (Working Group 2 Indonesia Mental Health System Development Taskforce, 2009):

1. Mental health programmes are not a priority. This can be seen in the policies of national, province and local decision-makers, including within health facilities. Mental health is neither in the main programme nor among the main indicators of health development.
2. Different bureaucratic systems between primary care (under the Health Office), general hospitals and mental hospitals.
3. Problems with health workers in the general health service, including low capacity, interest and motivation to deliver mental health management, high workloads and high turnover.
4. Distortion in the community's belief that a mental hospital is the only one able to provide mental health services, and not primary or secondary care. This view sometimes gets affirmation from the allocation of resources (human and infrastructure).
5. The condition of the infrastructure, and that medical supplies, particularly drugs in primary care, are very limited in terms of types and quantity. The unavailability of the same medication in primary care as in the hospital, when patients are back-referred to primary care, forces them to go back to mental hospitals to continue treatment.

Beside a mental health service that is integrated into the general health service, to answer the needs of various community mental health services there are a number of initiatives from the community to develop community-based mental health services. These services can be formal or informal. Examples of community-based mental health service are (Working Group 2 Indonesia Mental Health System Development Taskforce, 2009):

1. Recovery houses for victims of domestic violence.
2. Command posts for psychosocial support for victims of disaster.
3. Shelters for mental health recovery that are medical-, spiritual- or traditional-based.
4. Sheltered workshops.
5. Shelters for the elderly, orphanages and shelters for the psychotic homeless, etc.

It is important to give attention to the development of these forms of community participation. Regulation and supervision are needed because low quality of services and even mistreatment often happens because of ignorance and limited resources.

Another community-based service that has been developed in Indonesia is the Mental Health Alert Village *(Desa Siaga Sehat Jiwa)*. Its programme focuses on promotion and prevention. The Mental Health Alert Village relies on mental health cadres who are supervised by primary care health workers. The cadres are expected to provide early detection and intervention to community members who have mental health problems. In its development, the Mental Health Alert Village, especially in Aceh, has managed to play various roles, such as (Yessi, 2014):

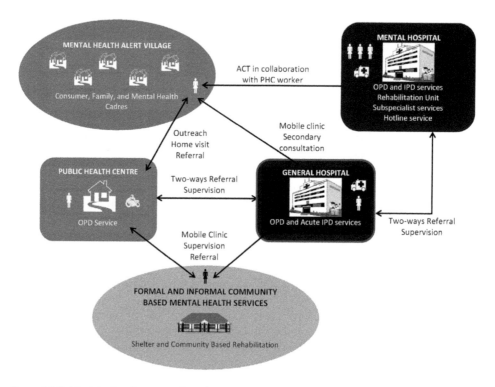

Figure 18.3 Model of an integrated service system in Indonesia

1. Improve knowledge and awareness of mental health problems.
2. Reduce stigma and discrimination towards people with mental illness.
3. Improve the mental health status of the community with existing resources.
4. Increase community capacity for and participation in supporting the recovery process of people with mental disorder.
5. Develop self-help groups and consumer and family organizations for people with mental illness.

Reviewing the existing models of services, an inter-service integration model (Figure 18.3) can be developed by revising the referral system, cooperation agreements, case management systems, mobile clinics and assertive community treatment (ACT) of higher complexity.

Health security system in Indonesia

Until 2013, people's awareness of the importance of having health insurance was low, as shown by the percentage of out-of-pocket health expenditures, which was 75.1 per cent in 2012 (The World Bank, 2014). The risk of catastrophic expenditure in this situation is high, especially for people with severe mental illness who tend to move downwards in their socioeconomic status. Therefore, a good health finance system needs to be developed to share the risks and to protect people (Thabrany, n.d.).

The government of Indonesia, in concurrence with the country's philosophical basis and principles to secure the lives of all citizens, had organized various health insurance schemes to ensure access to quality health service for every citizen. In principle, there were two types of health insurance (Thabrany, n.d.):

1. Health insurance for civil servants, retirees, veterans and private sector employees. The providers are PT Asuransi Kesehatan – ASKES (Persero) and PT Jaminan Sosial Tenaga Kerja – JAMSOSTEK (Persero).
2. Health insurance for the poor and nearly poor through *Jaminan Kesehatan Masyarakat (Jamkesmas)* (National Social Health Insurance) and *Jaminan Kesehatan Daerah (Jamkesda)* (Provincial Social Health Insurance).

Each scheme had its own procedures and policies which made it difficult to monitor and control cost and quality of health services. In addition, there were private health insurance providers; however, their coverage was low (Figure 18.4).

Since the enactment of Law number 40/2004 on National Social Security System (*Sistem Jaminan Sosial Nasional/SJSN*), the government has started to develop a unified National Health Security System (*Jaminan Kesehatan Nasional* – JKN) (Ministry of Health, Republic of Indonesia, 2013a). The law stipulates the application of the social insurance mechanism in five social security programmes: health insurance, work accident insurance, old age pensions, public pensions and life insurance. The aims are to ensure social protection and welfare for all Indonesian citizens, to fulfil their appropriate basic life necessities whenever they have to face problems resulting from loss or reduction of income due to sickness, accidents, losing jobs, old age or reaching pensionable age (National Development Planning Agency, 2013).

On 1 January 2014 the National Health Security System was put in effect. The existing schemes were merged into one national health insurance system, except the local governments' Social Health Insurance schemes that will be merged in a later stage. It is envisioned that universal coverage will be reached by 2019 from the current coverage of 63 per cent of the population

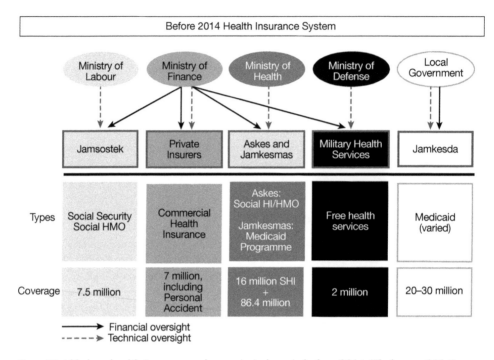

Figure 18.4 Various health insurance schemes in Indonesia before 2014 (Thabrany, 2014)

(about 123 million people). The benefits package is comprehensive including prevention and promotion, primary to tertiary care, out and inpatient services. The benefits package also covers the mental health service (Ministry of Health, Republic of Indonesia, 2013b).

Members who are enrolled in the national social health insurance scheme include everyone who has paid contributions/premiums or for whom they have been paid. Contributions for people below the poverty line are paid by central and/or local government, for formal workers contributions are shared by employees and employer as a percentage of salary/wage, and for informal workers paid as a nominal/flat rate (Mboi, 2013).

For mental health, JKN covers various services including out and inpatient services at primary, secondary and tertiary levels. This could encourage primary and secondary care to provide mental health services. Theoretically, JKN also ensures a better referral system and better drug procurement down to primary care level, although implementation has yet to be observed (Ministry of Health, Republic of Indonesia, 2013c).

In terms of service accountability, the system requires each service provider to develop clinical pathways, service guidelines, and standard operating procedures to ensure quality of service. JKN covers inpatient services for people with disability for up to three months. Potentially, this will facilitate revitalization of the rehabilitation programme in mental hospitals (Ministry of Health, Republic of Indonesia, 2013d).

JKN is only at its early stages, there are issues that need to be addressed, for instance:

1. The payment rate is too low, especially for outpatient services resulting in: (a) service providers having difficulties in using better and newer medicines with lower side-effects and sometimes even having to choose whether to use all the funds for medicine or for laboratory examinations; (b) lower quantities of medicine being prescribed which will force

the patient and family to come back more often to get their prescription refilled. Only schizophrenia, which is considered a chronic disease, can be covered for a one-month supply of medicine (Ministry of Health, Republic of Indonesia, 2013d).

2. Currently, treatment for intoxication, withdrawal and rehabilitation of substance abuse is not covered, because it is seen as an act of deliberate self-harm (Ministry of Health, Republic of Indonesia, 2013d).

3. Homeless people, especially homeless psychotics, and prisoners are not covered by the scheme yet. There should be a better enrolment mechanism for marginalized groups of people, since people with mental disorders are prone to being neglected, living on the streets and involved in criminal acts because of their illness (Ministry of Health, Republic of Indonesia, 2013d). This situation needs a strong intersectoral approach and collaboration that goes beyond service provision alone.

Although there are many things to be improved, the process to deliver quality services has made a good start. The involvement of government, service providers, professional organizations, and consumer and family organizations is very important in the process of monitoring and evaluation, and developing recommendations for the improvement of this new financing system.

Training for the mental health workforce

Human resources in mental health consist of health workers with competency in mental health, such as doctors, psychiatrists, nurses, psychiatric nurses; other professionals, for instance psychologists, social workers, occupational therapists; and other workers that are trained in mental health (Ministry of Health, Republic of Indonesia, 2014).

Data from the Badan Pengembangan dan Pemberdayaan Sumber Daya Manusia Kesehatan (BPPSDM) (2013) showed that the number of doctors in Indonesia was 42,398 (17/100,000 population), there were around 800 psychiatrists (0.33/100,000 population) and nurses numbered 296,126 (123/100,000 population) (Badan Pengembangan dan Pemberdayaan Sumber Daya Manusia Kesehatan (BPPSDM), 2013; Badan Pusat Statistik [Statistics Indonesia], 2012). This number, especially for psychiatrists, is not sufficient to achieve the optimum mental health status for the people of Indonesia. The situation is aggravated by the unequal distribution of health workers, with more than 48 per cent in Java and Bali Islands. The issue is not only about the number, but also the competency and capacity of health workers, which is determined by the quality of training and education.

Teaching of psychiatry in medical education

Until 2010 there were 72 medical study programmes in Indonesia with 5,000 new graduates per year. These study programmes consisted of 31 government and 41 private schools, but only 76 per cent of them were accredited (Konsil Kedokteran Indonesia [Indonesian Medical Council], 2012a). This indicates that medical education is not well-standardized. Based on that, in 2012 the Indonesian Medical Council established two guidelines for medical education organization, the Standard for Medical Professional Education (Standar Pendidikan Profesi Dokter) and the Standard for Indonesian Doctor's Competencies (Standar Kompetensi Dokter Indonesia).

In these standards, the duration of medical education in Indonesia ranges between 10 and 11 semesters, followed by a one-year internship programme (pre-registration training) that consists of eight months in general hospital and four months in public health centres (Konsil Kedokteran

Indonesia [Indonesian Medical Council], 2012b; Kementerian Kesehatan Indonesia, 2010). The content of the curriculum comprises biomedical science, clinical medicine, medical humanities and public health/preventive medicine/community medicine. In the pre-clinical stage (semesters 1–6), psychiatry is included in the modules on empathy and humanities, neuroscience, research, evidence-based medicine, religion and spiritualism, reproductive health, neurology and psychiatry, geriatrics, and growth and development (Konsil Kedokteran Indonesia [Indonesian Medical Council], 2012b). The goal is to have a comprehensive and patient's-needs-oriented medical education.

In the clinical stage, psychiatric teaching varies between three and five weeks. (Konsil Kedokteran Indonesia [Indonesian Medical Council], 2012b). Most of the psychiatric rotation for medical students is done in general hospitals and mental hospitals, only a few centres have it in community service settings. This approach was taken for the reason that there is limited availability of psychiatrists as teachers or tutors, and they are mostly not working in primary care.

As a consequence, students did not get the chance to learn about the mental health problems that they will encounter in primary care settings, in terms of types of cases, types of medicine available and infrastructures. Furthermore, this leads to a feeling of incapability of doctors in primary care to deliver mental health services.

To overcome this, since 2005, starting from a mental health programme for Tsunami survivors in Aceh, some psychiatric training centres have conducted a training programme for doctors in primary care, who are known as 'GP+' after training. The Directorate of Mental Health, Ministry of Health, Republic of Indonesia has developed standard training modules for doctors and nurses. Practically, this is an adaptation of the WHO *mhGAP Intervention Guide* (World Health Organization, 2010). The modules cover screening for mental health problems; diagnostic classification of mental disorders, and recording and reporting systems; depression, anxiety and psychotic disorder; mental disorders of children and adolescents; and dementia. The modules can be adjusted to form a training programme of three to five days according to the needs and capacity of the sub-national government to organize them. The addition of a module on tiered supervision was expected to ensure continuity of the learning process, and increase the motivation and ability of doctors in primary care to provide mental health care.

Training of psychiatrists

Until 2013, training centres for psychiatrists were limited to nine public faculties of medicine with an average number of graduates per year of 39. The number of psychiatrist graduates per year for the last ten years can be seen in Figure 18.5 (Kolegium Psikiatri Indonesia [Indonesian College of Psychiatry], 2013a).

Psychiatric training has eight semesters and ends with the National Board Examination. In order to increase the number of psychiatrists in Indonesia, the government collaborated with the Indonesian College of Psychiatry to develop new training centres and to provide scholarships (national or provincial) for doctors to take psychiatry as their specialization. This effort should be accompanied by promoting psychiatric education to medical students, taking into account that psychiatry is still highly stigmatized, considered not financially promising and is the last choice for specialization (Kolegium Psikiatri Indonesia [Indonesian College of Psychiatry], 2013b).

Psychiatry sub-specialization training

Up to 2013 there was only one sub-specialization training programme in Indonesia, the child and adolescent psychiatry training programme in the Department of Psychiatry, Faculty of

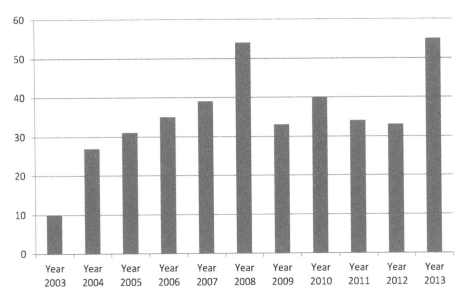

Figure 18.5 Number of graduates from the psychiatric training programme in Indonesia per year in the last 10 years (2003–2013)

Medicine, University of Indonesia. This sub-specialization training began in 1976 and has 39 graduates in all of Indonesia; certainly this is still a small number and the programme needs to be developed further (Department of Psychiatry, Faculty of Medicine, University of Indonesia, 2013).

Because of the great need for sub-specialist consultants in psychiatry to develop the teaching in training centres and expand the sub-specialization, in 2011 the Indonesian College of Psychiatry took the decision to acknowledge and formalize the sub-specialists title for psychiatrist consultants from training centres who met criteria based on their interest and track record in a specific area of sub-specialization and peer evaluation. This was a one-time decision to kick-start a process of developing sub-specialization training programmes.

After the first batch of sub-specialist consultants in psychiatry, a number of four-semester training curriculums have been developed for sub-specialization in geriatric psychiatry, forensic psychiatry, addiction psychiatry and medical psychotherapy (Department of Psychiatry, Faculty of Medicine, University of Indonesia, 2013).

Nursing education

Most of the nurses in Indonesia are general nurses with an academy level of nursing education (Diploma 3/D3). Since the year 2000, nursing education in Indonesia aims for higher levels, from D3 (academy) to doctorate level.

It has been estimated that in 2020 the need will be for one million nurses in Indonesia, so that in the next six years Indonesia has to produce more than 700,000 nurses. This has led to the establishment of many new nursing schools, but there are still only 100,000 academy and bachelor graduates of nursing per year.

In 2010 there were 288 nursing academies providing D3 level (academy) nursing education, 77.2 per cent of them were in Java and Sumatera Islands, and only 17 per cent of them were

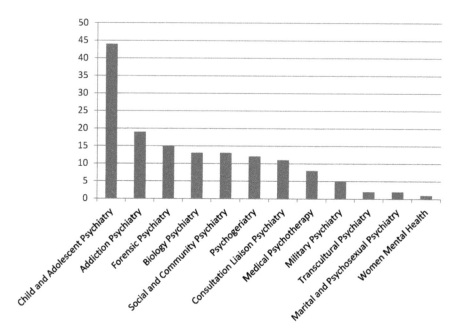

Figure 18.6 Number of psychiatric sub-specialist consultants in Indonesia in 2013 (Kolegium Psikiatri Indonesia [Indonesian College of Psychiatry], 2013c)

accredited. A similar picture could be seen in bachelor level nursing training. Only one of 308 centres had grade A accreditation (Directorate General of Higher Education, Ministry of Education and Culture, Republic of Indonesia (Direktorat Jenderal Pendidikan Tinggi Kementerian Pendidikan dan Kebudayaan RI), 2010). This raises questions about the quality of nursing graduates. Therefore, in 2010, the Ministry of Education in collaboration with the Indonesian Nursing Association developed a Standard of Education and a Standard of Competencies for Nurses.

The six-semester education for D3 nursing stresses the achievement of competency in nursing care of patients with psychosocial problems and patients with mental disorders. The competencies to be achieved are the ability to conduct a nursing assessment, formulate a nursing diagnosis, develop a nursing plan, implement various therapy modalities (stress management, supportive psychotherapy, health education, etc.), carry out collaborative work, carry out a nursing evaluation and create a nursing record (Politeknik Kesehatan III Kementerian Kesehatan RI [Health Polytechnic III, Ministry of Health, Republic of Indonesia], 2013/2014).

The bachelor degree in nursing (Strata 1/S1) is ten semesters and within its programme are materials related to mental health: nursing for adult patients, concept of self, stress and coping, disaster management, nursing for child patients, nursing for elderly patients and nursing for urban health problems. For the master's in nursing programme (Strata 2/S2), mental health is offered as an elective topic in the special interest programme. There are four study programmes that provide a master's in nursing, three of which are in Java.

Nurse specialist in mental health is a two-semester specialization programme after achieving a master's in nursing (S2). Competencies for its graduates are the ability to deliver advanced nursing care for advanced mental health nursing cases, to supervise general nurses and to develop knowledge and services in Indonesia. There are only three study programmes for nurse specialists in mental health, all in Java and Sumatera with ten new graduates per year in total. To overcome this, a huge investment in budgets and time is needed (Faculty of Nursing, University of Indonesia, 2013).

Considering the scale of mental health problems in the community, the fact that more than 50 per cent of nurses are in primary care, the insufficient quality and quantity of mental health education during formal training, and the high cost of further education in mental health, there is a great need for additional training in mental health for nurses, especially those who are working in primary care so they can provide nursing care in the community.

After 2005, in the aftermath of the Aceh Tsunami, a special training course on community mental health nursing was developed (basic, intermediate and advanced levels). Topics given in this course are community mental health nursing; communication in the mental health nursing service; community organization; disaster and crisis intervention; nursing care for children with violent behaviour and depression; nursing care for adult patients with social withdrawal, hallucination, delusion, violent behaviour, low self-esteem, suicidal behaviour and self-care deficit; nursing care for elderly patients with depression and dementia; recording and reporting; and monitoring and evaluation. One interesting aspect of this training model is the system of tiered supervision done by local facilitators, health offices and central facilitators. This supervision system ensures quality and continuity of knowledge and skills acquired from the training. Currently, more than 1,500 primary care nurses have been trained in 18 provinces in Indonesia (Kelompok Keilmuan Keperawatan Jiwa FIK-UI, Forum Komunikasi Keperawatan Jiwa Jakarta, Direktorat Kesehatan Jiwa Masyarakat Depkes RI, Direktorat Keperawatan Depkes RI, WHO, 2005).

Other mental health workers that have to be considered as the result of the training of community mental health nurses are mental health cadres. Ideally, each public health centre has at least two community mental health nurses and each nurse has to train and supervise 10–15 mental health cadres. Mental health cadres are resources within the community (community, religious and women leaders, consumers and families) for health-promotion and prevention activities. The presence of mental health cadres is the start of the development of Mental Health Alert Villages (Keliat, 2014).

The scope of the work of mental health cadres covers early detection, community (including consumer and families) mobilization to participate in mental health education and rehabilitation activities, home visits to patients who are independent, case referral to public health centres, and recording of activities and development of the mental health condition of patients (Desa Siaga Sehat Jiwa [Mental Health Alert Village], 2013; Suparyanto, 2011).

Peoples' perceptions about mental disorder according to traditional, cultural and spiritual values and beliefs

There is little research on traditional, cultural and spiritual views on the cause of mental illness in Indonesia, but there are a number of studies on mental disorders in disaster-affected communities or on restrained or confined people with mental illness, which show us that a cultural and spiritual aspect was the background to that treatment. Another indication is the popularity of traditional or faith-based healing shelters for people with mental disorders.

In a study by the Department of Psychiatry, Faculty of Medicine, University of Indonesia – Ciptomangunkusumo Hospital in Garut District, West Java, after the earthquake of 2009, people associated symptoms of mental disorders mostly with severe mental illness, i.e. schizophrenia; only a few understood that depression and anxiety are also mental disorders. According to the people of Garut, causes of mental illness are life problems, illicit substances, birth-related defects, accidents and also inbreeding. Other causes are supernatural forces, witchcraft, lack of faith or belief in God and the sins of the family. These causes are not different from what Kline saw in the people of Indonesia in 1963 (Diatri and Maramis, 2009; Kline, 1963).

Because of this kind of understanding, people with mental disorders are not brought to health facilities to get treatment. The first thing that people do is take care of the person with mental disorder by themselves, including hiding them in their house (shut in a room or in temporary restraint or confinement). This will go on for a minimum of two weeks. If the family cannot handle the patient anymore, they will bring him or her to traditional or religious healers (Diatri and Maramis, 2009).

These traditional and religious healers use various methods, most of them involve prayer, verses from holy scripts, mantras, advice and herbal remedies; but a few of them also mix these methods with medication.

Other research from the Department of Psychiatry, FMUI, in a traditional shelter for the mentally ill in Bekasi, West Java, in 2013, revealed that families bring a member who has a mental disorder to a traditional healer for various reasons, including when medical treatment is not affordable or perceived as not bringing substantial improvement to the patient. From this we can see that, not only do traditional beliefs and methods cause treatment delay, but like a circle, traditional methods are also chosen as the last resort whenever it is felt that medical treatment is not helping (Rossalina, 2014).

The research in Bekasi also showed that more than 70.4 per cent of the clients in the shelter were not from Bekasi, some of them were even from other islands. It will be interesting to study further the reasons why families brought a person so far away from home to seek 'treatment'. Will this lead to the inability of families to take care of the patient when he or she comes home? (Pitawati, 2014).

Most of the clients in Bekasi (43.3 per cent) had stayed in the shelter for more than one year. Their family stated that the condition of the family member had much improved and that they did not look as slow as they did when still on medication. On the other hand, people with mental disorders who were in the shelter said that they did not receive mental health services for their illness, moreover they developed physical health problems like skin disease and diarrhoea because of the poor living conditions in the shelter (Pitawati, 2014).

When traditional healing practices were not helping and the condition of the person with mental disorder did not improve or caused disturbance to the community, then the case was brought to village officers (the village chief or security personnel). The decision of village officers varied, some suggested that the patient should be brought back to the traditional/religious healer, some suggested bringing the patient to primary health care facilities or hospital. The role of the village officer in accessing health services is important, especially to get coverage by the health insurance scheme for the poor. This help is very significant according to families, because they are always worried about the costs related to medical services. The initial management of people with mental disorder by the community is depicted in Figure 18.7 (Diatri and Maramis, 2009).

Research by Rahardjanti in 2006 showed that the time to get psychiatric treatment for a first psychotic episode on average was 32.53 weeks (SD 47.26). This was an improvement on the 77.47 weeks in 1992. The research also revealed that only 10 per cent of the research participants went directly to the mental health services and more than 60 per cent chose traditional and religious healers. The most common reason for this was families considering mental disorder happened because of spirits or supernatural reasons. More than 60 per cent of families stated that they have negative feelings towards the psychiatric service, they were worried about the electric shock method or they did not want the patient to be with other persons with mental disorder (Rahardjanti, 2006).

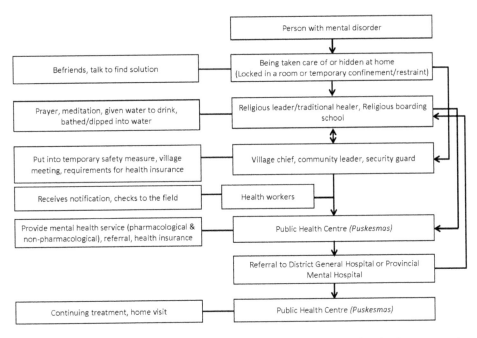

Figure 18.7 Initial management pathway for people with mental disorders in the community in Indonesia (Diatri and Maramis, 2009)

In Indonesia there is less stigma toward mental illness compared with other Asian countries (Kline, 1963). Maltreatment of people with mental disorder happened not because of stigma but because of lack of knowledge and wrong perceptions about the cause and ways to handle the problem. Research in Garut supported this and found that the community actually felt sorry for the patient and wanted to help, but did not know how to, especially when the person with mental illness did something dangerous (Diatri and Maramis, 2009).

The consequence was that if the person was not disturbing or troubling their surroundings, the community usually kept quiet; but whenever the person showed strange, disturbing or aggressive behaviour, then friends, neighbours, police or doctors would insist on bringing the person to a health facility; this is in accordance with Law Number 36/2009 on Health. Another concrete form of the community's help is a pool of voluntary contribution village funds that are used to help with transportation costs to hospital, the cost of home care, or as initial capital for income-generating activities by a person recovering from mental illness. This community initiative was incorporated by Ministry of Internal Affairs Decree on Alert Village, which has mental health in its programmes (see the section on the mental health service system in Indonesia) (Diatri and Maramis, 2009; Rahardjanti, 2006).

Improving access to health services and increasing understanding of mental illness by the community will influence health-seeking behaviour, treatment compliance and satisfaction with services. The enhancement of knowledge of families, village officers, health cadres, religious leaders, community leaders, women leaders and health workers is very important in primary health care. Together with quality improvement of mental health services, people's acceptance of mental health services will increase compared with traditional approaches, the effectiveness of which has not been proved and often violates the rights of people with mental disorders.

Special issues for psychiatry in Indonesia

This section will cover two issues: the development of the mental health system in Aceh in the aftermath of the 2004 Tsunami and the *Pasung*-Free Indonesia Programme.

Aceh mental health system development after the Tsunami

The Province of Aceh (previously Nanggroe Aceh Darussalam) has a population of 4,597,300 in a 56,770.81 km² land area. It has 23 Districts (18 *Kabupaten*/Regency and 5 *Kota*/City) and 289 Sub-districts *(Kecamatan)* (Pemerintah Provinsi Aceh, 2014).

Aceh suffered from more than 30 years of conflict between the Free Aceh Movement (*Gerakan Aceh Merdeka/GAM*) and the Indonesian military. According to official estimates, more than 30,000 people died as a result. A peace agreement on 15 August 2005 ended this long conflict.

Mental health service delivery prior to the Tsunami was done only through the province's sole mental hospital, located in the capital city of Banda Aceh. This mental hospital was institutional in nature, with one part-time and two full-time psychiatrists. It had 220 beds, with the occupancy rate usually exceeding 100 per cent. Public Health Centres (primary care) and District General Hospitals (secondary care) had limited to non-existent capacity to deliver mental health services. People had to pay out-of-pocket for the health care received.

The Tsunami of 26 December 2004 caused around 165,000 casualties and close to 400,000 people were displaced. Fifty-three of the province's 244 health facilities were destroyed or severely incapacitated.

More than 100 local and international agencies arrived in Aceh. They offered a wide range of mental health and psychosocial support services of different qualities. Their presence helped create new awareness and demand within the population for community-based mental health care. However, the vast majority of agencies planned to stay only through the initial emergency period and most had nothing planned to ensure that care would continue in the longer term. After they left, there would be gaps in services and support.

The Ministry of Health Indonesia and the World Health Organization provided leadership to develop sustainable community-based mental health services. Specific actions were based on WHO's Recommendations for Mental Health in Aceh (World Health Organization, 2005).

The overall objective was to integrate mental health into the province's primary health care (PHC) system. The programme would rely on community mental health nurses to deliver mental health care.

Training modules were developed for nurses and for doctors in primary care. The task for nurses in the community was to provide nursing intervention in the community. A team from the Faculty of Nursing, University of Indonesia, led by Budi Anna Keliat, developed a three-level training approach: Basic (care for people with severe mental disorder), Intermediate (work with the community) and Advanced (prevention and promotion). The Ministry of Health and the Department of Psychiatry, Faculty of Medicine, University of Indonesia developed a training module for doctors on primary care psychiatry (Prasetiyawan *et al.*, 2006).

Initially, training and supervision were implemented in the 11 most-affected districts of Aceh. Ten PHCs were selected from each district, each of which chose two nurses for training. A total of 110 PHCs and 220 nurses participated. These nurses were responsible for providing mental health services in their communities (Maramis, 2006).

WHO supported the Government of Indonesia in initiating the programme and funded the initial round of training. The Asian Development Bank (ADB) and the United States Agency for International Development (USAID) joined in to help in this development of community-based mental health services. CBM, an international non-governmental organization, supported training for community-based mental health services in five districts of Aceh and also collaborated with district health offices to develop sustainable PHC-based mental health services in those areas (World Health Organization, 2013).

The Norwegian Red Cross, the Asian Development Bank (ADB) and WHO advocated open wards, instead of locked wards in Banda Aceh Mental Hospital. A pilot project showed the applicability of this approach. The management of Banda Aceh Mental Hospital conducted short-term training programmes for their doctors and nurses.

In Jantho General Hospital in the District of Aceh Besar, the first psychiatric acute care unit was established with USAID-supported construction and staff training and ADB-funded training module development. This unit delivers short-term care for people with severe mental disorders who cannot be treated in the community because of the severity of their symptoms. The goal is to stabilize them and then refer them back to their PHC. This is a model for providing acute inpatient mental health care in a district general hospital. Two other inpatient units were established subsequently: (1) in Cut Nyak Dien General Hospital in Meulaboh, West Aceh, with support from CBM, this unit covers the west coast of Aceh; and (2) in Datu Beru General Hospital in Takengon, Central Aceh, this was an initiative by the local government to cover the central region of Aceh (World Health Organization, 2013).

Currently, mental health services are available in 90.4 per cent of the 302 public health centres in Aceh, with 136 GP+ (doctors who have been trained in mental health) and 491 community mental health nurses. The number of mental health trained doctors and community mental health nurses decreased quite substantially because some of them had already left. On the other hand, since 2007 the number of Mental Health Alert Villages increased three-fold to 1,049 (15.5 per cent of all villages) and the number of mental health cadres increased two times (5,735 persons). Aceh now has 14 psychiatrists with six out of 23 general hospitals providing acute psychiatric beds (Government of Aceh, Provincial Health Office, 2013).

Pasung-Free Indonesia Programme

The practice of *pasung* towards people with mental illness can be found all over Indonesia. '*Pasung*' in the Indonesian language refers to the physical restraint or confinement of 'criminals, crazy and dangerously aggressive people' (Broch, 2001). In its development, the term *pasung* was narrowed down to those with mental disorders in the community. Furthermore, *pasung* is not only about physical freedom but also something to do with right to access health services that will improve the function of people with mental disorder.

A number of studies in Indonesia have shown that the act of *pasung* was initiated by families to protect the patient, family and community from the violent behaviour of people with severe mental disorder (schizophrenia); most of them are 20–30 years old, male, with the duration of being in *pasung* between a few days to more than 20 years. More than 76 per cent of them had once been in contact with the health service but could not continue their treatment for various reasons, one of which was low quality of the health service (Minas and Diatri, 2008; Puteh *et al.*, 2011).

Acknowledging the impact of *pasung* on physical, occupational, social and humanitarian aspects of care, the government of Indonesia announced the *Pasung*-Free Indonesia Programme (*Program Indonesia Bebas Pasung*) on World Mental Health Day, 10 October 2010. This programme was meant to free people with mental disorder from the act of *pasung*, and to prevent *pasung* and re-*pasung* (Directorate of Mental Health, Ministry of Health, Republic of Indonesia, 2010).

Table 18.2 Actions to achieve *Pasung*-Free Indonesia

1. Protecting the rights of people with mental disorder	• Study and review current international and national laws and regulations, like the Human Rights Law 1999 and the Health Law 2009 • Support the establishment of a Mental Health Law (currently at the stage of final review between parliament and the government of Indonesia) • Advocate local legislation, like provincial regulations, governors' orders, and mayor/head of districts' orders • Develop national and sub-national policy, guidelines and standards

2. Increasing the knowledge and skill of mental health stakeholders	• Advocacy to stakeholders in mental health
	• Increase knowledge and capacity of stakeholders on mental health and *pasung* issues
	• Increase capacity of health workers in:
	  a. Promotion of mental health and prevention, early detection and intervention of mental disorders
	  b. Case outreach
	  c. Management of mental disorders, including psychiatric emergencies
	  d. Management of mental disorders in the community
	  e. The referral system
	  f. Rehabilitation (physical, psychological and social)
	• Develop cascade supervision from tertiary, secondary and primary care levels

3. Increasing the quality of mental health services at all levels	• Develop two-way reporting and service provision for *pasung* cases, involving the community and all levels of services • Build mental health services at primary care level in the form of mental health clinics, home visits, community-based rehabilitation, educational programmes, prevention of mental disorder and promotion of mental health programmes • Develop mental health services at secondary level in the form of acute psychiatric units in general hospitals • Develop a comprehensive mental health service with physical rehabilitation at tertiary level and community mental health outreach (mobile clinics) • Develop two-way referral systems • Develop infrastructure and supplies, including medications, at each level of service
4. Providing sufficient financing for the mental health programme	• Map and utilize various funding resources, either from government or non-government, central or local sources, for mental health programmes • List the main services, like home visits and referral, as a basis of prioritizing funds allocation • Calculate unit costs to determine the amount of the financing package

Table 18.2 continued

	• Optimally utilize national social health insurance for mental health • Gather community funds as a form of solidarity with people with mental disorder
5. Increasing cross-sectoral and cross-programme collaboration and coordination in mental health	• Map the role of each sector and programme in the *Pasung*-Free Programme • Conduct planned and continuous advocacy • Develop and revitalize mental health working groups at national, province and district levels • Develop collaboration agreements with various partners • Provide opportunities for all stakeholders to collaborate under the government's coordination
6. Empowering consumers, families and the community in the mental health effort	• Collaborate with the media to provide access to information • Train community, religious and women leaders, and health cadres, including consumers and families to become mental health cadres • Develop Mental Health Alert Villages that have programmes for promotion and prevention (early detection and early intervention for emergencies), recording and reporting, and community-based rehabilitation • Develop self-help groups and consumers' and families' organizations • Empower consumers and families in planning and monitoring the *Pasung*-Free Programme
7. Increasing research, monitoring and evaluation in the mental health programme	• Develop recording and reporting systems to prevent double entry of data • Develop the capacity of cadres and health workers in recording and reporting • Improve the capacity of cadres and health workers in conducting research to identify and solve problems

The goals will be achieved through various actions (Table 18.2) (Directorate of Mental Health, Ministry of Health, Republic of Indonesia, 2010; Directorate of Mental Health, Ministry of Health, Republic of Indonesia, 2011; Diatri *et al.*, 2012).

Since its launch, 23 of 33 provinces in Indonesia have been implementing the *Pasung*-Free Programme. Approximately 35.5 per cent of *pasung* cases in the community have been found and 82.6 per cent of them have been managed appropriately. Provinces with stronger community mental health programmes have higher achievement rates compared with those that are focused on facility-based services (mental hospitals) (Directorate of Mental Health, Ministry of Health, Republic of Indonesia, 2014).

Currently, the focus is mainly on case finding and case management, but later it should be on the continuity of this programme. The *Pasung*-Free Indonesia Programme is an important entry point for developing a better mental health system in Indonesia.

References

Aceh Provincial Health Office, 2013. *Mental Health Database*. Banda Aceh: Aceh Provincial Health Office.

Arsawakoi [Indonesian Mental Hospital and Drug Dependence Hospital Association], n.d. *Sejarah RSJ dan RSKO [History of Mental Hospital and Drug Dependency Hospital]*. [Online] Available at: http://arsawakoi.wordpress.com/sekilas-info-2/sekilas-info/ [Accessed 17 March 2014].

Asian Center for the Progress of Peoples, 2007. *Indonesia Country Profile*. [Online] Available at: www.acpp.org/uappeals/cprofile/Indo%20Country%20Profile.pdf [Accessed 16 February 2014].

Badan Pengembangan dan Pemberdayaan Sumber Daya Manusia Kesehatan (BPPSDM) [Board for the Development and Empowerment of Human Resources for Health], 2013. *Data Bank Badan PPSDM*. [Online] Available at: http://bppsdmk.depkes.go.id [Accessed 12 April 2014].

Badan Pusat Statistik [Statistics Indonesia], 2012. *Badan Pusat Statistik*. [Online] Available at: www.bps.go.id [Accessed 12 April 2014].

Broch, H. B., 2001. The villagers' reactions towards craziness: an Indonesian example. *Transcultural Psychiatry*, 38(3), 275–305.

Department of Psychiatry, Faculty of Medicine, University of Indonesia, 2013. *Kurikulum Pendidikan Program Spesialis-2 [Curriculum of Specialist-2 Education Programme]*. Jakarta: Department of Psychiatry, FMUI.

Desa Siaga Sehat Jiwa [Mental Health Alert Village], 2013. *Desa Siaga Sehat Jiwa Blogspot*. [Online] Available at: http://desasiagasehatjiwa.blogspot.com/2013/12/materi-kader-dan-kader-kesehatan-jiwa.html [Accessed 17 April 2014].

Diatri, H., 2013. *Tebet Public Health Centre Database 2009–2010*. Jakarta.

Diatri, H. and Maramis, A., 2009. *Garut Earthquake Survivors Need Assessment: Qualitative Report*. Jakarta: Department of Psychiatry, Faculty of Medicine, University of Indonesia.

Diatri, H. *et al.*, 2012. *Pasung Free Indonesia Program Log Frame*. Melbourne (Victoria).

Directorate General of Health Services, Ministry of Health, Republic of Indonesia, 2013. *Hospital Online Database*. [Online] Available at: http://202.70.136.52/rsonline/report/report_by_catrs.php [Accessed 27 April 2014].

Director General of Health Services, Ministry of Health, Republic of Indonesia, 2014. *Mental Health Development Plan: Challenges and Solutions*. Bandung: Third Community Psychiatry National Conference, 27 March 2014.

Directorate General of Higher Education, Ministry of Education and Culture, Republic of Indonesia (Direktorat Jenderal Pendidikan Tinggi Kementerian Pendidikan dan Kebudayaan RI), 2010. *Potret Ketersediaan dan Kebutuhan Tenaga Perawat [Portrait of the Availability and Needs of Nurses]*. Jakarta: Kementerian Pendidikan dan Kebudayaan RI.

Directorate of Community Mental Health, 2001. *National Mental Health Policy 2001–2005*. Jakarta: Department of Health, Republic of Indonesia.

Directorate of Mental Health, Ministry of Health, Republic of Indonesia, 2008. *Structure of Mental Health System in Indonesia*. Jakarta.

Directorate of Mental Health, Ministry of Health, Republic of Indonesia, 2010. *Pasung Free Indonesia Program Roadmap*. Bogor (West Java).

Directorate of Mental Health, Ministry of Health, Republic of Indonesia, 2011. *Guideline of Pasung Free Program*. Jakarta.

Directorate of Mental Health, Ministry of Health, Republic of Indonesia, 2014. *Pasung Free Baseline Data*. Jakarta.

Faculty of Nursing, University of Indonesia, 2013. *Buku Panduan Pendidikan [Education Guide]*. Jakarta: Faculty of Nursing.

Government of Aceh, Provincial Health Office, 2013. *Mental Health Data*. Banda Aceh.

Government of Aceh, n.d. *Qanun Aceh Nomor 4 Tahun 2010 [Aceh Provincial Regulation Nbr 4 Year 2010]*. [Online] Available at: www.bphn.go.id/data/documents/10pdaceh004.pdf [Accessed 15 August 2011].

Indonesian Parliament, n.d.a. *DPR-RI Undang-Undang*. [Online] Available at: www.dpr.go.id/uu/uu1966/UU_1966_3.pdf [Accessed 4 March 2014].

Indonesian Parliament, n.d.b. *Undang-Undang Nomor 23 Tahun 1992 tentang Kesehatan [Law Nbr 23 Year 1992 on Health]*. [Online] Available at: www.dpr.go.id/id/undang-undang/1992/23/uu/KESEHATAN [Accessed 4 March 2014].

Indonesian Parliament, n.d.c. *Undang-Undang Nomor 36 Tahun 2009 tentang Kesehatan [Law Nbr 36 Year 2009 on Health]*. [Online] Available at: www.dpr.go.id/id/undang-undang/2009/36/uu/KESEHATAN [Accessed 10 March 2014].

Keliat, B. A., 2014. *Community Mental Health Nursing Programme in Aceh and Indonesia* [Interview]. (April 2014).

Kelompok Keilmuan Keperawatan Jiwa FIK-UI, Forum Komunikasi Keperawatan Jiwa Jakarta, Direktorat Kesehatan Jiwa Masyarakat Depkes RI, Direktorat Keperawatan Depkes RI, WHO, 2005. *Basic Course on Community Mental Health Nurse Module*. Jakarta.

Kementerian Kesehatan Indonesia, 2010. *Peraturan Menteri Kesehatan Nomor 299 Tahun 2010 tentang Penyelenggaraan Program Internsip dan Penempatan Dokter Pasca Internsip [Minister of Health Decree Nbr 299 Year 2010 on Internship Programme and Deployment of Doctors Post-Internship]*. [Online] Available at: http://hukor.depkes.go.id/up_prod_permenkes/PMK%20No.%20299%20ttg%20Penyelenggaraan%20Program%20Internsip%20dan%20Penempatan%20Dokter%20Pasca%20Internsip.pdf [Accessed 14 April 2014].

Kline, N. S., 1963. Psychiatry in Indonesia. *The American Journal of Psychiatry,* 119, 809–15.

Kolegium Psikiatri Indonesia [Indonesian College of Psychiatry], 2013a. *Data Lulusan*, Jakarta: Kolegium Psikiatri Indonesia.

Kolegium Psikiatri Indonesia [Indonesian College of Psychiatry], 2013b. *Kurikulum Pendidikan Dokter Spesialis Kedokteran Jiwa Indonesia [Curriculum for the Training of Psychiatrists in Indonesia]*. Jakarta: Kolegium Psikiatri Indonesia.

Kolegium Psikiatri Indonesia [Indonesian College of Psychiatry], 2013c. *Consultant Database,* Jakarta: Kolegium Psikiatri Indonesia.

Konsil Kedokteran Indonesia [Indonesian Medical Council], 2012a. *Standar Kompetensi Dokter Indonesia [Standard of Indonesian Doctor's Competencies]*. [Online] Available at: http://www.kki.go.id/assets/data/arsip/SKDI_Perkonsil,_11_maret_13.pdf [Accessed 1 April 2013].

Konsil Kedokteran Indonesia [Indonesian Medical Council], 2012b. *Standar Pendidikan Profesi Dokter [Standard of Education for Medical Profession]*. [Online] Available at: www.kki.go.id/assets/data/arsip/Final_SPPDI,_21_Maret_2013.pdf [Accessed 1 April 2013].

Mangaweang, L., 2014. *Government Policy Related to Mental Health Services in General Hospital*. Bandung: Third Community Psychiatry National Conference, 26 March 2014.

Maramis, A., 2006. After the Tsunami, building back for better mental health in Aceh. *ASEAN Journal of Psychiatry,* 7(1), pp. 45–8.

Maramis, W. F. and Maramis, A. A., 2009. *Catatan Ilmu Kedokteran Jiwa [Lecture Notes on Psychiatry]*. 2nd ed. Surabaya: Airlangga University Press.

Mboi, N., 2013. *Moving Towards Universal Health Coverage in Indonesia*. Jakarta: Ministry of Health, Republic of Indonesia.

Minas, H. and Diatri, H., 2008. Pasung: Physical restraint and confinement of the mentally ill in the community. *International Journal of Mental Health Systems,* 2, 8.

Ministry of Health, Republic of Indonesia, 2013a. *Buku Pegangan Sosialisasi Jaminan Kesehatan Nasional (JKN) dalam Sistem Jaminan Sosial*. Jakarta: Ministry of Health, Republic of Indonesia.

Ministry of Health, Republic of Indonesia, 2013b. *Buku Pegangan Sosialisasi Jaminan Kesehatan Nasional (JKN) dalam Sistem Jaminan Sosial [Handbook for the Socialization of National Health Insurance Programme]*. Jakarta: Ministry of Health, Republic of Indonesia.

Ministry of Health, Republic of Indonesia, 2013c. *Ministry of Health Regulation Nbr 69 Year 2013 on Standard Tariffs of Health Services at Primary and Referral Level in the Implementation of Health Insurance Program*. Jakarta: Ministry of Health, Republic of Indonesia.

Ministry of Health, Republic of Indonesia, 2013d. *Ministry of Health Regulation Nbr 71 Year 2013 on Health Service in National Social Health Insurance [Peraturan Menteri Kesehatan Republik Indonesia Nomor 71 Tahun 2013 tentang Pelayanan Kesehatan pada Jaminan Kesehatan Nasional]*. Jakarta: Ministry of Health, Republic of Indonesia.

Ministry of Health, Republic of Indonesia, 2014. *Daftar Isian Masalah Rancangan Undang-Undang Kesehatan Jiwa [Problem List of the Draft of Mental Health Law]*. Jakarta: Ministry of Health, Republic of Indonesia

Ministry of Internal Affairs, 2013. *Buku Induk Kode Data Wilayah 2013 [Area Data Code Registry 2013]*. [Online] Available at: www.kemendagri.go.id/pages/data-wilayah [Accessed 2 March 2014].

National Development Planning Agency, 2013. *Social Protection Policy and the Development of Health Security Payer Agency*. Jakarta: National Development Planning Agency.

National Institute of Health Research and Development, 2008. *Report on National Basic Health Research (Riskesdas) 2007*. Jakarta: The National Institute of Health Research and Development, Ministry of Health, Republic of Indonesia.

Pemerintah Provinsi Aceh, 2014. *Pemerintah Provinsi Aceh: Geografis*. [Online] Available at: http:// acehprov.go.id/index.php/profil/read/2014/01/30/11/geografis-aceh.html [Accessed 10 April 2014].

Pitawati, D., 2014. *Health and Dependency Status Profile of Galuh Foundation's Clients December 2013–January 2014*. Jakarta: Department of Psychiatry, Faculty of Medicine, University of Indonesia.

Politeknik Kesehatan III Kementerian Kesehatan RI [Health Polytechnic III, Ministry of Health, Republic of Indonesia], 2013/2014. *Program Praktik Keperawatan Jiwa II [Mental Health Nursing II Practice Programme]*. Politeknik Kesehatan III Kementerian Kesehatan RI.

Pols, H., 2006. The development of psychiatry in Indonesia: From colonial to modern times. *International Review of Psychiatry,* 18(4), 363–70.

Portal Nasional RI, 2010. *The Geography of Indonesia*. [Online] Available at: www.indonesia.go.id/en/ indonesia-glance/geography-indonesia [Accessed 16 February 2014].

Prasetiyawan, P., Viora, E., Maramis, A. and Keliat, B. A., 2006. Mental health model of care programmes after the Tsunami in Aceh, Indonesia. *International Review of Psychiatry,* 18(6), 559–62.

Puteh, I., Marthoenis, M. and Minas, H., 2011. Aceh Free Pasung: Releasing the mentally ill from physical restraint. *International Journal of Mental Health Systems,* 5, 10.

Rahardjanti, N. W., 2006. *Duration of Psychiatric Health Seeking Behaviour in First Episode Psychotic Patients*. Jakarta: Department of Psychiatry, Faculty of Medicine, University of Indonesia.

Rossalina, 2014. *Galuh Foundation Capacity Building Need Assessment: Qualitative Report*. Jakarta: Department of Psychiatry, Faculty of Medicine, University of Indonesia.

Statistics Indonesia, 2011. *Sensus Penduduk 2010 [Indonesian Census 2010]*. [Online] Available at: http://sp2010.bps.go.id/ [Accessed 18 February 2014].

Suparyanto, 2011. *Kader Kesehatan*. [Online] Available at: http://dr-suparyanto.blogspot.com/2011/07/ kader-kesehatan.html [Accessed 17 April 2014].

Thabrany, H., 2014. *Health Care Financing and HCF Reform in Indonesia*. Jakarta: Center for Health Economics and Policy Analysis, University of Indonesia.

Thabrany, H., n.d.a. *Indonesia Health Insurance History*. [Online] Available at: http://staff.ui.ac.id/system/ files/users/hasbulah/material/babisejarahasuransikesehatanedited.pdf [Accessed 27 April 2014].

Thabrany, H., n.d.b. *Indonesian Health Insurance History*. [Online] Available at: http://staff.ui.ac.id/system/ files/users/hasbulah/material/babisejarahasuransikesehatanedited.pdf [Accessed 27 April 2014].

The World Bank Group, 2014. *Indonesia Overview*. [Online] Available at: www.worldbank.org/en/ country/indonesia/overview [Accessed 1 March 2014].

The World Bank, 2014. *Out of Pocket Expenditure*. [Online] Available at: http://data.worldbank.org/ indicator/SH.XPD.OOPC.ZS [Accessed 24 April 2014].

UNDP, 2013a. *Explanatory Note on 2013 HDR Composite Indices*. [Online] Available at: http://hdr.undp. org/sites/default/files/Country-Profiles/IDN.pdf [Accessed 1 March 2014].

UNDP, 2013b. *Human Development Report 2013, The Rise of the South: Human Progress in a Diverse World*. New York: United Nations Development Programme.

van der Kroef, J. M., 1951. The term Indonesia: Its origin and usage. *Journal of the American Oriental Society,* 71(3), 166–71.

Working Group 2 Indonesia Mental Health System Development Taskforce, 2009. *Indonesia Mental Health Service System*. Jakarta.

World Health Organization, 1994. *A User's Guide to the Self Reporting Questionnaire (SRQ)*. Geneva: World Health Organization.

World Health Organization, 2005. *WHO Recommendations for Mental Health in Aceh,* Geneva: World Health Organization.

World Health Organization, 2010. *mhGAP Intervention Guide for Mental, Neurological and Substance Use Disorder in Non-specialized Health Settings: Mental Health Gap Action Programme (mhGAP)*. Geneva: World Health Organization.

World Health Organization, 2013. *Building Back Better: Sustainable Mental Health Care after Emergencies*. Geneva: World Health Organization .

Yessi, S., 2014. *Mental Health Service Development in Aceh Province*. Banda Aceh: Aceh Mental Health Technical and Coordination Meeting, January 2014.

19

Malaysia

Thambu Maniam and Lai-Fong Chan

Geography

Malaysia is a South East Asian nation consisting of two parts. Peninsular Malaysia, also called Malaya, is at the southernmost tip of the Asian mainland. The East Malaysian states of Sabah and Sarawak (Malaysian Borneo) lie across the South China Sea on the eastern part of the island of Borneo. Malaysia has land borders with Thailand, Indonesia and Brunei, in addition to maritime borders with the Philippines, Singapore and Vietnam. The land area is approximately 330,000 square kilometers, and situated about two degrees north of the equator. Peninsular Malaysia is more highly developed and urbanized compared to East Malaysia.

The climate is equatorial, generally hot and humid throughout the year. The months of November through January are wetter months with rains from the northeast monsoon.

Malaysia used to be an agricultural economy, and at one time the world's largest exporter of tin and natural rubber. But over the last 20 years it has been transformed into an industrialized nation, with manufacturing of computer parts becoming a major economic activity. The oil and gas industries besides palm oil exports are major contributors to the economy. According to the United Nations system of classification of economic zones, Malaysia is placed in Zone 2 among upper-middle-income countries. The average annual household income in 2012 was Ringgit Malaysia (RM) 60,000 (US$1 = 3.2 RM). In 2012 the Gini Coefficient (an index of income distribution inequality, ranging from 0 to 1, with a value of 1 indicating complete inequality) was 0.43 (Department of Statistics Malaysia, 2014a). The unemployment rate is 3.0 percent and life expectancy is 72 years for men and 77 years for women (Department of Statistics Malaysia, 2014b). The nation is working towards becoming a developed country by the year 2020. The population is 30,000,000. Slightly over half the population are Malay Muslims; the Indigenous peoples of Sabah and Sarawak, Chinese and Indians make up the rest. Foreign workers, who provide much needed migrant labor, make up almost 8 percent of the population. Major religions practiced in the country are Islam, Buddhism, Christianity and Hinduism.

Malaya gained its independence from the British in 1957. In 1963, the Federation of Malaysia was formed consisting of Malaya, Singapore, Sabah and Sarawak. Singapore subsequently left the Federation in 1965. Malaysia is a constitutional monarchy practicing the Westminster system of parliamentary democracy. The capital city is Kuala Lumpur. A new federal administrative center has been set up in Putrajaya.

Mental health policy

In the provision of public health services, Malaysia has an outstanding record among developing countries. Infant mortality and maternal mortality rates have been drastically reduced since independence. However, the provision of mental health services has lagged behind somewhat. The Malaysian National Health Policy was developed in 1998. Key areas addressed included issues of accessibility and comprehensiveness of mental health services, integration with general health services, multi-sectorial and community involvement, human resource development, quality improvement and research activities. There was also an emphasis on protecting the rights of individuals with mental illness through legislation (Asia–Australia Mental Health, 2008).

In terms of legislative provisions, the Mental Health Act (MHA) was introduced in 2001 and the corresponding Mental Health Regulations were implemented in 2010. This new legislation, which replaced archaic laws such as the Mental Disorder Ordinance 1952 (Peninsular Malaysia), Lunatic Ordinance 1951 (Sabah) and Mental Health Ordinance 1961 (Sarawak), was designed to improve the provision and delivery of mental health care services in Malaysia. Under the MHA 2001, patients' rights are more protected to a certain degree, i.e. patients must be told what their rights are with respect to hospitalization, and there are certain provisions for consent for treatment. Patients admitted involuntarily, and those under isolation or restraint in any form have been accorded greater protection and care. However, the bar that is set for involuntary compulsory treatment is rather low. The MHA is still less liberal than in the West, for instance in terms of consent to electroconvulsive therapy (ECT) (Fifa and Maniam, 2011).

Psychiatric epidemiology

Mood and anxiety disorders

The National Health and Morbidity Survey (NHMS) in 2006 (Maniam *et al.*, 2008) found that 11.2 percent of adult Malaysians in the general population had some form of psychiatric morbidity based on the 28-item General Health Questionnaire (GHQ). The same survey showed that the prevalence of suicidal ideation was 6.3 percent (Maniam *et al.*, 2013). In 2011, the NHMS administered face-to-face interviews using the validated Malay version of the Mini International Neuropsychiatric Interview (MINI) (Firdaus *et al.*, 2012) and found the following prevalence rates: general anxiety disorder – 1.7 percent, current and lifetime major depressive disorder – 1.8 percent and 2.4 percent respectively (Abdul Kadir *et al.*, 2011). In another study the rate of depression among the elderly in an urban population in the state of Selangor, Malaysia was found to be 6.3 percent (Mohd *et al.*, 2005). Significant factors for elderly depression were identified as female gender, Indian ethnicity, chronic illness, functional disability and cognitive impairment.

Suicidal behavior

Suicide has been a public health concern in Malaysia for many years. In terms of suicidal behavior, the NHMS 2011 used interviewer-administered questions from the WHO SUPRE-MISS Questionnaire. The prevalence estimates for suicidal attempts, plans and ideation were 0.5 percent, 0.9 percent and 1.7 percent, respectively (Maniam *et al.*, 2014). The authors have discussed the reasons why these rates could be underestimates. Socio-demographic risk factors associated with suicidal behavior included younger age, female gender and Indian ethnicity. Suicidal ideation was significantly associated with a diagnosis of current generalized anxiety disorder, while suicide plans and attempts were significantly associated with a past history of major depressive disorder. Self-reported suicidal ideation yielded a higher rate in 2006 (6.3 percent) compared to face-to-face interview in 2011, possibly due to the stigma and strong social disapproval associated with suicidal behavior in Malaysian society (Maniam *et al.*, 2014). There is no general agreement on what the Malaysian suicide rate is. It has variously been reported to be as low as 1.6 (Hayati *et al.* 2008) and estimated to reach 13 per 100,000 (Maniam, 1995). The reason for this discrepancy has been discussed elsewhere (Maniam and Chan, 2013).

In 2010 the Malaysian Ministry of Health (MOH) drew up a national suicide prevention plan (Ministry of Health Malaysia, Disease Control Division, 2010). The plan, known as the National Strategy and Action Plan for Suicide Prevention has had a difficult time being born, and has been implemented in part only. It calls for collaboration between the public and private sectors including such volunteer non-government organizations such as the Befrienders (akin to the Samaritans in other countries).

Schizophrenia

The National Health Mental Registry (NHMR) reported the first-contact incidence of schizophrenia as five cases per 100,000 population/year from 2003 to 2005 (Aziz *et al.*, 2008). This figure is lower compared to the AESOP study in the UK that reported rates of 7.2–20.1 cases per 100,000 population/year calculated from the incidence of schizophrenia cases who made first contact with mental health services (Kirkbride *et al.*, 2006). The NMHR data was collected from reported cases of DSM-IV schizophrenia who presented at government hospitals and public health facilities. Cases seen in private hospitals and clinics would be missed. The mean duration of untreated psychosis (DUP), a significant prognostic factor in schizophrenia, was 28.7 months. This figure is slightly shorter than the average DUP of 31.25 months in low- and middle-income countries but much longer than the mean DUP of 15.35 months in high-income nations (Large *et al.*, 2008). The relatively low first-contact incidence of schizophrenia and the long DUP may be a reflection of the traditional beliefs about mental illness that still predominate over biological and medical explanatory models, especially among the more rural population in Malaysia.

Children and adolescents

The NHMS 2011 showed a prevalence of 20 percent for psychiatric morbidity among Malaysians aged 5–16 years of age. These included developmental disabilities, and emotional and behavioral disorders (Kadir *et al.*, 2011). The field of child and adolescent psychiatry is still underresourced in this country with very small numbers of child and adolescent psychiatrists struggling to meet the needs of a population with a large proportion of young people.

Mental health systems

The first psychiatric hospital in Malaysia was set up in 1911, during British colonial rule. Then called the Central Mental Hospital, it was later renamed Hospital Bahagia Ulu Kinta (HBUK). At its peak there were over 4,000 patients, but in recent years the patient population has been reduced to well below 2,000.

In 1933, another psychiatric hospital was set up in Tampoi, catering to the southern states of Malaya. There are also two other psychiatric hospitals in East Malaysia, one each in Sabah and Sarawak.

Following the recommendations of Cunningham Dax, the WHO mental health consultant, decentralization of psychiatric services was implemented in the 1970s. More psychiatric units were set up in general hospitals. Most psychiatric services were initially custodial in nature. Earnest efforts have been made to rectify this state of affairs. In the state of Perak, where HBUK is situated, follow-up clinics were set up in community halls and temples to make these more accessible to the people. Nursing homes were started, helping to reduce the inpatient population, and contributing significantly to deinstitutionalization and decentralization of services. Subsequently community services began to be set up, and took off with greater sense of purpose after the visit and recommendations of the third WHO consultant in the 1990s.

Community services have grown rapidly since the turn of the century (Ruzanna and Marhani, 2010). Many large psychiatry departments have set up community psychiatry units providing home services both for acute and long-term care, and have supported employment, thereby reducing re-admission rates.

Addiction is an issue of major concern in Malaysia. In the 1970s opiate addiction became widespread. It was a time of major social change in the country. Rural–urban migration was gathering speed. With rapid urbanization the relative security of village life and support of extended families fell away. In the late 1980s HIV infection gained a foothold in the intravenous drug using community, and became a major concern in the 1990s. The introduction of the death penalty for drug pushers made no discernible dent in the rate of drug abuse. Whereas initial efforts to curb the drug use problem were somewhat punitive, with court-mandated compulsory detentions and use of the "cold turkey" method of detoxification, over the past two decades the relevant authorities have adopted new approaches. There is greater openness to needle exchange programs and encouraging safer sex practices, which had earlier been frowned upon for religious reasons in this conservative society. Methadone substitution therapy was also introduced (Hussain Habil, 2001).

More recently amphetamine-related substances have begun to replace heroin as the drug of choice. Initially methamphetamine use was noted mainly in people who frequented clubs and karaoke joints, but it has now spread to street drug users.

Psychiatry training

The University of Malaya Medical Centre (UMMC) started the first psychiatry postgraduate training program in 1973, followed by the Universiti Kebangsaan Malaysia Medical Centre (UKMMC) in 1985, and then Universiti Sains Malaysia (USM). Most of the psychiatrists currently practicing in this country have been trained in these universities. Other universities have also set up training programs, following the formation of a National Conjoint Board for Psychiatry. The Conjoint Board determines the curriculum and conducts postgraduate examinations. Subspecialty training is conducted both locally as well as by sending psychiatrists to developed countries, mostly to countries in the (British) Commonwealth.

Most of the public medical universities have foundation departments of psychiatry. Undergraduates typically receive 8–10 weeks of exposure to the theory and practice of psychiatry. At the end of their course they are tested on psychiatry long cases or short cases besides answering theory questions.

The psychiatrist–population ratio in 1987 was one psychiatrist to 350,000 people. This has narrowed to approximately 1:100,000, with the aim of achieving the WHO recommended ratio of 1:30,000. Most of the psychiatrists work in urban areas and in universities. Though Malaysia generally has an excellent public health system with good access to health care, the same cannot be said for the population of Sabah and Sarawak, especially with respect to specialist psychiatric care. Currently, there are about 40 general hospitals in Malaysia with specialist psychiatry services but not all of them provide separate inpatient services for acutely ill psychiatric patients.

In Malaysia, patients are not registered with their own GPs, and there is no specific or formal catchment area that hospitals are responsible for. Patients may choose which hospital they want to go to, and who they want to see. It is not uncommon for a patient to cross two or three state borders to see a psychiatrist of their choice, by-passing numerous hospitals along the way.

The new Mental Health Act provides for inpatient private psychiatric care even for involuntary patients. However, the hospitals providing such care must be registered for this and adhere to the provisions of the Act.

Funding

Much of the cost of treating psychiatric patients is borne by the public purse. There is no insurance coverage for psychiatric illness, apart from some special group health insurance schemes taken out by employers for their staff. These are for outpatient treatment. The National Health Financing Scheme is in the process of being set up. The details have, at present, not been made public. How people with mental illness will fare under this scheme is as yet unclear.

Social/explanatory model(s) about mental illness: traditions, values, beliefs

Traditional beliefs about causes and treatment of psychiatric illness still predominate in Malaysia. Razali *et al.* (1996) found that significantly more psychiatric patients among the Malay community in Kota Bahru, Kelantan, who believed in supernatural causes for their psychiatric disorder consulted with a *bomoh* (Malay traditional healer) and had poorer psychiatric treatment adherence. In addition, a significant treatment delay was associated with prior *bomoh* consultation (Razali and Najib, 2000). However, a more recent study among patients with first-episode psychosis in a more urbanized area in the capital city of Kuala Lumpur did not find any significant association between treatment delay and consultation with traditional healers (Phang *et al.*, 2010). About a third of patients were recommended by at least one traditional healer to seek medical help for their psychotic illness. Whether such findings point towards a potential collaborative role for traditional healers in the management of first-episode psychosis, as suggested by Phang *et al.* (2010), remains to be further explored.

In the past the elderly, the mentally ill and the disabled were generally cared for at home by family members. In recent years mental health workers and other medical professionals have noted that there is an increasing trend to place the chronically ill and the disabled in nursing homes. Part of the reason for this development is that, with increasing urbanization, family structures have changed. The extended family system with three generations living together has given way to the nuclear family. Both parents work outside the home. Children are often cared for during the day by foreign maids or babysitters. Hence, it has become difficult to look after the ill and the infirm at home. In many cases this has given rise to, among elderly parents, a sense of being rejected and abandoned. Moreover, those in the lower middle class generally only have access to small apartments in urban areas. Lack of space necessitates seeking alternative care arrangements. Consequently, private nursing homes have mushroomed. Many do not have proper programs for residents. The good well-run homes tend to be too expensive for the average middle class family.

Topics of specific/special concern

Stigma towards people with mental illness remains a significant challenge in Malaysian society. Efforts to improve public awareness about mental illness need to be stepped up. A cross-cultural study (Loo et al., 2012) showed that Malaysians might not be very well versed in correctly identifying cases of mental disorders and recognizing the need to seek professional help. In addition, more needs to be done in terms of social advocacy for mental health issues. For example, people with mental illness often struggle with the lack of a "safety net" in the form of adequate social support and resources, i.e. financial, housing, etc. Programs that focus on support for care-givers and families of people with mental illness are spearheaded by the community psychiatry arm of government hospitals as well as non-governmental organizations, though these programs tend to be somewhat sporadic.

An important milestone was achieved in 2008 when patients with severe mental illness were able to officially register their disability status with the government welfare services. This provided access to some, albeit meager, measure of financial aid as well exemption from payment of certain health-care costs in government hospitals, e.g. payment for inpatient care.

A more recent issue of concern has arisen with regard to funding for the provision of care for the mentally ill. Many employers in the private sector have been covering the cost of treatment for their employees. However, with the introduction of Health Maintenance Organizations (HMOs) employers have contracted out such services. Some HMOs have begun to restrict general practitioners from claiming for treating depression and other common psychiatric disorders seen in primary care. This discourages patients from continuing their antidepressant treatment, since they would have to pay out of their own pocket. The only other alternative for them is to turn to the public sector hospitals which are already overcrowded. There is still a lack of insurance coverage for people diagnosed with mental disorders.

The psychiatric profession in the country is concerned about the training in psychiatry for undergraduates in private medical schools. In the last 10 years, private medical education has mushroomed. But the shortage of trained teaching staff has been a major problem which could affect the quality of training. At the moment a solution to this does not appear to be in sight.

There has been accumulating evidence that the Indian community in Malaysia is showing high levels of social distress. Common indices of social distress such as higher suicide and attempted suicide rates, school dropout rates, alcoholism, domestic violence, gangsterism and higher rates of incarceration have been noted to be increased among Indians. They also occupy the highest ranks among those with mental illness. A concerted effort to help this community needs to be put in place.

From a legal standpoint, efforts need to be made to decriminalize suicide attempts, which are currently still listed as a chargeable criminal offense. Much more needs to be done in terms of advocating for more resources and funding as well as prioritizing mental health issues among policy-makers.

Finally, there is a great need for human resource development not only in terms of psychiatrists. There are too few subspecialists in child and adolescent psychiatry and psycho-geriatrics. Clinical psychologists are a rare breed. The Ministry of Health, which is by far the largest provider of health services for the nation, has only a handful of clinical psychologists. Whole states have none. There are indications that the authorities have become more aware of this and have begun to respond, though the fruits are yet to be seen. The need for trained psychiatric nurses and psychiatric social workers is equally great and as yet remains unmet.

In conclusion, psychiatry and mental health services have come a long way since independence half a century ago – emerging from the shadows of psychiatric institutions hidden away in remote areas far from polite society. Psychiatry's increasing popularity among young doctors assures its future. As an example, in the year when the first author began his training in psychiatry there were a mere two trainees in the local training program. This year there were 70 applicants, whereas only 50 training positions were available.

References

Abdul Kadir, A.B., Ang, K.T., Azizul, A., Firdaus, M., Jasvindar, K., Lim, C.H. (2011) Mental health problems in adults. In: Kaur, G., Kaur, J., Nalachakravarthy, O., Norzawati, Y., Fadzilah, K., Helen Tee, G.H. (eds). *National Health and Morbidity Survey 2011 (NHMS 2011). Vol. II: Non-Communicable Diseases*. Kuala Lumpur: Institute for Public Health (IPH).

Asia–Australia Mental Health (2008) Asia-Pacific Community Mental Health Development Project (APCMHD): Summary Report (Malaysia). Suarn S., Cheah Y.C., Ruzanna Z., Marhani M. (eds). Melbourne: Asia–Australia Mental Health. http://aamh.edu.au/__data/assets/pdf_file/0011/408593/MalaysiasCountryReport.pdf (this is part of a larger report on Asia Pacific countries, accessible at: http://issuu.com/asialink/docs/apcmhdp_report2011).

Aziz, A.A., Salina, A.A., Kadir, A.A., Badiah, Y., Cheah, Y.C., Hayati, A.N. (2008) The National Mental Health Registry (NMHR). *The Medical Journal of Malaysia*, 63, 15–17.

Department of Statistics Malaysia (2014a) Putrajaya. www.statistics.gov.my/portal/download_Bulletin_Bulanan/files/BPBM/2014/MAC/MALAYSIA/02Population.pdf (accessed 23 July 2014).

Department of Statistics Malaysia (2014b) Putrajaya. www.statistics.gov.my/portal/images/stories/files/LatestReleases/vital/Vital_Statistics_Malaysia_2011.pdf (accessed 23 July 2014).

Fifa, R. and Maniam, T. (2011) The Role of Law in Electroconvulsive Therapy: A Comparative Analysis of Laws in the United States, Australia and Malaysia. Paper presented at the XXXII International Congress on Law and Mental Health, Humboldt University, Berlin, Germany, 17–23 July 2011.

Firdaus, M., Kadir, A.B., Mazni, M.J., Azizul, A., Salina, A.A., Marhani, M. (2012) A preliminary study on the specificity and sensitivity values inter-rater reliability of Mini International Neuropsychiatric Interview (MINI) in Malaysia. *ASEAN Journal of Psychiatry*,13(2),157–64.

Hayati, A.N., Abdullah, A.A. and Sham, M.M. (2008) National Suicide Registry Malaysia: Preliminary Report July to December 2007. Kuala Lumpur: Institute for Public Health.

Hussain Habil, M. (2001) *Managing Heroin Addicts Through Medical Therapy*. Kuala Lumpur: University of Malaya Press.

Kirkbride, J.B., Fearon, P., Morgan, C., Dazzan, P., Morgan, K., Tarrant, J. (2006) Heterogeneity in incidence rates of schizophrenia and other psychotic syndromes: findings from the 3-center AeSOP study. *Archives of General Psychiatry*, 63(3), 250–8.

Large, M., Farooq, S. and Nielssen, O. (2008) Duration of untreated psychosis in low and middle income countries: the relationship between GDP and DUP. *British Journal of Psychiatry*, 193, 272–8.

Loo, P.W., Wong, S. and Furnham, A. (2012) Mental health literacy: a cross-cultural study from Britain, Hong Kong and Malaysia. *Asia-Pacific Psychiatry*, 4, 113–25. doi: 10.1111/j.1758–5872.2012.00198.x

Maniam, T. (1995) Suicide and undetermined violent deaths in Malaysia, 1966–1990: evidence for the misclassification of suicide statistics. *Asia-Pacific Journal of Public Health*, 8, 181–85.

Maniam, T. and Chan, L.F. (2013) Half a century of suicide studies – a plea for new directions in research and prevention. *Sains Malaysiana*, 42(3), 399–402.

Maniam, T., Abdul Kadir, A.B., 'Abqariyah, Y., Lim, C.H., Nurashikin, I., Salina A.A. (2008) Psychiatric morbidity in adults. In: Institute for Public Health (IPH) (eds) *The Third National Health and Morbidity Survey (NHMS III) 2006*, Vol. 2. Malaysia: Ministry of Health.

Maniam, T., Karuthan, C., Lim, C.H., Kadir, A.B., Nurashikin, I., Salina A.A. and Jeevitha, M. (2013) Suicide prevention program for at risk groups: pointers from an epidemiological study. *Preventive Medicine*, 57(Supplement), S45–6.

Maniam, T., Marhani, M., Firdaus, M., Kadir, A.B., Maznid, M.J., Azizul, A., Salina, A.A., Fadzillah, A.R., Nurashikin, I., Ang, K.T., Jasvindar, K. and Noor Ani, A. (2014) Risk factors for suicidal ideation, plans and attempts in Malaysia – results of an epidemiological survey. *Comprehensive Psychiatry*, 55(Supplement 1), S121–5.

Ministry of Health Malaysia, Disease Control Division (2010) *National Strategy and Action Plan for Suicide Prevention*. Putrajaya: Ministry of Health.

Mohd, S., Sidik, R.L., Aini, M. and Mohd, N. (2005) The prevalence of depression among elderly in an urban area of Selangor, Malaysia. *The International Medical Journal*, 4(2), 57–63.

Phang, C.K., Midin, M. and Aziz, S.A. (2010) Traditional healers are causing treatment delay among patients with psychosis in Hospital Kuala Lumpur: fact or fallacy? *ASEAN Journal of Psychiatry*, 11(2), 206–15.

Razali, S.M. and Najib, M.A.M. (2000) Help-seeking pathways among Malay psychiatric patients. *International Journal of Social Psychiatry*, 46(4), 281–9.

Razali, S.M., Khan, U.A. and Hasanah, C.I. (1996) Belief in supernatural causes of mental illness among Malay patients: impact on treatment. *Acta Psychiatrica Scandinavica*, 94 229–33. doi: 10.1111/j.1600–0447.1996.tb09854.x

Ruzanna, Z. and Marhani, M. (2010) Assertive Community Treatment (ACT) for patients with severe mental illness: experience in Malaysia. *Malaysian Journal of Psychiatry*, 17(1), 73–8.

20

The Philippines

*Paul V. Lee, Salvador Benjamin D. Vista and
Victoria Patricia C. De la Llana*

Country/location geography

The Philippines is an archipelago, composed of 7,107 islands, and is located between latitude 4°23'N and 21°25'N and longitude 116°E and 127°E. Its length is 1,850 kilometers, its breadth is 965 kilometers. The Pacific Ocean on the east, the West Philippine Sea on the west and north, and the Celebes Sea on the south surround the archipelago. The country is divided into 14 regions, 73 provinces and 60 cities (Philippine Information Agency, 2005).

Mental health policy

The National Mental Health Policy, also known as Administrative Order No. 8 s. 2001, was signed by then Secretary of Health Manuel Dayrit. This aims to improve mental health and integrate services for those with mental disorders. The implementation was to be guided by the following principles: leadership, collaboration and partnership, empowerment and participation, equity, standards for quality mental health services, human resource development, health service delivery system, mental health care, stability and sustainability, information system, legislation, as well as monitoring and evaluation.

In order to provide policy guidelines and procedures for establishing mental health programs at national and local levels, Administrative Order No. 2007–0009, entitled "Operational Framework for the Sustainable Establishment of the Mental Health Program" was established in March 9, 2007 and signed by then Health Secretary Dr Francisco Duque.

This Administrative Order aimed to reduce mental health prevalence; reduce mortality from suicide and intentional harm, reduce the risk of mental disorder through the promotion of mental health in the general population, and to improve the quality of life of those suffering from such conditions.

The National Mental Health Program is focused on four sub-programs, which include Wellness of Daily Living, under the National Center for Disease Prevention and Control, Extreme Life Experience under the Health Emergency Management Staff – National Center for Mental Health, Substance Abuse and Other Forms of Addiction, and Mental Disorders.

This Order was amended in the year 2012, where it was stated that a National Program Management Committee (NPMC) shall be organized in the Department of Health in order to "ensure coordination and sustainability of the National Mental Health Program."

In 1995, the National Health Insurance Act was established in order to make health care available at a more affordable cost. The Philippine Health Insurance Corporation at the time listed "outpatient psychotherapy and counseling for mental disorders" and "drug and alcohol abuse or dependency treatment" as part of the list of "Excluded Personal Health Services." In 2012, the Republic Act 10606 amended this section, instead only stating that "the Corporation shall not cover expenses for health services which the Corporation and the Department of Health (DOH) consider cost-ineffective through health technology assessment," and "the Corporation may institute additional exclusions and limitations as it may deem reasonable in keeping with its protection objectives and financial sustainability." It has expanded to include mental health care, but is restricted to acute inpatient care for severe mental illness (World Health Organization, 2007).

In response to a growing drug use problem in the country, the Comprehensive Dangerous Drugs Act (RA 9165) was formulated in 2002 to prevent drug abuse problems, which are considered a major cause of mental illness among the economically productive age group.

In 2009, Senator Juan Ponce Enrile filed Senate Bill No. 3509, called the National Mental Health Act of 2009, entitled "An Act Providing for a National Mental Health Care Delivery System, Establishing for the Purpose the Philippine Council for Mental Health and Appropriating Funds Therefor." It has undergone its first reading by congress, and its status is currently pending in the legislative branch of government.

The Commission on Human Rights included the mentally disabled as one of the sectors to be protected in the Philippine human rights plan in 1995. Some community-based inpatient psychiatric units, residential psychiatric facilities and a hospital have been reviewed. Also, there was an institution which reported at least one day of training, meeting or working session on human rights protection of patients. "Twenty-one percent of community in-patient psychiatric units and community residential facilities had such training" (World Health Organization, 2007).

Psychiatric epidemiology

A 1989 study done by the University of the Philippines Department of Psychiatry in a rural area 45 kilometers from Manila found that 34 percent of those with mental disorders had social problems. In a 1993–1994 collaboration between the Regional Health Office of Region IV and the University of the Philippines Psychiatrists' Foundation, Inc., a population survey for mental disorders was done in both rural and urban settings in three provinces of the said region. Results showed that the prevalence of mental disorders was 35 percent, with the three most common diagnoses among adults being psychosis (4.3 percent), anxiety (14.3 percent), and panic (5.6 percent). For children and adolescents, the five most common diagnoses included enuresis (9.3 percent), speech and language disorder (3.9 percent), mental sub-normality (3.7 percent), adaptation reaction (2/4 percent), and neurotic disorder (1/1 percent) (Conde, 2004).

In the year 2000, a survey by the National Statistics Office, the primary statistical arm of the Philippine government, found that mental illness was the third most common form of disability in the country. According to this disability survey, prevalence rates were found to be 88/100,000. In the same year, psychiatrists accomplished what was called a Baseline Survey for the National Objectives for Health, which found that more frequently reported symptoms of an underlying mental health problem were sadness, confusion, forgetfulness, no control over the use of cigarettes and alcohol, and delusions. On commission from the Department of Health, the Social Weather

Station, a private social survey institute, found that 0.7 percent of total households have a family member with a mental disability (Administrative Order 2007–0009-A, 2012).

The Department of Health – National Epidemiology Center conducted a study on the prevalence of mental health problems in 2006. This survey was limited to government employees from 20 national agencies in Metro Manila. It was found that among 327 participants, 32 percent had "experienced a mental health problem at least once in their lifetime." The three most prevalent diagnoses included specific phobias (15 percent), alcohol abuse (10 percent), and depression (6 percent). "Males were more likely to have substance-related problems than females." Mental health problems were significantly associated with individuals aged 20–29 years old, with large families and low educational attainment (Administrative Order 2007–0009-A, 2012).

A literature review of local studies and sources of information regarding suicide in the Philippines was done by Redaniel et al. in 2011. It was found that suicide rates were higher for both males and females in the 15–24-year-old age range, with males having a second peak at 65 years old and older. It also showed that 58–77 percent of non-fatal self-harm patients are female. The majority of these cases are single, but 61–84 percent of them were found to be in a relationship. A 1989 study showed that 78.7 percent of patients who attempted suicide had adjustment disorders, 7.1 percent had schizophrenia, and 6.2 percent were described to have manic depression. Self-poisoning was shown to be the most common method of self-harm, with family and relationship problems being the most common reasons for self-harm (Redaniel et al., 2011).

A 2013 study on the medical and sociodemographic data on self-harm showed that patients who consult for self-harm tend to be female, aged 18–25 years old, single, heterosexual, employed or studying (college undergraduate), and Roman Catholic. Most of these patients have low incomes. The most common method employed is ingestion of a poisonous substance. Most often, these patients had no previous history of self-harm, or past medical or psychiatric illness. Also, there is no notable family medical or psychiatric history, or substance use history. The self-harm episode is usually triggered by problems with the patient's romantic partner. The Axis I diagnosis tends to be an adjustment disorder, Axis II diagnosis was deferred, the Axis III diagnosis mostly comprises conditions brought about by the self-harmful act, an Axis IV description of interpersonal relationship problems, and an Axis V Global Assessment of Functioning rating of 11–20. Patients are more often than not improved when discharged from the emergency department (De la Llana and Vista, 2013).

Mental health systems

History

The care of the mentally ill in the Philippines began in the nineteenth century, when a Spanish sailor presented with behavioral changes. On the request of his commander, the sailor was brought for care to Hospicio de San Jose, a charitable institution that catered to orphaned children and the elderly.

Since then, many others who were considered mentally ill have come to Hospicio de San Jose for treatment. Because of their increasing numbers, new buildings were constructed to accommodate more and more patients. When these proved to be insufficient, another facility was built in the city of Cavite. By 1897, Hospicio de San Jose had 548 patients with mental illness.

In the year 1904, San Lazaro Hospital was established to accommodate the increasing number of patients. In 1905, the new hospital housed 50 male patients and 19 female patients. By 1906, it had expanded to house 250 patients.

In the year 1918, the City of Manila built its own hospital dedicated to mental health, the Sanitarium in San Juan del Monte, Rizal. Dr Telesforo Ejercito was the first head of the hospital, which housed 265 patients. This was later transferred to San Pedro, Makati, under the leadership of Dr Ramon Syquia.

In 1925, through the Public Works Act 3258, an "insane asylum" was constructed. The facility was built on 64 hectares of land in Barrio Mauway, Mandaluyong, Rizal, 11 kilometers from Manila.

In 1928, the 379 patients crowded into San Lazaro Hospital were moved to the new hospital, which was called "Insular Psychopathic Hospital," now known as the "National Center for Mental Health." Since then, the government has tirelessly worked towards the development of this institution. While construction and maintenance work in the facility were constant, there were simply too many admissions and too few discharges of patients. In 1941, P$1,600,000 was allocated for the construction and furnishing of a new building as a solution for overcrowding. This project was begun, but never finished as the Second World War erupted.

The hospital endured, even through the Japanese Occupation. By 1942, 3,156 patients were confined, and a total of 2,062 patients were admitted within the next three years. When the American forces liberated the facility on February 9, 1945, there were only 307 inpatients left – 2,191 were discharged and sent home, while 2,624 died. Common causes of death were starvation and lack of medications; others were tortured and killed by the Japanese and hospital staff for suspected insurgency against the invaders. As years passed, more and more patients suffering from mental conditions were admitted.

In 1955, 300 patients were moved to a former "Quarantine Station" in Mariveles as a solution to overcrowding. This was closed due to management problems, but reopened in 1963 after restructuring in order to improve facilities and overcrowding of 8,000 patients in buildings constructed to accommodate 2,500 patients. Also part of the overcrowding solution was to distribute patients to facilities in the provinces as well. Paulino J. Garcia, then the Minister for Health, directed the opening of branches of the hospital in various regions and provinces.

The National Center for Mental Health was established on December 17, 1928. Dr Elias Domingo was the first to hold the title of chief of hospital and his term was from 1928 to 1935. It current leader holds the position of Medical Center Chief.

In light of needs of the mental health care system of the country, then Department of Health Secretary Alfredo Bengzon created a task force under the leadership of Dr Baltazar Reyes. This task force established a Crisis Intervention Service (CIS). Another committee was established, called a "Discharge and Follow-up Committee," led by Dr Sergia Abueva.

The National Mental Hospital became known as the National Center for Mental Health through Ministry Circular No. 125 S. 1986, and Memorandum Order No. 48 from the Office of the President. In accordance with these, procedures under the CIS were implemented under the leadership of Dr Brigida Buenaseda. The Discharge and Follow-Up Committee also conducted patients who could be looked after outside the hospital to their homes. Through these innovations, the hospital's inpatient population decreased from over 4,000 patients in 1986, to around 2,000 in the 1990s.

The National Center for Mental Health remains the primary government-run institution for the care of mentally ill patients.

Psychiatric training in the Philippines

The University of the Philippines was established in 1908, and what was formerly known as the Philippine Medical School became the UP College of Medicine. When the Philippine General

Hospital opened in 1910, two American physicians, Dr Almond T. Gough and Dr Samuel Tretze, taught psychiatry. Medical students did brief rotations in the Insane Department of San Lazaro Hospital. When the Psychopathic Hospital was opened, the students did two-week rotations there.

The Faculty of Medicine and Surgery in the University of Santo Tomas was established in 1871, before the UP College of Medicine. However, it initially did not have psychiatry as part of its formal curriculum. Fourth-year medical students did short rotations in the Insular Psychopathic Hospital. Instruction in both institutions was done in English, using American textbooks (Yap, 1995).

From 1917 to 1919, Dr Elias Domingo, then Chief Resident of the Department of Medicine in the Philippine General Hospital, was sent to Pennsylvania, USA, through a Rockefeller scholarship in order to train in psychiatry. He became the first Filipino psychiatrist.

In 1978, the Department of Psychiatry in the Philippine General Hospital created a specialized section that dealt with psychiatric problems of children and adolescents named the Section of Child and Adolescent Psychiatry. Dr Cornelio G. Banaag, Jr, was the first child psychiatrist in the country. A fellowship training program in this subspecialty was later established.

The University of the Philippines College of Medicine adopted a community orientation in its curriculum; in line with this, a fellowship training program in Social and Community Psychiatry was established in 1989 by Dr Lourdes L. Ignacio.

In the 1970s and 1980s, the consultation psychiatry service had been open to the other departments in the hospital under the supervision of Dr Baltazar Reyes, Jr, and Dr Lourdes Lapuz. After the 1985 establishment of the Pain Clinic, the Department of Psychiatry was formally invited to form a liaison with the unit. The Section of Consultation–Liaison Psychiatry was organized by Dr Jercyl Demeterio, and the fellowship training program in Consultation–Liaison Psychiatry was established in 1990. Later, liaison programs with the burn unit, pulmonology department, colorectal cancer and polyp study group, anesthesia department, renal transplant department, cancer institute and otorhinolaryngology department were established.

In the 1990s, a 7.8 magnitude earthquake struck Luzon, and Mount Pinatubo erupted, which is considered one of the larger volcanic eruptions in the twentieth century. The psychiatry department actively participated in the psychosocial rehabilitation of the victims of these natural disasters. Psychiatry residents made psychosocial interventions, trained other health workers in mental health, developed local materials on the disaster, and forged linkages with government and non-government organizations (Reyes, 1968).

Government resources

The Department of Health Resources for Mental Health includes 5,865 beds in ten psychiatric hospitals/wards nationwide (Table 20.1). There are five regional mental health facilities with outpatient services, but there are no mental health inpatient services in Region I, Caraga, and the Autonomous Region of Muslim Mindanao. There are 12 beds for every 200,000 Filipinos. There are also Drug Treatment and Rehabilitation Centers (Table 20.2). There is a proposal to upgrade existing DOH mental health facilities and hospitals, establish psychiatric departments or units in regional hospitals and medical centers, establish acute and chronic care psychiatric facilities (110 beds) in strategic areas nationwide, and develop community mental health services.

In terms of human resources, there is one psychiatrist for every 200,000 people. As of 2010, there were 432 psychiatrists registered with the Philippine Psychiatric Association; the Philippine population is 94,013,200. The National Program Management Committee for the National

Mental Health Program at the Department of Health and the Regional Mental Health Team in the Council for Health and Development are the entities assigned to implement the National Mental Health Policy at national and regional levels. Current activities include a possible change of location of the National Center for Mental Health, construction of mental health facilities to serve rural areas, and training in the delivery of mental health care and psychosocial support for non-physicians, such as nurses and midwives (Vicente, 2013).

Table 20.1 Department of Health (DOH) hospitals with psychiatric and mental health facilities in the Philippines

Region	DOH Hospital with psychiatric facilities	Inpatient (bed capacity)	Outpatient service
Cordillera Administrative Region	Baguio General Hospital and Medical Center	40	Yes
1	Ilocos Training and Regional Medical Center	None	Yes
2	Cagayan Valley Regional Medical Center	200	Yes
3	Mariveles Mental Hospital (Bataan General Hospital)	500	Yes
4	None (but there is an LGU [local government unit]-operated mental hospital, Cavite Center for Mental Health and outpatient service in Batangas Province)	250	Yes
5	Bicol Medical Center	200	Yes
6	Western Visayas Medical Center (Pototan Mental Health Unit)	65	Yes
7	Vicente Sotto Memorial Medical Center	60	Yes
8	Schistosomiasis Control and Research Hospital	10	Yes
9	Zamboanga City Medical Center	40	Yes
10	Northern Mindanao Medical Center	None	Yes
11	Davao Medical Center	350	Yes
12	Cotabato Regional Medical Center	None	Yes
13	None	None	
Autonomous Region in Muslim Mindanao	None	None	
National Capital Region	National Center for Mental Health	4,200	Yes
	Total inpatient beds	5,865	
	Ratio of beds per 200,000 population = 12 beds/200,000 population		

Source: Vicente (2013)

Table 20.2 Treatment and rehabilitation centers of the
Department of Health in the Philippines

Name of facility	Bed capacity
Camp Bagong Diwa Treatment and Rehabilitation Center, Taguig	1,000
Ilagan, Isabela	100
Pilar Bataan	100
Tagaytay	300
Malinao, Albay	100
San Fernando, Camarines Sur	100
Pototan, Iloilo	100
Cebu City	300
Argao, Cebu	200
Dulag, Leyte	100
Cagayan de Oro	100
Caraga	100
NCMH Detox	60

Source: Vicente (2013)

Social/explanatory model(s) about mental illness

Traditionally, explanatory models of disease and illness in general were related to inanimate objects or to natural and supernatural phenomena. Mental illness might be due to "angry deities whom the victims have displeased," witches or *mangkukulam* who chant incantations or prick dolls, or devilmen or *mangangaway* who pray to Satan to cause symptoms (Yap, 1995), or even spirits possessing the patient. These are apparent in the use of the terms "*kulam*" or "*sapi*" as explanations for behavioral changes.

Treatment involved bringing the mentally ill to churches, as well as traditional healers called *manggagamot, hilot, arbularyo,* or *medico* for consultation. Maneuvers included incantations and prayers, breathing in steam, or a ritual called *tawas.*

Even today, the mentally ill who come for consultations in city hospitals mention a visit to a traditional healer prior to consulting a psychiatrist trained in formal medical schools. While it is very common to consult traditional healers prior to consulting a psychiatrist, it also happens that patients request hospital discharge against medical advice, or are lost to follow-up in the outpatient clinics in order to consult traditional healers.

Topics of interest specific to the Philippines

Overseas Filipino Workers (OFWs) are considered assets in the Philippine economy with dollar remittances to the country for their families, and have been for decades. However, there are documented psychosocial costs of this economic advantage for both the OFWs and the families left behind.

For the OFWs themselves, they experience "adverse or harsh social and cultural conditions" in the countries where they work, as well as "homesickness and detachment from the family and breakdown of marital ties that often result" (Conde, 2004). They cope through spirituality, a strong social support network of other OFWs, "and in the thought that the sacrifices they are making in being separated from their families are matched by the improvements in their socioeconomic conditions" (Conde, 2004).

In a series of case studies on OFW families done by Carandang *et al.* (2007), certain themes were noted, which centered on psychosocial stresses encountered by the family left behind by the OFW, changing family roles and responsibilities, coping with the absence of loved ones, and facing the fact that their lives did not improve in spite of working abroad.

The Department of Health, through the Overseas Workers Welfare Assistance (OWWA) has introduced policies to prevent mental illness and maintain mental health among OFWs. Pre-departure policy includes neuropsychiatric screening of potential OFWs, and those found to be symptomatic will not be certified to leave for employment. A pre-departure seminar is also required, where OFWs are briefed as to what to expect in their country of employment, and even coping strategies are discussed.

> A memorandum of agreement has been signed among the Department of Health, the Department of Labor and Employment, as well as the Department of Social Welfare and Development to appoint social welfare officers in Philippine consulates who can provide counseling and social welfare assistance. Physicians in several consulates have been trained by the Department of Health to identify and manage disorders among the overseas workers.
>
> Conde, 2004

Other advocacy groups

Currently active to various degrees of service, training and research are:

- Philippine College of Psychopharmacology: an organization formed by psychiatrists and neurologists whose main objective is to advocate for the optimum use of psychopharmaco-logic agents through service, training and research activities. Current activities include regular scientific fora, educational activities, and research projects.
- Group for Addiction Psychiatrists in the Philippines: an advocacy group organized by addiction psychiatrists and composed of physicians and rehabilitation workers who meet regularly to share new knowledge and experiences in the treatment of addictions. The group has generated consensus guidelines in methamphetamine-related disorders, and is currently working towards treatment guidelines for alcohol-related disorders.
- Child and Adolescent Psychiatrists of the Philippines, Inc.: a subspecialty group of the Philippine Psychiatric Association. It regulates training and certification as well as overseeing the conduct of services and research nationwide.
- World Association for Psychosocial Rehabilitation: promotes the principles and goals of psychosocial rehabilitation. This organization holds regular training and research activities for professionals and clients

References

Administrative Order 2007–0009-A (2012) *Operational Framework for the Sustainable Establishment of the Mental Health Program.* Department of Health, Philippines.

Carandang, M.L., Carandang, C and Sison, B.A. (2007) *Nawala ang Ilaw ng Tahanan: Case Studies of Families Left Behind by OFW Mothers.* Anvil Publishing, Manila, Philippines.

Conde, B. (2004) 'Philippines mental health country profile', *International Review of Psychiatry*, 16(1–2), 159–66.

De la Llana, V. and Vista, S. (2013) 'The medical and sociodemographic profile of patients seen in the PGH psychiatry service for self-injurious behavior from January to June 2013, Unpublished paper.

Philippine Information Agency (2005) *General Profile of the Philippines*. Available from: http://archives.pia.gov.ph/?m=6&subject=philinfo&item=geography [accessed 9 May 2014].

Redaniel, M. *et al.* (2011) 'Suicide in the Philippines: time trend analysis (1974–2005) and literature review, *BMC Public Health*, 11, 536.

Reyes, B.V. (1968) 'History of the department of psychiatry in the college of medicine, UP.' Manual of the Structural and Functional Organization of the Department of Psychiatry, UP–PGH Medical Center.

Vicente, B.A. (2013) *Mental Health*. Lecture notes, distributed in 2014.

World Health Organization (2007) *WHO–AIMS Report on Mental Health System in the Philippines*. WHO, Manila.

Yap, M.R. (1995) *Through the Years: History of Philippine Psychiatry*. Available from: www.philpsych.ph/about-us/ppa-history [accessed 6 May 2014].

21

Republic of Singapore

Leslie Lim Eng Choon and Shi-Hooi Poon

Geography

Singapore is a highly urbanised, island city-state in Southeast Asia, located at the southern tip of the Malayan peninsula between Malaysia and Indonesia. It has a total land area of 714.3 square kilometres (275.8 square miles) and measures forty-nine kilometres (thirty miles) from east to west and twenty-five kilometres (sixteen miles) from north to south (Department of Statistics Singapore, nd).

The island is situated 1° north of the equator. Its climate is characterised by uniform temperature and pressure, high humidity and abundant rainfall. The average annual rainfall is around 2,340 mm (92.1 in.). Monsoons are expected from mid-November till early March and from mid-June till early September when heavy downpours are expected to be frequent (National Environment Agency – Meteorological Services, nd).

Although temperatures are fairly constant, they can vary from a minimum of 23°C (73.4°F) to a maximum of 32°C (89.6°F), with May generally considered the hottest month of the year (National Environment Agency – Meteorological Services, nd). Relative humidity varies from 60 per cent in the mid-afternoon to 90 per cent in the early morning. There are more than 300 parks, and four nature reserves. Almost 50 per cent of the country is covered in greenery. Because of this, Singapore is also commonly known as the 'Garden City' (National Parks Board, nd).

Economy

Since independence in 1965, Singapore has experienced rapid economic expansion, to the extent that the city-state has been transformed from third to first world status in a matter of decades. Singapore's strong economic performance reflects the success of its open and outward-oriented development strategy. Over the years, the composition of Singapore's exports has evolved from labour-intensive to high value-added, such as consumer electronics, pharmaceuticals, chemicals and information technology products. In addition, Singapore is also a hub for financial services (The SGS market, nd). From 2000 to 2010, the GDP nearly doubled, rising from S$163 billion to S$304 billion. Real GDP per capita also rose rapidly at a compounded rate of nearly 12 per cent per annum (p.a.), while inflation and unemployment rates averaged less than 2 per cent p.a. and 3 per cent p.a. respectively, during this period. As a result of its healthy fiscal position and consistent budget surpluses over the years, Singapore has attained a high level of foreign reserves and the strongest sovereign credit rating for long-term foreign-currency debt in Asia (The SGS market, nd).

Population

The population of 5.3 million comprises Chinese, Malays and Indians, and other races. There are 3.8 million citizens and permanent residents, and 1.5 million non-residents (*The Year Book of Statistics Singapore*, 2013). The Chinese form the majority 74.17 per cent, Malays 13.3 per cent and Indians 9.2 per cent. About 83 per cent live in government-built housing board (also termed 'HDB') flats, 11 per cent in condominiums and private apartments and 5.8 per cent make their abode in landed properties (bungalows, semi-detached and terraced houses). Almost 90 per cent of dwellings are owner occupied (*The Year Book of Statistics Singapore*, 2013).

Mental health systems

Healthcare services have advanced in tandem with the nation's progress since colonial days, which will be elaborated below.

Colonial experiences

Early psychiatry in Singapore was quintessentially an outpost of British psychiatry, modified by local conditions and cultural influences (Ng, 2001). Since the founding of modern Singapore by Sir Stamford Raffles in 1819, the island has rapidly flourished by providing commercial gateways between the East and West. The influx of Western influences has shaped the development of mental health services; while the migration of people from varying backgrounds has contributed to a melting pot of diverse ethnicities, thus creating a unique local culture of its own. Mental health development was a harsh, yet inspiring process shaped by multiple influences (Ng, 2001).

In the years preceding 1841, patients suffering from mental illnesses were labelled 'insane', and confined to the 'Convict Gaol'. These people were completely neglected, looked after by convicts, and often left to die.

A revolutionary initiative was put in place when a 30-bed 'Insane Hospital' was built in 1841. Although patients did not receive treatment or medical care, they were placed in a suitably hygienic and spacious environment. Patients also enjoyed a rudimentary form of occupational therapy in the form of basket weaving. Treatment in the form of purgatives and stimulants was introduced in 1847.

The compound surrounding the 'Insane Hospital' (later renamed 'Lunatic Asylum'), soon saw new buildings rapidly developed to house the burgeoning number of patients. These growing numbers were in part due to increased awareness of mental illness and the inability of family members to care for them adequately. They were also a result of increased immigration in the face of a booming economy. Services were gradually expanded to include a female ward in 1867; and in 1888, the first psychiatrist – Dr W. Gilmore Ellis, arrived in Singapore to take over the reins and oversee the running of the Lunatic Asylum. The hospital was eventually moved to relatively larger compounds where psychiatric patients could engage in farming and gardening as part of their rehabilitation.

Advances in psychiatric care in Singapore did seem promising at that point in time. Unfortunately, Singapore succumbed to the Japanese Occupation between 1942 and 1945. The premises of the Lunatic Asylum were converted for military use. Patients were either sent home, or were discharged to St John's Island where they mostly perished from starvation. When the Japanese Occupation ended in 1945, the Lunatic Asylum returned to its original purpose of housing and treating psychiatric patients. By this time, the number of remaining patients had dwindled to a shadow of what it was before the war (Ng, 2001).

The ensuing peace led to rapid improvements in the care and treatment of patients. New therapies such as electroconvulsive therapy and insulin coma therapy were brought in by the British. Pharmacological therapies were gradually introduced and incorporated into standard care as well.

In 1951, several radical changes were made. For one, the names 'Mental Hospital' and 'Lunatic Asylum' were abolished in an attempt to reduce stigma as well as to show respect and sensitivity to patients suffering from mental disorders. This also reflected increased awareness of mental illnesses, and the need for effective treatment in helping these patients. The Lunatic Asylum was also renamed Woodbridge Hospital, taking its name from a bridge some distance away from the institution. This served as the main provider of psychiatric services in Singapore for many subsequent years.

Since the setting up of Woodbridge Hospital, a one-stop mental health facility where all patients could seek help, there was no pause in the development of mental health services in Singapore. The Departments of Social Work, Occupational Therapy, Psychological Services and Rehabilitation were set up in quick succession. Satellite clinics were set up in various parts of the island nation for the convenience of residents living in the neighbourhood.

In the 1970s, voluntary welfare organisations were formed to help people with mental health needs, including a home for intellectually disabled children, and a 24-hour hotline (by the Samaritans of Singapore). A clinic catering specifically for children and adolescents (the 'Child Guidance Clinic') was also started. Services catering to specific subgroups of patients, such as military personnel and forensic populations were started.

Owing to overwhelming positive feedback from the public as well as increased utilisation of services in Woodbridge Hospital, satellite psychiatric departments were opened in various general hospitals in Singapore very soon after – thus introducing the important concept of liaison psychiatry. Various subspecialty departments were started across the island, including addiction medicine, emergency psychiatry and early psychosis intervention.

Following the establishment and success of multiple hospital-based services, policy-makers started looking into the extension of mental health care into the community, thus founding the community psychiatry movement. This was a turning point for mental health care in Singapore. Services providing home visits to the elderly, and partnership with family physicians served to meet the needs of patients and caregivers alike. It also promoted community awareness of mental conditions and reduced the social stigma associated with psychiatric illness (Ng, 2001).

Service delivery model and patterns of referral

Patients are currently assessed in the primary care setting by general practitioners (GPs) or government polyclinic doctors before being referred to tertiary centres where they are seen by psychiatrists. Some GPs may choose to treat minor psychiatric conditions and refer them to specialist services should the patient fail to improve.

Services currently available

In 2007, the National Mental Health Blueprint (NMHB) was introduced. It was a five-year, government-funded project, spearheaded by the Ministry of Health. Various segments of this plan are still ongoing while other sectors have been improved upon. This plan reviewed the entire spectrum of mental health and mental illness with a view to preserving mental well-being and promoting mental resilience (primary prevention) (National Mental Health Blueprint Singapore, 2007–2012). A total of $157 million has been spent on this programme so far. The various aspects of the programme are discussed below.

Mental health promotion

A number of initiatives are in place to raise awareness and understanding of the importance of mental well-being. Programmes are also designed to help people understand the symptoms of mental disorders and improve accessibility of professional services, as well as reduce discrimination and stigma against people suffering from such problems. These initiatives aim to target different segments of the population, using outreach efforts targeted at schools, workplaces and the general community.

Integrated mental health care

Using the biopsychosocial model for the care of mental health needs of the Singapore population, it is essential to integrate tertiary services from our main psychiatric institution with primary care and community services to improve access and reduce stigma. Various integrated mental health care teams have been formed to promote early detection and treatment of mental health problems in the community, targeting different demographic groups. These include the Response, Early Intervention and Assessment in Community Mental Health (REACH) Team (which targets children and adolescents in schools), the Community Mental Health Team (intended for adults) and the Community Psychogeriatric Programme. There are also separate programmes targeting people suffering from psychosis – the Early Psychosis Intervention Program (EPIP) as well as the Community Health Assessment Team (CHAT, which caters to youths before the onset of mental illness).

Integrated hospital teams

Liaison services in restructured hospitals have also expanded their services to serve patients admitted under medical or surgical departments. These services harness the expertise of multidisciplinary teams. The remits of some of these specialised teams include managing the psychiatric aspects of irritable bowel syndrome, postnatal depression, psychosocial trauma, depression and distress in diabetes, post-stroke depression as well as psychological aspects of HIV infection. These services contribute to the holistic management of certain high-risk conditions involving screening for mental illness and providing early intervention or treatment if needed.

Mental health–general practitioner partnership

This is a programme aimed at getting GPs involved in the care and management of stable psychiatric patients in the community. The scheme allows patients to seek psychiatric treatment at convenient locations (usually near their homes or work places) and at convenient times. This results in the correct siting of care and better allocation of resources; so that tertiary institutions can cater to more acutely ill patients rather than spend their time reviewing patients whose conditions have stabilised (National Mental Health Blueprint Singapore, 2007–2012).

Following the overwhelming success of the NMHB, the Community Mental Health Strategy was launched in 2012. This policy serves to further address the needs of psychiatric patients (and those at risk of developing psychiatric illness) and develop the services to care for and support them. Some of the key initiatives include Community Resource and Engagement Support Teams (CREST) – which aim to provide psychoeducation and encourage early help-seeking; Community Intervention Teams (COMIT) and Assessment Shared Care Teams (ASCAT) – which encourage community treatment of psychiatric patients. These services will be gradually developed and expanded in the next five years (Chong, R. *et al.*, 2012).

Mental health policy

Mental health policies in Singapore have come a long way since the first legislation relating to the detention of persons of unsound mind was introduced in 1889. This was known as the Straits Settlement Ordinance No. VIII of 1889. Over the years, with new regulations added on, mental health policies have gradually evolved into the current policies we have today (Ng, 2001).

Detention and compulsory treatment

Involuntary detention of a mentally disordered person in Singapore is currently regulated by the Mental Health (Care and Treatment) Act 2008 [MH(CT)A 2008] (AGC Singapore, nd). This supersedes the preceding Mental Disorders and Treatment Act (Chapter 178 of the 1985 Revised Edition). This Act serves to guide the admission, detention, care and treatment of mentally disordered persons in designated psychiatric institutions in Singapore. The main psychiatric institution in Singapore is the Institute of Mental Health/Woodbridge Hospital where most involuntary patients are admitted.

First, a designated medical practitioner at Woodbridge Hospital, having diagnosed a person to be suffering from a mental disorder, and who is of the opinion that he/she should receive inpatient treatment, or continue inpatient treatment at a psychiatric institution, can invoke the powers of the Act.

Admission and detention for treatment can be classified into five different categories, named Form 1 through to Form 5. The endorsement of these forms allows persons assessed to be mentally unsound to be detained in the psychiatric institution for inpatient assessment and treatment. The duration of detention ranges from 72 hours to six months and up to an additional twelve months – renewable by a magistrate each year, if deemed necessary.

The MH(CT)A 2008, unlike the Mental Health Act in the United Kingdom, does not allow for appeals against compulsory detention and treatment. However, concessions for home leave are granted if it is judged beneficial to the patient's recovery. Two independent visitors make this decision after a thorough assessment of the patient.

Visitors to the psychiatric institution comprise a team of independent specialist psychiatrists and mental health workers who do not work in the psychiatric institution. Their scope of duties includes regular inspection of the psychiatric institution at regular intervals, review of patients admitted under the MH(CT)A 2008 and assessing whether they continue to pose a danger to themselves or others, thus requiring further treatment.

At any time point, if a patient has been deemed fit for discharge by the treating psychiatrist and/or two visitors – one of whom must be a medical practitioner, he/she can be discharged from the psychiatric institution.

One should note that while the MH(CT)A 2008 allows for enforcement of psychiatric care, it does not apply to medical care of patients who are unable to make decisions on their own as a result of an underlying medical condition (e.g. delirium), or a psychiatric condition that may cloud their judgement. Under such circumstances, clinical decisions are made in accordance with the Mental Capacity Act.

Link between mental health and prison systems/populations

The Singapore prison system has facilities for psychiatric assessment and treatment of prisoners known to suffer or who are suspected to be suffering from any psychiatric illness.

Persons suspected to have committed a crime and who are deemed to be suffering from a mental disorder, can be remanded in Woodbridge Hospital for a forensic psychiatric assessment. Patients can also be remanded in Woodbridge Hospital under the Criminal Procedure Code. These patients are treated by attending psychiatrists in the hospital, and are assessed by the board of visitors at least every six months.

Psychiatrists also assist Singapore's judiciary system as expert witnesses during court proceedings. Outpatient forensic assessments, often requested by lawyers and/or the Singapore police, are conducted in the psychiatric institution or by specialists in the private sector.

Specialised psychiatric care is also available in the Singapore prison system, staffed by a team of trained psychiatrists, psychologists and nurses. Also, firm psychiatric care plans after release from prison are put in place to ensure proper continuity of care and treatment.

Psychiatric epidemiology

In line with promoting mental health care and addressing the needs of patients and caregivers, the Singapore Mental Health Study was conducted from 2009 to 2010 (Chong, S.A. *et al.*, 2012a). The aim of this cross-sectional epidemiology survey was to analyse the rates of major mental disorders in the country and their associated risk factors so as to better allocate resources for service provision. In addition, this study also looked into the impact of psychiatric disorders on patients and their caregivers, as well as access and barriers to receiving adequate care. The diagnoses of mental disorders in adults aged 18 and above were established using the World Mental Health Composite International Diagnostic Interview (WMH–CIDI; Kessler and Ustun, 2004).

The study found that the lifetime prevalence of at least one affective, anxiety or alcohol use disorder was 12 per cent of the population; while the 12-month prevalence was 4.4 per cent. The most prevalent 12-month disorder was major depressive disorder (MDD). Only 2.5 per cent of the population suffered from two or more mental disorders (Chong, S.A. *et al.*, 2012a).

Of the affective disorders, the lifetime prevalence of dysthymia was 0.3 per cent, the lifetime prevalence of bipolar disorder was 1.2 per cent and the distribution between affected men and women was more or less equal (1.3 per cent vs 1.2 per cent). The lifetime prevalence of MDD was 5.8 per cent. The 12-month prevalence of MDD was 2.2 per cent compared to that of 0.6 per cent for bipolar disorder.

The combined lifetime prevalence of the two most common anxiety conditions, generalised anxiety disorder (GAD) and obsessive–compulsive disorder (OCD) was 3.6 per cent. The prevalence of OCD was higher than GAD, at 3.0 per cent compared to 0.9 per cent. The 12-month prevalence of OCD and GAD were 1.1 per cent and 0.4 per cent respectively.

The lifetime and 12-month prevalence rates of other major mental disorders are given in Table 21.1 (Chong, S.A. *et al.*, 2012a).

Table 21.1 Lifetime and 12-month prevalence of psychiatric disorders in Singapore (Chong, S.A. *et al.*, 2012a)

Disorder	Lifetime prevalence % (SE) % (SE)		12-month prevalence	
Major depressive disorder	5.8	(0.4)	2.2	(0.2)
Dysthymia	0.3	(0.1)	0.3	(0.1)
Bipolar I and II disorders	1.2	(0.2)	0.6	(0.1)
Generalised anxiety disorder	0.9	(0.2)	0.4	(0.1)
Obsessive compulsive disorder	3.0	(0.3)	1.1	(0.2)
Alcohol abuse	3.1	(0.3)	0.5	(0.1)
Alcohol dependence	0.5	(0.1)	0.3	(0.1)
Any disorder	12.0	(0.6)	4.4	(0.3)
Co-morbidity	2.5	(0.3)	0.9	(0.2)

Mental health workforce training and internship system

Postgraduate training in psychiatry

In recent years, there has been a greater realisation of the importance of developing mental health services in Singapore. As part of the National Mental Health Blueprint, resources have been allocated to increase the number of psychiatrists. The Division of Graduate Medical Studies has been organising the Master of Medicine in Psychiatry postgraduate examinations since 1985 (Division of Graduate Medical Studies, National University of Singapore, nd). Since May 2010, the Ministry having teamed up with the Accreditation Council for Graduate Medical Education in the United States will be initiating American-style residency programmes whereby trainees (also known as Residents) have to undergo a five-year period of training. At the end of the five years, Residents have to sit an 'exit' exam to determine their fitness to become specialists. Successful candidates attain the Associate Consultant grade and they can subsequently be promoted to Consultant grade after a couple of years.

Mental health training for family physicians

In addition, a training programme leading to the Graduate Diploma in Mental Health was launched to train family physicians to better manage psychiatric patients in the community. This 12-month programme aims to equip family physicians with skills in detection and treatment of minor mental health problems, such as mild anxiety or depressive disorders in the community.

Health Manpower Development Plan

Additional funds were also injected to add impetus to the mental health Health Manpower Development Plan (HMDP), a programme established by the Ministry of Health, Singapore. This programme serves to provide sponsorship for doctors and allied health professionals to pursue postgraduate training and or to upgrade their clinical skills. Successful applicants are sent to overseas institutions of their choice (National Mental Health Blueprint Singapore, 2007–2012).

Social/explanatory model(s) about mental illness

Models of mental illness

Although such concepts are rarer in modern-day society, the idea that mental illnesses arise from spirit possession is still accepted by Singaporeans from more traditional backgrounds. Many patients still seek help from spiritual healers in the first instance when they develop psychiatric symptoms.

The Malays

Malay patients attribute mental disorders to the brain being overheated, thus causing violent and angry behaviour (Laderman, 1993; Ng, 2001). Those affected usually seek help from traditional Malay healers (or *bomohs*) who generally judge illnesses as being caused by physical factors, supernatural factors (e.g. possession by evil spirits) and predispositions (Razali *et al.*, 1996). Many Malays believe in witchcraft and black magic, and regard abnormal behaviour as the work of supernatural powers (Ng, 2001).

Razali and Najib (2000) observed that in Malay societies where the extended family are housed under one roof, the strength of social support and the belief in supernatural causes of mental conditions were strongly associated with the decision to seek treatment with a *bomoh* in preference to Western psychiatric treatment, which is perceived as ineffective in such situations (Razali and Najib, 2000; Razali *et al.*, 1996).

Witchcraft is also believed to play an aetiological role in illness, with the victim being the target of a spell being cast on his/her food and drink. The *bomoh*'s role is to identify the motive and, if possible, name the perpetrator of the attack (Razali, 1995). Treatment may require the *bomoh* to enter into a trance, exorcise the spirits afflicting the patient, recite verses and prayers from the Koran, and examine the horoscope (Razali, 1995).

The Chinese

A study of Chinese patients seeking help from a psychiatric department in a teaching hospital in Singapore found that 36 per cent of them had consulted a spiritual or traditional healer before going to the hospital. There is apparently no association between educational level and help-seeking from traditional healers (Kua *et al.*, 1993).

The Chinese traditional healer is the *sinseh*, who prescribes herbs, and advises on the correct balance of food and the use of talismans and charms (Gwee, 1968). The Chinese subscribe to the theory of *yin* and *yang* in which *reh* (heat or warmth) is caused by an excess of *yang* and *leng* (cold) – the result of excess *yin* over *yang* in the body. Medications are prescribed to increase the level of *reh* in conditions with an excess of *yin* or deficiency of *yang* (Rin, 1965). *Yin–yang* imbalance is believed to result in anger, insanity, numbness, speech disturbances or wildness (Rin, 1965). Any physiological excess can lead to physical exhaustion and bowel problems, as well as poor appetite or impaired sexual functioning (Kua *et al.*, 1993).

Qi is considered to be the energy flowing throughout the body. Any loss or obstruction of *Qi* is judged to be deleterious to one's health. A deficiency of vitality results in neurotic symptoms. According to traditional belief, nocturnal emissions and habitual masturbation result in loss of *jing* (semen), an essential source of energy (Rin, 1965). Through the exercise of self-discipline, will-power to remain stoic in the face of adversity and positive thinking, health is maintained (Kua *et al.*, 1993).

The Indians

The Indians adhere to Ayurveda, the classical Sanskrit system of medicine based on ancient texts written in North India from the time of Christ till AD 1000 (Trawick, 1992). The teachings of Ayurveda encompass the names and activities of the humours, the qualities of different times, places and types of weather, and the types of food and their effects on the body (Trawick, 1992). In depression, according to Ayuverda, the subject experiences a widespread burning sensation (Trawick, 1992). Insanity is thought to be the result of inappropriate diet, disrespect towards the gods and teachers; and mental shock the consequence of excessive fear, joy and faulty bodily activity (Bhugra, 1992).

Thus, native healers such as the Chinese medium and Hindu priest may be sought by those experiencing psychological problems, who then visit places of worship (e.g. temples) for their treatment (Ng, 2001). It appears that exercising faith in traditional treatment or healing has resulted in favourable results, where as many as nearly one quarter of those with psychoneurosis reported feeling better after praying to deities widely regarded as possessing healing powers (Satija et al., 1981; Ng et al., 2008).

Help-seeking

Owing to a preference for traditional healers over established psychiatric services, it is not surprising that in a previous community survey, it was found that although 37 per cent of households affirmed a preference for seeking psychiatric help if they should develop a psychiatric illness, only 6 per cent of persons diagnosed with psychiatric disorders were receiving psychiatric treatment (Ng et al., 2003). This trend towards low rates of help-seeking was replicated in a subsequent local community survey of 2002–2003 (Ng et al., 2008). A large proportion of adults with depressive and anxiety disorders did not seek help. Not surprisingly, those who sought help did so when their anxiety and depressive symptoms resulted in functional disability, the strongest independent predictor of help-seeking (Chong, S.A. et al. 2012b).

Patients with mental health problems receive affordable primary care treatments from general practitioners or subsidised specialist care in the public psychiatric services (one large psychiatric institute and five general hospital psychiatric departments). However, it was reported that the main determining factors for seeking help were not health service system factors, such as availability and access to primary and specialist care, but personal and social factors (Chong, S.A. et al., 2012b).

A possible explanation is that perceptions of distress, suffering and the thresholds for seeking help vary among individuals with the same level of illness severity, and they also vary within the same individual at differing points in time. Such concerns and apprehensions are, nevertheless, surmountable (Chong, S.A. et al., 2012b).

Help-seeking rates have increased from 6 per cent (Ng et al., 2003) to 32 per cent (Chong, S.A. et al., 2012b). The Singapore Mental Health Study has found that of those diagnosed with psychiatric disorders who sought help, 15.7 per cent consulted mental health professionals, 8.4 per cent saw their GPs and 7.6 per cent turned to spiritual healers (Lee, 2013).

Topics of interest specific to Singapore

In spite of the immense developments in terms of policies and service provision in the realm of mental healthcare in Singapore, there are still a multitude of challenges mental health professionals and patients face regularly. Some of these are as follows.

Stigma

Stigma continues to be a major problem. Patients seen at the general hospitals are often reluctant to be transferred to the state psychiatric hospital, Woodbridge Hospital. Another reminder of the harsh realities of stigma is that in any job application, questions are asked about the health status of the applicant, with responses indicated with a 'tick' in the relevant boxes. In particular, should an applicant tick 'yes' to the query about past psychiatric illness, the chances of being accepted for employment are practically non-existent.

Mental health laws

Although there are powers of compulsory detention and treatment, these can only be implemented in Woodbridge Hospital. All patients admitted to general hospitals are voluntary patients. Should the patient become acutely agitated and in danger of causing harm to himself/herself or to others, a transfer to Woodbridge Hospital becomes necessary.

In Singapore, we do not have community treatment orders (CTOs) whereby patients with a serious mental disorder are required to accept psychiatric treatment while living in the community, with the aim of preventing relapse, hospital readmission and incarceration (Lee, 2013).

Role of voluntary welfare organisations

There are two major voluntary welfare organisations that provide community-based rehabilitation of mentally ill patients, i.e. Singapore Association for Mental Health (SAMH) and the Singapore Anglican Community Services (SACS). Some of the services SAMH provides include counselling, a group home, social clubs, and a day activity and rehabilitation centre. The SACS offers supported residential care with an emphasis on education and vocational training, with Hougang Care Centre adopting a clubhouse model, and Simei Care Centre preferring the social enterprise model (Sengupta *et al.*, 2012).

The authors observe deficiencies in collaboration and cooperation between health and social service sectors, with each sector having different models of mental health and illness, and different value systems. For instance, social workers, trained to identify strengths and skills, often take issue with the medical model which focusses more on pathology and, to a lesser extent, on social factors that impact on people's lives (Sengupta *et al.*, 2012). Inter-sector networking meetings between the psychiatric and social service agencies have often been arranged on a piecemeal and ad hoc basis, usually when there are disagreements or other urgent matters to discuss. These gaps in regular communication have negative consequences, resulting in poorly integrated and fragmented services and poor understanding between service providers (Lee, 2013).

Conclusion

Development of modern psychiatry in Singapore has come a long way since its early colonial beginnings. Despite introduction of various policies and services over the years, the landscape is still evolving. The successful management of mental disorders should parallel the monumental task of increasing societal awareness of mental illness, debunking myths surrounding mental illness and reducing the size of stigma, thereby achieving earlier detection, earlier treatment and an improved prognosis for all mentally ill individuals. At the same time the aim is to strengthen inter-sectorial links between social welfare and clinical services, such that with better lines of communication, patients will have access to early intervention and effective crisis management, and enjoy a better quality of life in the community.

References

AGC Singapore (nd) Attorney-General's Chambers. http://statutes.agc.gov.sg/. Accessed 14 Sept. 2013.

Bhugra, D. (1992) 'Psychiatry in ancient Indian texts: a review', *History of Psych.*, iii: 167–86.

Chong, R., Tan, W.M., Wong, L.M. and Cheah, J. (2012) 'Integrating mental health: the last frontier?', *Int. J. of Integrated Care*, (12: 28 September, URN:NBN:NL:UI:10-1-113825/ijic 2012–198, www.ijic.org/.

Chong, S.A., Abdin, E., Vaingankar, J.A., Heng, D., Sherbourne, C., Yap, M., Lim, Y.W., Wong, H.B, Ghosh-Dastidar, B., Kwok, K.W. and Subramaniam, M. (2012a) 'A population-based survey of mental disorders in Singapore', *Ann. Acad. Med. Singapore*, 41: 49–66.

Chong, S.A., Abdin, E., Vaingankar, J.A., Kwok, K.W. and Subramaniam, M. (2012b) 'Where do people with mental disorders in Singapore go to for help?' *Ann. Acad. Med. Singapore*, 41: 154–60.

Department of Statistics Singapore (nd). www.singstat.gov.sg. Accessed 12 Sept. 2013.

Division of Graduate Medical Studies, National University of Singapore (nd). http://medicine.nus.edu.sg/dgms/. Accessed 14 Nov. 2013.

Gwee, A.L. (1968) 'Koro – its origin and nature as a disease entity', *Singapore Med. J.*, 9: 3–6.

Kessler, R.C. and Ustun, T.B. (2004). The World Mental Health (WMH) Survey Initiative version of the World Health Organization (WHO) Composite International Diagnostic Interview (CIDI). *Int. J. Methods Psychiatr. Res.*, 13: 93–121.

Kua, E.H., Chew, P.H. and Ko, S.M. (1993) 'Spirit possession and healing among Chinese psychiatric patients', *Acta Psychiatr. Scand.*, 88: 447–50.

Laderman, C. (1993) *Taming the wind of desire: psychology, medicine, and aesthetics in Malay shamanistic performance.* California: University of California Press.

Lee, C. (2013) 'Community psychiatry', in *Essential guide to psychiatry*, Singapore: Pearson.

National Environmental Agency – Meteorological Services (nd). http://app.nea.gov.sg/data/mss/pdf/26March07.pdf. Accessed 18 Oct. 2013.

National Mental Health Blueprint Singapore (2007–2012), Ministry of Health, Singapore.

National Parks Board (nd). www.nparks.gov.sg/cms/. Accessed 18 Oct. 2013.

Ng, B.Y. (2001) *Till the break of day: a history of mental health services in Singapore 1841–1993*, 1st edn, Singapore: Singapore University Press.

Ng, T.P., Fones, C.S. and Kua, E.H. (2003) Preference, need and utilization of mental health services, Singapore National Mental Health Survey. *Aust. N.Z. J. Psychiatry*, 37(5): 613–19.

Ng, T.P., Jin, A.-Z., Ho, R., Chua, H.-C., Fones, C.S.L. and Lim, L. (2008) 'Health beliefs and help-seeking for depressive and anxiety disorders among urban Singaporean adults', *Psych. Services*, 59: 105–8.

Razali, M.S. (1995) 'Psychiatrists and folk healers in Malaysia', *World Health For.*, 16: 56–8.

Razali, S.M. and Najib, M.A.M. (2000) 'Help-seeking pathways among Malay psychiatric patients', *Int. J. Soc. Psychiatry*, 46: 281–9.

Razali, S.M., Khan, U.A. and Hasanah, C.I. (1996) 'Belief in supernatural causes of mental illness among Malay patients: impact on treatment', *Acta Psychiatr. Scand.*, 94: 229–33.

Rin, H. (1965) 'A study of the aetiology of koro in respect to the Chinese concept of illness', *Int. J. Soc. Psychiatry*, XI(1): 7–13.

Satija, D.C., Singh, D., Nathawat, S.S. and Sharma, V. (1981) 'A psychiatric study of patients attending Mechandipur Balaji Temple', *Indian J. of Psychiatry*, 23: 247–50.

Sengupta, S., Leong, J.Y. and Lee, C. (2012) 'Community psychiatry in Singapore,' in B.S. Chavan, N. Gupta, P. Arun, A. Sidana and S. Jadhav (eds) *Community mental health in India*. New Delhi: Jaypee Brothers Medical Publishers (Pvt) Ltd.

The SGS market (nd). www.sgs.gov.sg/The-SGS-Market/ The-Singapore-Economy.aspx. Accessed 12 Sept. 2013.

The Year Book of Statistics Singapore (2013) http://www.singstat.gov.sg/publications/publications_and_papers/reference/yearbook_of_stats.html. Accessed 12 Sept. 2013.

Trawick, M. (1992) 'Ayurveda, cosmopolitan medicine and other traditions in South Asia', in C. Leslie and A. Young (eds) *Paths to Asian medical knowledge*. Berkeley: University of California Press.

Section 6

Thailand and nearby countries

Overview

Pichet Udomratn

Thailand and the four nearby countries of Cambodia, Lao PDR, Myanmar and Vietnam (CLMV) are part of Southeast Asia and the Association of Southeast Asian Nations (ASEAN). However, these five countries are also part of the Great Mekong River Subregion (GMS) and have much in common in their cultures and beliefs because in the past they belonged to the same kingdom.

In this section, each chapter will focus on various aspects of psychiatry and mental health.

In Thailand, psychiatry has developed in many ways. The Mental Health Care Bill which was approved in 2008 was similar to legislation enacted in Western countries, in that all persons in need of psychiatric treatment either will be able to access it voluntarily or will be brought to a hospital for evaluation and compulsory treatment. The top three prevalence rates of mental disorders in Thailand are alcohol-use disorders, major depressive disorder and generalised anxiety disorder. Although the suicide rate has been a major public health concern in the country for some time, especially when it peaked at 8.6 per 100,000 in 1999, after the National Suicide Prevention Strategies were implemented the rate dropped to 5.9 per 100,000 in 2010.

From the Cambodia chapter, readers will learn about mental health development in this country after four decades of civil war from 1960 to 1998. Western-style mental health services were started in the 1990s through international aid. A mental health service has been set up in many general hospitals, together with mental health units in health centres. Anxiety and depression are the main psychiatric conditions found in Cambodia. Numerous challenges still exist, as in many developing countries.

From the chapter on Lao PDR, readers will learn about the mental health policy and the national mental health strategy to be in place by the year 2020. Currently, there is no specific mental health legislation in Lao PDR but legal provisions concerning mental health are included in welfare disability and general health legislation. The five most common mental disorders are neurosis, psychosis from infectious disease, depression, schizophrenia and substance abuse. Mental health services are now expanded to the provincial and community levels. While reducing the stigma of mental illness is very challenging in this country, interventions from traditional healers are used as alternative therapies for some patients.

From the Myanmar chapter, readers will learn about mental health policy and mental health services in that country. A strategy to reduce the treatment and services gap for mental disorders by 20 per cent by the year 2020 has been implemented. The common mental disorders are psychoses, anxiety disorders and depressive disorders. Attempts have been made to shift mental health care from hospital settings to community settings to ensure effective care. Although the mental health sector had a low priority in the health system in the past, nowadays the mental health sector has been upgraded to medium priority. Many aspects of progress will give a better opportunity for the development of mental health care in this country.

In the chapter on Vietnam, mental health policy and mental health systems are described. Currently, there are no specific legal rights for the mentally ill but the government agencies are in the process of developing them. Alcohol abuse, depression and anxiety are the three main conditions found in Vietnam. Community-based approaches have been adopted as a means of delivering rehabilitation to patients. Mental health provision in Vietnam suffers from many limitations, but there is a plan to promote mental health and provide a better service that is comprehensive, accessible and cost-effective.

In conclusion, Thailand and nearby countries have faced common challenges (for instance, an insufficient number of mental health workers). Furthermore, general practitioners are not confident in assessment and management of psychiatric patients, and so training is required. Patients and their families have a poor understanding of psychiatric disorders, and the stigma of mental illness is still a major issue. However, a number of strategic plans have been implemented in these countries. Better psychiatry and mental health can be expected in the future.

22

Mental health system in the Kingdom of Cambodia

Kim Savuon and Keo Sothy

Geography

Cambodia is one of the oldest countries in South East Asia. Officially known as the Kingdom of Cambodia, it is a constitutional monarchy with a multi-party democracy. The Kingdom of Cambodia shares its borders with the Kingdom of Thailand in the west, the People's Democratic Republic of Lao in the north, and the Socialist Republic of Vietnam in the east; it has a coastline to the south-west, on the Gulf of Thailand.

Cambodia has seen considerable socio-economic progress in recent years, accompanied by improvements in many health indicators. The economy has expanded by over 10 percent per year in recent years and poverty has declined but, despite this, 35 percent of the population still remained below the poverty line in 2006 (latest figures available). Many more families are susceptible to being tipped into poverty, especially in times of personal health crisis, sometimes due to health costs for themselves or their families. This creates many challenges in ensuring universal access to quality health care, alleviated only in part by such additional measures as health equity funds, an embryonic system of social health insurance, decentralization of the health system, and the contributions of health non-governmental organizations (NGOs).

Various key geographical, economic and demographic indicators are:

- The total land surface is 181,035 km^2
- The country is divided into one municipality, 24 provinces and 26 cities
- The total population is 15,053,112
- The main religion is Buddhism
- The currency is the Riel (US$1 = 4,000±100 Riels)
- Around 15 percent of the population can be classified as urban, and the remaining 85 percent as rural
- The male/female sex ratio is 96/100
- The annual population growth rate is 1.54 percent
- Life expectancy at birth for males is 60 years and for females 63 years
- The adult literacy rate is 89 percent among men and 86 percent among women
- Government expenditure on health care is 5.92 percent of GDP and per capita per year amounts to US$25.0
- GDP per capita is US$739.

National priorities for health

The Ministry of Health set three priorities for the health sector to cover the period 2008–2015:

1. To reduce maternal, newborn and child morbidity and mortality and to increase reproductive health
2. To reduce morbidity and mortality of HIV/AIDS, malaria, TB and other communicable diseases
3. To reduce the burden of non-communicable diseases and other health problems (diabetes, cardiovascular diseases, cancer, mental illness, substance abuse, accidents and injuries, eye care, oral health, etc.).

History

Cambodia was in a state of civil war from 1960 to 1998 and during this period nearly two million people were killed through torture, deprivation of food, forced labor and disease. The country's economy, health system, education system and other fundamental structures were completely destroyed by the Khmer Rouge regime of 1975–79, now infamous for the genocide stemming from its policy of social engineering. That regime also saw the long-term dissolution of family and community structures as well as cultural, medical, educational and art infrastructures. Almost all the literature that accounts for mental health training and services references this history in a similar manner. There is a call to incorporate specifically Cambodian criteria for trauma-related disorders, such as "*baksbat*" and "*Ivinh Chu Chot*" (bitter–sour–bitter) experiences.

Even after the Khmer Rouge regime fell, Cambodia continued to suffer from civil war and unofficial economic sanctions and received emergency aid only from a few Eastern-bloc countries. After the Paris Peace accord in 1991, Cambodia slowly and steadily returned to peace under the United Nations Transitional Authority of Cambodia (UNTAC, 1992–93). After peaceful democratic elections in 1998, 2003 and 2008, the Kingdom of Cambodia is now becoming a prosperous and developing nation. The survivors of the Khmer Rouge regime and civil war have endured exceedingly high levels of stress and collective trauma, which have had a severe impact on mental health. Currently, Cambodia is striving to improve the physical health of the nation by reducing infant and maternal mortality and meeting the HIV/AIDS crisis with meager resources. But demand for mental health care is huge and the psychosocial well-being of families and communities all over Cambodia is the cornerstone of sustained development. The loss of over a quarter of the population (the losses were especially high among the Cambodian intelligentsia); remaining landmines and unexploded bombs; massive destruction of infrastructure, the health care and education systems, as well as religious and cultural legacies; the extreme dehumanized brutality of the Khmer Rouge regime, and the search for the reasons for such brutality and better understanding of what happened and why; along with profound and multiple traumatic experiences have left Cambodia as a deeply traumatized society.

Mental health service development

Inevitably such massive psychosocial trauma in the last few decades, with virtually no Western-style mental health services has raised major issues in development and acceptance of mental health problems. Currently, there is no mental hospital in the country. Since 1993, Cambodia has seen numerous international aid, development and training programs, including a few initiatives related to mental health. In 1994 the Canadian Marcel Roy Foundation for the Children of Cambodia started a Center for Child and Adolescent Mental Health (CCAMH currently supported by Caritas-Cambodia) at the Cheychumneas Referral Hospital, Kandal province. In the same year, the International Organization for Migration (IOM), supported by the Norwegian Council for Mental Health, started the Cambodian Mental Health Training Project (CMHTP) to train ten Cambodian doctors as psychiatrists. Psychiatry was included only from 1995 in the medical curricula for doctors and nurses. In 1996, the Harvard Training Program in Cambodia (HTPC) started an outpatient department (OPD) for the mentally ill at Siem Riep Provincial Hospital, followed one year later by mental health training for 48 doctors and medical assistants.

Mental health policy

> The vision for every Cambodian is that they should live in harmony with optimum psychosocial well-being and socio-economic development to achieve a satisfactory quality of life as they wish.

The mental health policy of the Ministry of Health states that all Cambodians should have access to quality mental health services as well as health promotion, prevention, treatment and rehabilitation, and that these services should respect their dignity and rights and culture. The Cambodia mental health policy is mainly focused on community mental health. The policy parallels the WHO's mental health policy.

Policy direction

Key strands of the policy are to:

1. Make mental health services more responsive and closer to the public through the decentralization of service delivery and management, guided by the national *Policy on Service Delivery* and the policy on *Decentralization and Dilution (deconcentration)*.
2. Strengthen sector-wide governance, focusing on increased national ownership and accountability, harmonization and alignment, greater coordination and effective partnerships among all stakeholders.
3. Scale up access to and coverage by mental health services.
4. Improve quality in mental health service delivery and management through the establishment of and compliance with the national protocols, clinical practice guidelines and quality standards, and in particular the establishment of accreditation systems.
5. Increase the competency and skills of the mental health workforce, as well as their accountability, through strengthening allied technical skills and advanced technology, better training, career development, appropriate incentives, and good working environments.
6. Strengthen and invest in mental health information systems and mental health research for evidence-based policy-making, planning, monitoring performance and evaluation.
7. Increase investment in medical infrastructure and equipment and advanced technology, and improve the non-medical support services such as management and supply systems for drugs and commodities.
8. Promote quality of life and healthy lifestyles in the population by raising mental health awareness and creating supportive environments, including through strengthening institutional structures, financial and human resources, and information, education and communication (IEC) materials that promote mental health, behavior change and appropriate help-seeking for mental health problems.

9. Strengthen mental health interventions to deal with challenges relating to gender, mental health of minorities, school mental health, substance abuse, injury, occupational health, and disaster, through timely response, effective collaboration, and coordination with other sectors.
10. Promote effective public–private partnerships in mental service provision based on policy, regulation, legislation and technical standards.
11. Encourage community engagement with mental health service delivery, including in the management of mental health facilities and continuous quality improvement.
12. Systematically strengthen institutions at all levels of the mental health system to implement the policy agenda.

Organization of mental health services

Due to insufficient human resources and infrastructure for the provision of a specific mental health service, mental disorders are treated within the general health services, in general hospitals and health centers (Figures 22.1 and 22.2). Employed staff must have had some brief basic training in mental health.

Guidelines for mental health services in general referral hospitals

There are guidelines for mental health services in general hospitals. These include:

• General hospitals are responsible for diagnosis, care, and all forms of treatment of patients with mental problems, as referred from the health centers and the community.
• Patients presenting as psychiatric emergencies can be hospitalized for a short time and sent home with treatment and regular follow-up for a time, and then sent back to continue treatment at a health center or with families.
• Mental health education and continuing education are available at community level.
• There is close cooperation with other services at the referral hospitals and the health centers.

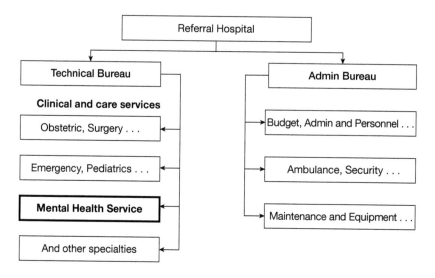

Figure 22.1 Mental health service within the structure of referral hospitals in Cambodia

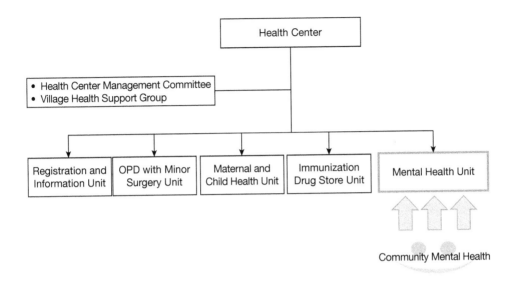

Figure 22.2 Mental health units within the structure of health centers in Cambodia

Facilities and resources of mental health services in referral hospitals

Each facility should have two units: first a psychiatric outpatient unit for assessment and intervention with an inpatient department for psychiatric emergency cases. The number of beds ranges from five to ten. In addition, some referral hospitals also have a rehabilitation center and other relevant services.

Staffing

The recommended staffing includes at least one psychiatrist/one GP and two nurses trained in basic mental health care along with psychologists or social workers as well as other staff as required.

Guidelines for mental health units at health centers

There are centrally agreed guidelines for service delivery related to mental health care in health centers. These include:

- Health centers should provide primary care, including mental health care, across the country. They should have, where possible, a physician and nurses trained in basic mental health care, in compliance with clinical mental health guidelines.
- They should offer on-going care for mentally ill patients transferred from referral hospitals or national hospitals. However; coverage of mental health services within national/referral hospitals and health centers does not meet demand, and they still do not cover all parts of the country.
- They should provide not only psychotropic medications but also community mental health education, and collaborate with local authorities, NGOs, village health support groups, traditional healers, and monks to conduct surveillance for severely mentally ill patients who may injure themselves or others. If this service is not available, such patients should be referred to a referral or national hospital.

- More specifically, they should educate communities, mentally ill patients and their families about mental health, and collaborate with relevant organizations to support and develop mental health activities at community level.
- Early detection of mental illnesses within communities is a responsibility of the health centers. They should also make home visits, as required and needed, to patients who have stopped treatment, and develop plans for engaging them in continuing treatment.

Interventions

As in many other countries, the therapeutic interventions (Somasundaram and van de Put, 1999; Somasundaram et al., 1999) typically used in the clinics are as follows:

- Pharmacotherapy such as TCAs, traditional neuroleptics, some anti-epileptic medication (carbamazepoine, phenobarbital)
- Crisis intervention
- Counseling
- Relaxation techniques.

However, in addition they should also offer traditional medicine, like that available through traditional healers (*Kru Khmer*), monks, village elders or mediums.

There is some emphasis on non-pharmacological forms of treatment for common psychosocial problems and appropriate referral for help. As 90 percent of Cambodians are Buddhist, psychosocial interventions that have been found effective in the Cambodian context include the formation of self-help groups for women who, for one reason or another, have lost their husbands, and the use of traditional Buddhist relaxation methods such as "mindful breathing" (*Ana Pana Sati*) and meditation.

Currently, patients and families pay for consultations, as there is no health insurance to cover psychiatric treatment, or in fact any form of medical treatment.

Psychiatric epidemiology

According to information from the Ministry of Health, the numbers of people accessing mental health services have increased so much year-on-year that demand has outstripped supply of resources. Inevitably the problem of access is worse for people in rural areas, and any treatment they do receive is mostly simply medication. Like in other countries, the groups especially vulnerable to mental health problems are the poor, the illiterate, those who abuse alcohol and other substances, and those subject to domestic violence and other forms of social injustice. Mental illness now represents a huge burden for Cambodia.

The University of Health Sciences is training at most ten postgraduate medical students in psychiatry every year and the medical health care school is providing some training to postgraduate nurses, but there is a lack of interest in the subject on the part of students. The Ministry of Health is responsible for providing basic mental health knowledge to staff in the hospitals and health centers.

The Department of Psychology at the Royal University of Phnom Penh found the following population rates of mental disorder: anxiety around 28 percent; depression 17 percent; rates of suicide 7 percent; rates of PTSD 3 percent; all forms of psychotic disorders 2 percent; and alcohol abuse 1 percent. All forms of disabilities among children under 15 years old was 23 percent whereas the total number of recorded drug users was 4,313 (in the year 2012).

Mental health system

Before 1975, Cambodia did have a psychiatric hospital, led by two psychiatrists who were trained in France, although not surprisingly it was overcrowded. The hospital was under central government control and was funded by the government as well. But in the aftermath of the Khmer Rouge regime the country had to start over again from nothing, including in the mental health field.

In 1979, the Faculty of Medicine in Phnom Penh was reopened. No foreign aid was available during this period. From 1979 to 1992 no specialized mental services were available. Families of people with mental problems used traditional healers (*Kru Khmer*), monks or fortune tellers to treat their relatives.

In 1994, with cooperation from NORARD (the Norway Development Agency), the Ministry of Health started to train mental health professionals and initially provided a psychiatric outpatient service in a general hospital in Phnom Penh. From that point, outpatient treatment services have expanded gradually. Psychiatric residents, and medical students at public and private universities have trained in psychiatry. By 2014, 52 psychiatrists, 45 psychiatric nurses, and more than 1,000 basic mental health physicians and basic mental health nurses have been trained thus far. There are presently eight outpatient units that provide specialist care and 40 outpatient units providing basic mental health care in 91 general referral hospitals (Tables 22.1 and 22.2). Twenty-four of the 1,026 health centers provide basic mental health care. In addition, several NGOs are working on mental health issues in some parts of the country.

The Khmer–Soviet Friendship Hospital in Phnom Penh has the biggest psychiatric outpatient department in the country. It is attended by patients from all over the country for consultation; a quarter of Cambodia's psychiatrists work there. This department provides training for medical students as well as for psychiatric residents.

Table 22.1 Summary of mental health human resources in Cambodia

Types of mental health professionals	Ministry of Health/ national hospitals	Referral hospitals	NGOs/ other	Total
Psychiatrists	19	6	14	45
Psychiatric nurses	15	25	5	45

Table 22.2 Summary of mental health service coverage in Cambodia

Types of mental services	National hospitals (7)	Referral hospitals (91)	Health centers (1,026)
Specialized			
Outpatient departments	2	8	—
Inpatient departments	1 (10 beds)	1 (6 beds)	—
Primary care	—	40	24
Child and adolescent mental health (outpatient department)	—	1	—
Rehabilitation centers	—	—	—
Total	2/7	49/91	24/1,026

Explanatory model(s) of mental illness

Culture is a major factor in both the explanation and the presentation of mental disorders. The use of cultural narratives and idioms has created uniquely Cambodian pathologies, although these appear to be disappearing gradually over time. Hallucinations and delusions often relate to local events and culture, but with bizarre twists such that the patient's thinking was no longer shared by others, showing the pathoplastic effect of the psychosis within the sociocultural context. Thus, paranoid ideas often involved the Khmer Rouge, Vietnam or the security forces. Ideas or experiences of spells or black magic corresponded to cultural beliefs. Hallucinations often involved local spirits or ancestors. Some believed they were Buddha. The diagnosis of psychosis was based more on abnormal, disorganized behavior.

Through its present survey, the Department of Psychology at the Phnom Penh Royal University found that the stigma against mental disorders remains strong (Cambodian Mental Health Survey, 2012). Cultural explanations and presentations of mental illness are rooted in basic traditional practices rather than a physical model of health. Cambodian people often use the following terms for mental illness:

- ឆ្កួត "*Chhkuot*" refers to psychotic features (crazy or mad) of a genetic nature, and so not amenable to cure. It involves black magic, or a spirit or putting thoughts in the patient's mind. If someone in the family suffers from *Chhkuot* she/he is typically locked in a room or cottage separate from the family. If they need help they are first sent to see traditional healers (*Kru Khmer*), monks or fortune tellers; psychiatric services are the last choice for them. Sometimes a ritual ceremony for ancestors is held to heal the patient.
- កម្ម "*Karma*" refers to suffering from a previous life. This is a Buddhist concept. People believe that mental problems are, from a religious perspective, "fate", part of the balance resulting from good and bad deeds. From this derives a strong spiritual and behavioral code of conduct. This explanation may have positive and negative effects. The positive effects include the person accepting what they face and experience. The negative effects include the person not acting properly to solve or improve the situation. For example, a poor family may think that they are poor because they had done a bad thing in a previous life, so they must accept this and not try to find a way to improve their situation. Thus, this external locus of control will also determine where and how they seek help.
- Animistic belief includes the concept of "unappeased" ancestors as the cause of mental illness. Angry ancestors are placated by ceremonies and offerings placed on the family's shrine.
- The Cambodian belief system incorporates the concept of luck and astrology. Thus, fortune tellers are frequently consulted.
- ខ្យល់គត "*Kyol koeu*" (wind overload) is an example of orthostatic irregularity often associated with panic disorder that can result from physical problems (e.g. nausea, palpitations, dizziness and low energy) and can be treated by readily available medications.
- Culturally specific panic attacks, ខ្យល់ចាប់ "wind attack" (*khyâl chab*) (e.g. orthostatically induced and neck-focused panic) lie at the center of the Khmer response to trauma/or severe stress. People suffer from psychosocial problems and they try to cope with physical symptoms rather than solve or discuss psychosocial problems.
- ខ្មោចសង្កត់ "*Khmaoch sângkât*'" ("ghost pushes down") is a form of sleep paralysis (SP), in which a demon acts upon an individual who is either falling asleep or waking. The experience causes paralysis, a sensation of a hand on the chest or neck, chest tightness and shortness of breath, and is interpreted as a sign of bad luck and imminent danger of dying. SP was clearly associated with trauma and PTSD in Cambodian and other cultures.

- "Weak heart" syndrome refers to anxiety, or ខ្សោយបេះដូង ("*khsaoy beh daung*"), which involves the belief that "excessive bodily wind" ("*kyol goeu*") causes a breakdown in heart function, with palpitations on slight provocation (e.g. orthostatic, an odor, being startled, exercise-induced palpitations).
- មិនគ្រប់ទឹក "*Min-krub teuk*" refers to intellectual problems or psychotic symptoms.
- "*Trov am Peou*" means getting action from another spirit. This concept is described as follows. When someone has a conflict or problems with other people (at work, relatives, friends, neighbors), if one of them gets mental problems then this patient's family believes those other people used witches to make the patient ill.
- មាយា "*Meayea*" means the patient sometimes feels bad, and is used to describe somatoform disorders.

Challenges faced by the public mental health services

The general challenges in relation to functional areas of the mental health system on both the "supply-side" and the "demand-side" are many and these include a fragmentation of activities, funding, monitoring and supervision, and administrative lines of authority; ineffective regulatory mechanisms; weak coordination between public and private (including not-for-profit) health services; difficult access to services due to geographical problems; and lack of information on mental health services available in remote areas. In addition, financial dependence on external donors for funding of health care in general, but mental health services in particular, and poor salary structures for staff working in the public sector prevent effective delivery of mental health services. Lack of human resources such as trained clinical psychologists working in the public mental health services and lack of rehabilitation centers for the chronic mentally ill further complicate service planning and delivery. A lack of psychotropic medication at all levels of mental health services, which in turn causes many patients to drop out of treatment is an important factor. A disproportionate spread of human resources in urban areas means that rural areas are underserved.

Inadequate skills and competencies and limited management capacity due to insufficient practical training and too few teaching staff, along with weak performance-related management (constraining increased productivity and quality of mental health services) and a lack of coordination in training activities (resulting in frequent absence of staff from their workplace), can contribute further to needs not being met. Despite efforts to improve the use of data in planning and monitoring, there is limited use of mental health information at all levels of the system. This is further compounded by a lack of coordination and collaboration among information providers within and outside the mental health system. Consequently, national health surveys or national surveys with health components are being conducted too close to each other to provide meaningful information for trend analysis. While a reasonably effective surveillance system exists for 12 notifiable diseases, case reporting and monitoring of key mental illnesses are weak. Mental Health Information System staff at local level have insufficient knowledge and skills and are poorly motivated, lacking information communication technology (ICT) software and hardware to manage data effectively, and conduct basic data analysis.

Like in many other countries in the region, the private sector's contribution to the mental health sector is growing in importance, but regulation remains weak.

Further institutional development is needed, including especially: aligning financial flows with managerial authority and accountability for outcomes; increasing managerial autonomy while ensuring accountability and maintaining the quality of the Mental Health Association of Cambodia; while at the same time providing it with more systems support and protection against changes in international funding priorities.

Activities of NGOs

The network of NGOs occupies an important place in the referral system. For example, a widow or a landmine victim with depression due to socioeconomic problems can be referred to an appropriate NGO for vocational training and introduction to various income-generating programs. On the other hand, NGOs seeing clients with mental problems can refer them to the mental health services. The Caritas-Cambodia Transcultural Psychosocial Organization (TPO) and Cambodia have been involved in setting up mental health services in selected provinces. A community-based approach was adopted in which grassroots workers were trained so that they would be able to tackle most basic problems of mental health in the villages.

Topics of interest specific to Cambodia

So now the big challenge for mental health professionals is to raise awareness of mental health issues with the people in the community. Other priorities include advocacy with health policy-makers and stakeholders along with patients and their carers and families. Obviously training primary health workers to take care of patients in the community is crucial. Mental health first aid is a good choice, because it is more affordable than the use of a health facility and reduces stigma and discrimination. Other topics which need further exploration include development of specializations such as forensic psychiatry, child and adolescent mental health, and rehabilitation psychiatry. For these services, and co-morbidity with substance abuse, a combination of health professionals and Buddhist monks may be helpful. In addition, more trained personnel for mental health and specific programs such as community suicide prevention are needed. Institutional development (establishment of a Department of Mental Health and a Research Center for Mental Health) is required to help develop research capacity and research activities.

Strategies for future mental health development

The key to delivering services which will be used and accepted by patients is to build on providing treatment in primary mental health care with access to psychotropic medication available at all levels of mental health service provision. In addition, appropriate mental health care in the community can be developed by providing education to the public on mental health awareness and mental health first aid, with active encouragement and involvement of the community, family and consumers to be involved in mental health care. A clear mental health policy, legislation and other guidelines are needed, which will also affect development of human resources for mental health directly as well as through links with other sectors, including NGOs. These community developments must be routinely monitored so that specific intervention programs (e.g. in suicide prevention) can be conducted, and both audit and research are encouraged.

Bibliography

Cambodian Mental Health Survey (2012). Royal University of Phnom Penh, Department of Psychology.
Health Strategic Plan (2008–2015) Ministry of Health, Cambodia.
Somasundaram, D. J., van de Put, W. A. C. M., Eisenbruch, M., and de Jong, J. T. (1999). Starting mental health services in Cambodia. *Social Science & Medicine*, 48(8), 1029–46.
Somasundaram, D. J., and van de Put, W. A. C. M. (1999). Mental health care in Cambodia. *Bulletin of the World Health Organization*, 77(3), 275–7.
World Health Organization (2010). *mhGAP intervention guide for mental, neurological and substance use disorders in non-specialized health settings: mental health Gap Action Programme (mhGAP)*. Geneva: WHO.

23

Mental health in the Lao People's Democratic Republic

Some secured changes

Chantharavady Choulamany

Country location

The Lao People's Democratic Republic (Lao PDR) is a landlocked country in Southeast Asia bordered by China, Vietnam, Cambodia, Thailand and Myanmar, with an area of 236,800 square kilometres. The plains region comprises large and small plains along the Mekong River. The country is crossed by many rivers and streams.[36] Around 70 per cent of the country is mountainous, with the most fertile land along the Mekong plains. The population was estimated at 6,514,432, with a density of 28 persons per square kilometre in 2012 [37] and an average household size of 5.9 people. Life expectancy is the lowest in Southeast Asia: life expectancy at birth for males is 62 years and for females is 64 years. The infant mortality rate is 42 per 1,000 live births and the under-five mortality rate is 79 per 1,000 live births, while the maternal mortality rate stands at 405 per 100,000 live births.[12] About 77 per cent of the population live in rural areas. The adult literacy rate is 73 per cent.[38]

The population includes 49 ethnic groups. These groups differ in their residential patterns, agricultural practices, forms of village governance, and religious beliefs. Approximately 67 per cent of the Lao population are Buddhists, 1.5 per cent are Christians, less than 1 per cent are Muslim and Bahai, and nearly 31 per cent are animists.[25]

The road system is not extensive. In the late 1980s, the Lao government adopted a programme of administrative and economic reform to move to a market-oriented system. It became a full member of the Association of South-East Asian Nations (ASEAN) in July 1997. It is classified as a middle-lower-income country by the Word Bank, but is one of the poorest countries in the East Asia and Pacific region, with 27.6 per cent of the population living below the poverty line. The Gross National Income (GNI) per capita was US$2,435 and average per capita income US$1,040 in 2012.[38]

The Lao PDR's development appears impressive. Poverty was reduced from 46 per cent in 1993 to 25 per cent in 2010. Rice is the staple food for all Laotians, and most families and villages produce enough for their own consumption.

The country is the most heavily bombed country in the world. During the second Indochina war (1964–73), the country was subject to over 580,000 bombing missions, and in addition saw many wide-ranging ground battles. Over 270 million cluster munitions were used, of which an estimated 80 million remained live, now buried in the Lao landscape after the war's end. All 17 provinces are contaminated with unexploded ordnance (UXO) – approximately 25 per cent of villages are affected. The legacy is therefore one of continuous death and injury, and disrupted socio-economic development. Tragically, UXO accidents still injure and harm approximately 300 people yearly. From 1964 to 2008, there were 50,000 UXO victims, a quarter of them children.[20] The correlation between UXO contamination and poverty is clear, with 42 of the 46 poorest districts affected.[38]

The health system is predominantly public, although a private alternative is growing. There are some private hospitals, around 1,865 private pharmacies and 254 private clinics, mainly in urban areas. The public health facilities consist of four central teaching and referral hospitals; five regional hospitals, including one teaching hospital; 16 provincial hospitals; 127 district hospitals; and about 746 health centres. A total of 5,081 hospital beds were available in 2005, giving a ratio of 0.9 beds per 1,000 inhabitants. As of 2011, per capita health expenditure amounted to US$38.8.[34] Of this amount, about seventy-eight per cent is out-of-pocket. Hospitals are highly dependent on patient fees for recurrent expenditure. Health insurance systems are nascent and the civil service scheme is being reformed. There are 2,660 regular high-level and mid-level medical staff at health-facility level, corresponding to 0.2 per 1,000 population, which is below the recommended WHO target of 2.5 per 1,000. Compared with international standards, the productivity of health workers is considered low.

Mental health policy

The National Mental Health Policy endorsed by the Minister of Health in October 2007 has four components: integration of mental health into general health care; equity of access to mental health services across different groups; human rights of people with mental illness; quality of mental health care services and management.[15] It provides vague guidance and direction for implementing mental health services at different levels by establishing the treatment network, developing human resources, financing, conducting research, management and monitoring.

To respond to this policy, BasicNeeds, the first British non-governmental organisation working in the mental health field in Lao PDR since 2007, began work in the country. The main goal of BasicNeeds is to improve the quality of life for those suffering from mental and/or epilepsy disorders by implementing the BasicNeeds Model of Mental Health and Development, which has been implemented in 13 other countries worldwide. Key components of the Model include: *community mental health* – enabling effective and affordable community-oriented mental health treatment services; *capacity building* – identifying, mobilising, sensitising, training stake-holders, including mentally ill people, their families and partner organisations, aiming to involve them in the development process; *sustainable livelihoods* – facilitating opportunities for affected individuals to gain or regain work, and so earn and contribute to the family and community, which will lead to self-reliance and social reintegration; *research* – generating evidence from the practice of mental health and development in the community, which will start to tackle the lack of awareness of mental health issues within the wider community and institutions, including the government; and *collaboration* – managing partnerships and relationships with stakeholders who are involved in implementing the model on the ground and/or responsible for policy and practice decisions, and providing an efficient administrative service, including financial and evaluation services, taking their resources as close to the field as possible.

Mental health problems are part of the global burden of disease. However, Lao PDR has been putting little effort into mental health. The existing policy has not yet been fully put into practice.[5] The only two mental health units are located in Mahosot Hospital and No. 103 Hospital, both in the centre of the capital city of Vientiane, and these serve the country's entire population. Geographic distance, poverty and an overall ignorance are thought to be associated with the low rates of admission to those facilities.[8]

Currently there is no specific mental health legislation. Legal provisions concerning mental health are included in welfare disability and general health legislation. In the eighth chapter of the Penal Law No. 12/NA, dated 9 November 2005, there are two articles related to the measures that may be applied by the court to mentally disturbed offenders (Article 54) and offenders addicted to alcohol or drugs (Article 55). These people should first be medically checked, then referred to psychiatric hospitals or a specific medical care centre for further psychiatric investigation and treatment. Then, once they have recovered from their mental illness or addiction, they should be brought back and sentenced by the court. The duration of medical treatment should be included when calculating the length of sentence.[19]

The existing mental health policy does not acknowledge United Nations Resolution 46/119, Principles for the Protection of Persons with Mental Illness and the Improvement of Mental Health Care (1991),[35] which is a detailed and comprehensive statement about the rights of persons with mental illness. The Resolution recognises: the right to informed consent; the right to protection from harm; prohibition of arbitrary or unnecessary isolation or physical restraint; the right to live, work, and receive treatment within the community; recognition of the patient's cultural background in order to achieve a more comprehensive reintegration into society; and use of the least restrictive environment maintaining and furthering the independence of the patients and promoting their participation in the community.

Most involuntary mental health consultations or admissions are upon the request of a third party (e.g. family members). There are no forensic beds or prison mental health facilities. The use of restraints or seclusion is conducted in the inpatient units only for patients deemed to be at risk of self-harm, and others during an acute psychotic episode. Data on prisoners with mental illness seeking treatment with mental health professionals and on their involuntary admission are unavailable.[17]

The results of a joint initiative between the Ministry of Health and BasicNeeds (from 2007 to the present) in community mental health and extended learning are being used to inform the development of the Lao mental health policy. The BasicNeeds programme is a way of developing a better response to UN Resolution 46/119.

The National Mental Health Strategy to the year 2020,[16] approved by the Minister of Health in March 2013, has five pillars: human resources development; establishment of a research culture and capacity in collaboration with domestic and international organisations; enhancement of mental health service delivery at national and local level; promotion of and advocacy for mental health; and the development of mental health policy and legislation. The strategy describes clear directives, objectives and expected outcomes for each pillar, with guidance on achieving each target.

Psychiatric epidemiology

From October 2012 to September 2013, at the mental health unit of Mahosot Hospital, 1,059 new outpatients were treated, of whom 71 were children. Mental disorders included anxiety disorder (29 per cent), psychosis due to infectious disease (e.g. pernicious malaria) (12 per cent), depression (7 per cent), schizophrenia (6 per cent) and substance abuse (4 per cent);[14] while epilepsy accounted for 14 per cent, psychosomatic disorder 7 per cent, neurological diseases 10 per cent and others 8 per cent. Among the 508 patients hospitalised, the diagnoses were anxiety disorder (18 per cent), schizophrenia (16 per cent), psychosis due to infectious disease (14 per cent), drug abuse (11 per cent), suicidal attempts (6 per cent), bipolar disorder (3 per cent), depression (3 per cent) and dementia (under 2 per cent).

At the mental health unit of No. 103 Hospital, over the same period, 675 patients were admitted, of whom 475 used drugs and 11 had epilepsy. Other diagnoses were schizophrenia (13 per cent), anxiety (5.5 per cent), psychosis related to substance abuse or malaria (2.7 per cent), depression (2 per cent), transitory hallucinations (0.9 per cent), psychosis related to brain trauma (0.6 per cent), bipolar disorder (0.5 per cent) and mental retardation (0.5 per cent).[21]

As of October 2013, the cumulative number of people with mental illness and/or epilepsy under the BasicNeeds-Lao programme was 1,520, of whom 980 were from Vientiane (the capital) and 540 from Borikhamxay; there was no significant gender difference in this respect. Among these patients, the diagnoses were anxiety (34 per cent), followed by schizophrenia (14 per cent), depressive psychosis (8 per cent), depression (7 per cent), mental retardation (5 per cent), substance abuse (4 per cent), bipolar disorder (2 per cent), epilepsy (25 per cent) and other problems (2 per cent).[6]

The emergency care unit of Mahosot treated 30 patients after a suicide attempt in the period 2005–2009, but this increased to 291 over the period 2009–2011.

An exploratory study on depression among 210 sixth-grade students (the last school grade) in 30 secondary schools in Vientiane in 2012, using the Beck Depression Inventory (BDI-II), showed that 24 per cent of them were depressed. Thus depression exists among Lao adolescents.[22] This proportion is slightly higher than among Thai adolescents in Bangkok, where the figure was 20 per cent.[24] The prevalence of clinical depression has no gender difference, which is similar to Iran.[28]

A retrospective study on relapses of schizophrenia at the Mahosot mental health unit analysed the clinical files of 52 patients with schizophrenia experiencing relapse(s) in 2012. It demonstrated that men had more relapses than women, with an average age of 30; 67 per cent were single; 56 per cent had finished secondary school and 43 per cent were unemployed. Forty per cent had just one relapse while 27 per cent had two; 15 per cent had three and about 6 per cent had four.[9]

In 2002, lifetime prevalence of methamphetamine (*Ya-Baa*) use among the young reached 42 per cent; the figure among bar staff was 34 per cent and among service women 14 per cent.[29] A survey conducted in 2003 by urine testing 14,260 students in 17 provinces showed that 3.7 per cent of students in urban areas had tried amphetamines; this increased to 27.6 per cent in 2005.[13] The prevalence of opium use was 0.42 per cent in the ten northern provinces among those aged 15 to 64. Seventy-two per cent of opium users treated with opium tincture in the community remained free of drugs.[30] As of 2009, an estimated 1.5 per cent of all drug users in Lao PDR were living with HIV. Injecting heroin increased in 2012, regrettably with little evidence of the use of sterile needles and syringes.[31]

A quarter of the 2,880 drug addicts treated at the Somsanga Centre in Vientiane were teenagers in 2012. The main drugs of use were *Ya-Baa*, heroin, alcohol and opium. The reasons for taking drugs included family problems and peer pressure. The relapse rate was 11 per cent in 2011,[26] which was lower than in 2003 (68 per cent).[10]

Forty children with autism are served by the Lao Association for Autism. Seventy-six per cent of Lao children aged from two to 14 are abused (psychological aggression or physical punishment) by an adult in their household, due to the belief that punishment is necessary to raise a child properly. The percentage of children experiencing violent discipline exceeds 60 per cent.[12] The effects of child abuse can appear in childhood, adolescence or adulthood and may affect various aspects of an individual's development (physical, cognitive, psychological, behavioural, self-esteem, attention disorders). Almost one half of Lao children are moderately stunted and 19 per cent severely stunted.[12] Under-nutrition may impair intellectual development, which in turn can significantly reduce future earning potential.[11] Unfortunately, no study on mental health problems related to these two issues has been done in Lao PDR.

Concerning dementia, mostly Lao families complain about their elders' memory impairment.

The prevalence of post-traumatic stress disorder (PTSD) is significantly higher among the injured UXO victims (10 per cent) than among the non-injured UXO victims (4 per cent) in Sepone district of Savannakhet province, a central part of the country.[27]

The Lao mental health workforce is extremely limited. Only 42 people work in mental health facilities: just two psychiatrists, a neurologist, 10 general practitioners, 18 nurses and 11 others. There are no psychiatric nurses, clinical psychologists, social workers or occupational therapists. There are 0.01 psychiatrists per bed and 0.26 nurses per bed in general hospital psychiatric inpatient units.[17]

So far, BasicNeeds-Lao has provided mental health/treatment training to 74 health staff and 101 village volunteers who are involved in mental health service delivery in their communities, in Vientiane and Borikhamxay province.

Between 1997 and 2007, 14 health staff from seven provincial hospitals received four months of training at the Mahosot mental health facility.

A rapid change in mental health care capacity has occurred since 2011. Four doctors from the Mahosot mental health unit received three months of advanced training in psychiatry at the Department of Psychiatry at Khonkaen University, Thailand; additionally, two nurses had four months of training in psychiatric nursing at Suan-Prung Hospital in Chiangmai, Thailand. One doctor attended a two-month mental health leadership training programme in Melbourne, Australia; and a doctor and a social worker had one month of mental health training in South Korea. The WHO supported the first mental health consultation workshop for developing postgraduate psychiatry and a training programme for research in public health psychiatry for Lao doctors in April 2013.

The mental health system

The psychiatric unit of No. 103 Hospital was established in 1978, with 14 beds, and staffed by two general practitioners and three nurses delivering both outpatient and inpatient care to serve soldiers with mental disturbances. Nowadays, it serves civil patients too. In October 2010 this unit was renovated. Currently it has ten wards, of which eight are isolation rooms for patients in acute psychotic states and two big wards for accommodating ten patients with minor mental disorders.

In 1979, psychiatry was taught at the University of Medicine in Vientiane to fifth-year medical students by a Russian psychiatrist (who left in 1982 due to the termination of his posting) and a Laotian, Associate Professor Sisouk Vongphrachanh. They also delivered psychiatric consultations at the outpatient unit of Mahosot Hospital in Vientiane on two mornings each week, not only to provide mental health services to people with mental illness and/or epilepsy, but also so that the medical students would have a place at which to practise their psychiatry. In early 1984, the author began her mental health on-the-job-training. Patients in an acute psychiatric episode were admitted at the internal medicine unit and followed by these doctors daily. In late 1984, a senior doctor undertook three-year psychiatry specialisation training in Hungary. Mental health treatment was sustained and delivered by a junior doctor. In 1987, the Director of Mahosot Hospital decided to create a proper mental health unit with four beds, staffed by the junior doctor, an assistant physician and a nurse. Both outpatient and inpatient mental health care were offered. By 1991, the author had specialised abroad in psychiatry. Since 1992 this small unit has expanded to 15 beds: two for patients in the acute phase and 13 for people with minor mental disorders.

As there is no specific psychiatric institution, mental health services are integrated into the Lao general health system. These services can be classified as: Tertiary Psychiatric Care (mental health units) at the two central hospitals; Secondary Psychiatric Care in seven provincial hospitals – namely Vientiane, Borikhamxay, Khammouan, Champassack, Luang Prabang and Oudomxay (providing only outpatient mental health services), and Savannakhet (delivering both outpatient and inpatient care since early 2013, supported by the Transition for Eastern Alliance, a Dutch organisation); Primary Mental Health Services in community settings, although these are in fact available in only 12 district hospitals, of which nine are in Vientiane and three in districts in Borikhamxay province under the BasicNeeds-Lao programme.[6]

The diagnosis of mental illness is based on the anamnesis provided by the patient and his/her carer and mental health status examination. Counselling and psychotropic medication are the two major treatment options at the central hospitals, while the BasicNeeds programme focuses on a bio-psycho-social approach. Social interventions include open support groups and the integration of stabilised individuals in employment programmes, to improve their quality of life, enhance their self-reliance and aid their social reintegration.

Home visits are offered to patients in the acute phase who cannot come to district hospital clinics under the BasicNeeds-Lao programme. Home visits focus on taking medication regularly, drug side-effects and the obstacles faced by patients. Carers who are unable to cope with a patient can ring district health workers and request a home visit from the mental health care service.[18] At each such visit, the health status and socio-economic situation of users and their families' attitudes are recorded. Mental health education is also provided.

No formal mental health referral system exists in the country, although physicians at the primary health care clinics do make referrals to a mental health professional. Where this is done, it is usually done verbally, rather than formally, in writing.[17] So far the BasicNeeds referral system has been for use only within its programme.

In Lao PDR, only 2.8 per cent of government expenditure in 2007 was on health care, although this had increased to 6.1 per cent by 2011 (Lao National Health Accounts 2006–7).[33] Budgets for the mental health units at the two central hospitals are integrated within the overall hospital budgets, so government expenditure on mental health cannot be calculated.[3] As there is no psychiatric hospital, less than 1 per cent of the health budget has been a ring-fenced budget for mental health.[17]

Some additional funding for mental health came from the WHO and Handicap International Belgium. The Handicap International Belgium funding was for a one-year pilot project. Funding supported the health clinic at a district hospital and, more specifically, self-support for UXO victims.[23] So far, BasicNeeds has allocated more than US$1 million for mental health work, including promotion, outreach, research and building social capital by working with lay members of the community.[6]

Additionally, district hospitals under the BasicNeeds-Lao programme can prescribe psycho-tropic drugs. Each district hospital has nearly US$100 per month for these medicines.

The Transition for Eastern Alliance financially supports the Nursing College in Savannakhet in developing a psychiatric nursing curriculum for nursing students, training of four health staff from the province and constructing a mental health facility in the provincial hospital. The last facility comprises six rooms, one of which will be used as an outpatient clinic, three for inpatients (each with six beds), another for psychiatric intensive care and a library room. The necessary equipment is also being supplied. The budget allocation for these activities is unknown.

Social and explanatory models of mental illness

Despite the importance of Buddhism to many Lao people (especially the Loum and Theung groups), animist beliefs are also common. The beliefs in *phi* (spirits) strongly correlate nature and community, and thereby provide an explanation for illness. Belief in *phi* is blended with Buddhism, especially at the village level, and some monks are respected as having the ability to exorcise malevolent spirits. *Phi* are everywhere and diverse, and may be connected to the earth, heaven, fire and water.

There is a popular belief that a human being is a union of 32 organs and that each one has a soul (*khwan*), so that there are 32 souls acting as protectors of different parts of the body. These *khwan* may often wander outside the body, causing an imbalance of the soul, which may lead to illness (e.g. physical or emotional weakness); alternatively, some bad spirits may enter the body.

The majority of Lao people indeed believe that bad demons cause psychosis, followed by having sinned in a past life, which may be connected with the occurrence of mental illness or with having a family member experience mental health problems or developmental disorders.[1,4]

Mental illness is also perceived by Lao people – and professionals especially – as brain damage, cognitive disorder (e.g. memory impairment, speech disturbances and hallucinations), affective-emotional disorder, or abnormal physical appearance (e.g. untidiness and dirtiness). Local folk representations of mental illness as a metaphorical understanding of mental disorder and theories of illness aetiology were discussed by Westermeyer in 1973.[32] Then, in 1981, two main folk categories were assessed and some comparability was found between folk and psychiatric diagnoses such as *baa* (insane). The term *phi baa* (evil spirit madness or ghost madness) is widely used in Lao PDR; it refers to major mental dysfunction and spirit possession (*phi*), inducing such symptoms as arguing, pacing, muteness or talkativeness, and incoherent ideas and thoughts. It is a common word for 'mad'.[8]

The Lao folk model of mental illness comprises 52 types of madness, including: instant violent behaviour or *baa ti*; slowness or *khon sa*; doing something which is not understandable or *baa sibo sibei*; euphoria or *baa muan*; depression or *seum sao*; delirium or *baa bay*; delirium and hallucination or *baa puang*; epilepsy or *baa mu* due to *phi* attacking and even destroying the brain, or the person eating under-cooked pork.[8]

A few types of *baa* are related to magic: magical diagram madness, caused by doing something wrong when wearing the magic thing, or *katha*, then breaking a taboo or lacking respect for the *katha* rules or *baa katha*; *dharma* (broken *dharma* madness, as *dharma* is difficult to reach for someone who is too ambitious and gets mad in a desire to study it, or *baa tham tek*); and addiction (alcoholic person or *baa khi lao*).

Some positive changes have been evident in Lao PDR since 2007. BasicNeeds-Lao has paid particular attention to involving the relevant authorities, first at central level and then at local level, and other potential partners right from the beginning of the programme's implementation in 2007, through a series of consultation meetings with policy-makers at the Ministry of Health to establish mutual understanding and confidence. Key stakeholders have been familiarised with the BasicNeeds model and development philosophy. The programme has also helped to establish a government-supported network of organisations working in mental health and development.[7] Partnership and dialogue between international organisations or institutions, NGOs and government staff in mental health activities are encouraged, in order to underpin sustainable development in mental health.

The ministerial mental health taskforce will be instrumental in the successful implementation of the national mental health strategy by 2020. It is in the process of getting approval from the

Minister of Health. It will be a focal point in coordinating with different organisations interested in mental health locally and internationally under the leadership of the Minister/Vice-Minister of Health.

In conclusion, trust must be built among all the partners. Working alone will not lead to success, especially in Lao PDR, where there is a scarcity of human resources in mental health, a poorly established mental health system and unfamiliarity with cross-sectoral partnerships.

The mental health services at present are expanding somewhat into provincial and community levels. Trained health staff have better knowledge and skills in interviewing, diagnosing and providing appropriate mental health care, including drugs, talking therapy and social activities to enable users to reintegrate within the community. Nowadays they feel more confident in delivering such services than they did in the past. Psychotropic drugs are included in the hospital drug funds, to ensure the continuity of drugs' availability. This demonstrates that provincial and district health authorities have put mental health work on their agenda.

Setting mental health services in the community is efficient and cost-effective, as it facilitates access.

Major challenges and alternative therapies

Interventions for mental illness are seen as a marginal activity within the Lao health care system. The existing services have been provided through the only two mental health units, both in the capital, Vientiane, from 1979 to mid-2007. The BasicNeeds-Lao programme is essentially starting from scratch in its work to develop genuinely community-based interventions. Outreach initiatives to provide early identification and intervention for at-risk groups at the community level find it very challenging to reach mentally ill people, but this costs less than bringing people to central hospitals. Although mental health issues are neglected and human resources in mental health are limited, community mental health services can be developed in a cost-effective and sustainable manner by mobilising all partners and ensuring strong monitoring and evaluation, from central to community level. This work would certainly augment patient recovery.

The remoteness of villages, the limited transportation and poverty prevent some patients, especially the poorest and their carers, from coming to hospital for regular mental health follow-up, thus disrupting their treatment (and prospects), and making them vulnerable to relapse and further poverty. However, policy-makers are influenced by the idea of extending community-based interventions.

Developing sustainable livelihoods for stable patients is challenging, as development is not seen as a priority within a community-based approach to mental health, with social interventions aiming to improve the quality of life of users and their families. By promoting the importance of livelihoods and the social aspects of mental health problems, the issues of poverty and social exclusion could be engaged.

Associated with the lack of statutory provision, patients are often discriminated against and excluded from their own communities.[5] Some are prohibited from eating with their families due to their poor hygiene, and some have been caged or chained by their families because of disturbed behaviour associated with mental illness.[1,2,4] After falling ill, many patients cannot earn a living, or drop out of school; friends generally stop socialising with them. Additionally, tension within the family is increased. Parents are the ones most affected by mental illness in a family member. The burden of care can be great; some quit their job to spend time with their mentally ill loved ones, leaving insufficient time for earning an income, which in turn leads to financial crisis within the family (as well as family disagreements). Carers feel depressed, hopeless, frustrated, worried and fearful; they may be left in debt or with no income.[1] The results of community consultation meetings in both Vientiane and Borikhamxay show that stigma and discrimination towards the mentally ill and their families exist in Lao PDR, as elsewhere. Individuals with mental health problems and their carers repeatedly ask the community to stop discriminating against them, and to accept and understand their circumstances.[2,4]

Work to reduce stigma is very challenging in Lao PDR but the BasicNeeds-Lao programme has already tackled this issue on various fronts (e.g. group work with patients, focused on raising confidence and overcoming psychological barriers to recovery and social development; the recruitment of patients who have recovered to lead an anti-stigma programme; and work with potential employers to reduce discrimination against those with mental illness).

As formal mental health services are inaccessible by the majority of people in the country, interventions from different traditional healers are used as alternative therapies; these healers include herbalists, faith healers and spirit mediums. Herbalists treat using natural plants and herbs, similar to homoeopathists in the West. For example, a *Mo ya* prescribes herbal medicine or traditional medicine.[8] Faith healers undertake pastoral work and perform religious rituals. They heal through prayer and counselling. Many individuals and families seek help with emotional challenges through spiritual practices, usually centred on the local Buddhist temple. Thus Lao people will find refuge, relief of symptoms and calm from Buddhism and meditation if they face fear of getting 'unluckiness', psychological problems and health problems. Religious treatment is seen as effective. It is believed that while evil spirits can cause illness, the presence of the good souls preserves health and a good fate. A traditional ceremony (or *Baci*) performed by people from the plain is believed to be effective.[8]

Spirit mediums, 'witch doctors' or 'diviners' acquire their healing powers through inheritance. They often use exorcism rituals to remove supernatural spirits. Some ethnic groups hold superstitious beliefs, and mainly rely on shamans to cure any health problem. The treatment techniques practised by superstitious healers are diverse. For mental illness, a magic ceremony is performed with traditional dance as an offering because a spirit wants to take the person as a step-child or spouse. The spirit medium will chase the bad spirit out by tying the mentally ill person's wrist with copper cord, in combination with traditional medicine. Some will tie a white string on the wrist, hit the mentally ill person with a bunch of thick candles and get them to drink holy water. A *Mo thiem* is considered to be the right type of medium to mediate communication between spirits of the dead and other human beings. A *Mo monh* will prepare amulets or a talisman; he can send spells then give holy water to drink and attach cotton strings to the wrists. A *Mo phi* is the healer with the closest relation to spirits and refers to them for healing practices and rituals. He can expel bad spirits (*phi*). Sometimes healers use abusive practices such as chaining a person who is delirious, whipping him, or burning his mouth to exorcise spirits.

References

1 BasicNeeds-Lao (2008) 'Baseline study report on community mental health in Vientiane capital', 1: 13, unpublished report.
2 BasicNeeds-Lao (2008) 'Report on community consultation meeting in Vientiane capital', unpublished report.
3 BasicNeeds-Lao (2009) 'Financing in mental health', unpublished report.
4 BasicNeeds (2010) 'Report on the community consultation meetings in Borikhamxay Province, unpublished report.
5 BasicNeeds-Lao (2012) 'Baseline study report on community mental health in Borikhamxay Province', 1: 6, unpublished report.
6 BasicNeeds-Lao (2013) 'Quarterly programme progress reports', unpublished report.
7 BasicNeeds-Lao (2013) 'Report on the alliance creation in mental health', unpublished report.

8 Bertrand, D. and Choulamany, C. (2002) 'Mental health situation analysis in Lao People's Democratic Republic', 3: 25; 4: 38; Annex 13: 60–1.

9 Bounlu, M. (2013) 'Study on relapse among patients with schizophrenia at the mental health unit, Mahosot Hospital', unpublished memoire, University of Health Sciences of Lao PDR, 4: 26–37.

10 Choulamany, C. *et al.* (2003) 'Evaluating the treatment of amphetamine-type stimulant in the mental health unit, Mahosot Hospital', unpublished paper, p. 20.

11 Jamison, D.T., Breman, J.G. and Measham, A.R. (2006) *Disease Control Priorities in Developing Countries.* 2nd edition. Washington (DC): World Bank. Chapter 28 Stunting, Wasting and Micronutrients Deficiency Disorders.

12 Lao Social Indicator Survey (LSIS) and Millennium Development Goals (MDG) Indicators, Lao PDR 2011–2012, pp. iii, xxii, 55, 238, 170.

13 LCDC, National Drug Control Master Plan (February 2009) *A Five Year Strategy to Address the Illicit Drug Control Problem in the Lao PDR (2009–2013).*

14 Mahosot Hospital, Mental Health Unit (2013) 'Data record 2012–2013'.

15 Ministry of Health, National Mental Health Policy (October 2007) pp. 7–9

16 Ministry of Health, National Mental Health Strategy by Year 2020 (March 2013), p. 11.

17 Ministry of Health and World Health Organization (2012) *WHO–AIMS Report on Mental Health System in Lao PDR*, pp. 13, 18, 20.

18 Morakoth, M. (2008) 'Practice of community mental health in Lao PDR: Seeking reliability and quality assurance in low and middle-income countries', Lao PDR: BasicNeeds, p. 9.

19 National Assembly (2005) 'No 09/NA, 09/11/2005, Law on Healthcare'.20 National Regulatory Authority for UXO/Mines Section Actor in Lao PDR (UXO–NRA). www.nra.gov.la/ uxoproblem.html. History and War. Accessed on 04/11/2013

21 No. 103 Hospital, Mental Health Unit (2013) 'Data record 2012–2013'.

22 Phanthavong, P. (2012) 'Exploratory study in depression among secondary school population of the sixth year in Vientiane Capital', unpublished thesis, Institut Francophone de Médecine Tropicale, Lao PDR, 7: 21.

23 Raja, S. *et al.* (2010) 'Mental health finance in Ghana, Uganda, Sri Lanka, India and Lao PDR', *International Journal of Mental Health Systems*, 4: 11.

24 Ruangkanchanasetr, S., Plitponkarnpim, A., Hetrakul, P. and Kongsakon, R. (2005) 'Youth risk behavior survey: Bangkok, Thailand', *Journal of Adolescent Health*, 36: 227–35.

25 Steering Committee for Census of Population and Housing (2005) 'Results from the population and housing census 2005', 1: 8, 3: 36

26 Somsanga Centre (2013) 'Presentation at the Mental Health Promotion Workshop, Vientiane Capital'.

27 Southivong, B. *et al.* (2011) 'A cross-sectional study of post-traumatic stress disorder and social support in Lao PDR', *Bulletin of the World Health Organization*, 91: 765–72.

28 Talaei, A. *et al.* (2009) 'A survey of depression among Iranian medical students and its correlation with social support and satisfaction', *Iran Journal of Psychiatry*, 4: 17–22.

29 UNODC (2002) 'Drug abuse among disco clients, service women and unemployed youth in Vientiane Capital', unpublished report.

30 UNODC (2011) 'Report of the independent external evaluation for community-based treatment using tincture of opium to target opium dependence in the Lao PDR', pp. 26, 29, 33, unpublished report.

31 UNODC. (2013) 'Patterns and trends of amphetamine-type stimulant and other drugs: Challenges for Asia and Pacific, Global Smart Programme', p. 84, unpublished report.

32 Westermeyer. (1973) 'Grenade amok in Laos, a psychosocial perspective', *International Journal of Social Psychiatry*, 19: 251–260.

33 WHO (2009) *Country Cooperation Strategy (CCS) in the Lao PDR, 2009–2011*, Geneva.

34 www.apps.who.int/gho/data/node.country.country-LAO. Global Health Observatory Data Repository. Western Pacific Region. Lao People's Democratic Republic statistics summary (2002–present). Accessed on 20/10/2013.

35 www.equalrightstrust.org/ertdocumentbank/UN_Resolution_on_protection_of_persons_with_mental_ illness.pdf, Office of the High Commissioners for Human Rights. Accessed on 23/10/2013.

36 www.na.gov.la/appf17/geography.html. About Laos. History in Brief. Accessed on 22/10/2013.

37 www.nsc.gov.la/images/population_2011–2012.pdf. Population_2011–2012, Lao Statistics Bureau. Accessed on 22/10/2013.

38 www.undp.org/content/lao_pdr/en/home/countryinfo/. About Lao PDR. Accessed on 22/10/2013.

24

Myanmar

Win Aung Myint, Soe Min and Thiha Swe

Country/location geography

The population of Myanmar in 2011–12 was estimated at 60.38 million. The life expectancy at birth is 60–64 years. The average life expectancy for urban males and females is 65.8 years and 70.8 years, respectively. And the average life expectancy for rural males and females is 64.3 years and 67.8 years, respectively (Ministry of Health, Myanmar, 2013). According to UN Statistics for 2008, as cited by the WHO (2011), the literacy rate is 96 per cent for men and 95 per cent for women. In Myanmar, neuropsychiatric disorders are estimated to contribute to 9.2 per cent of the global burden of disease (WHO, 2011).

The Republic of the Union of Myanmar is the westernmost country in South-East Asia, located on the Bay of Bengal and Andaman Sea. It is bordered on the east and northeast by the Lao People's Democratic Republic and the Kingdom of Thailand, on the north and northeast by the People's Republic of China, on the northwest by the Republic of India and on the west by the People's Republic of Bangladesh. Myanmar covers an area of 676,578 square kilometres on the Indo-China peninsular. It lies between latitude 09°32' N and 28°31'N and longitude 92°10' E and 101°11' E. It stretches 2,200 kilometres from north to south and 925 kilometres from east to west at its widest point.

The country is divided administratively into Nay Pyi Taw Union Territory and 14 states and regions. It consists of 70 districts, 330 townships, 84 sub-townships, 398 towns, 3,063 wards, 13,618 village tracts and 64,134 villages. Myanmar falls into three well-marked natural divisions: the western hills, the central belt and the Shan plateau on the east, with a continuation of this highland in the Tanintharyi. Three parallel chains of mountain ranges, running from north to south, divide the country into three river systems, the Ayeyarwady, Sittaung and Thanlwin (Ministry of Health, Myanmar, 2013).

Mental health policy

Development of a mental health law

There is a need to replace the outdated Lunacy Act, 1912, which did not, for example, cover patient rights. A draft of a new Mental Health Law has been prepared and is in the process of being enacted (it is hoped before 2015).

Governance

Mental health is specifically mentioned in the general health policy. A mental health component is included in the National Health Plan, which is revised and implemented every five years, most recently in 2011. This mental health plan has specific timelines for its implementation and funding has already been allocated for half or more of its items. The plan aims to shift mental health services and resources from hospitals to community facilities and to integrate mental health services into primary care.

Specific mental health legislation exists, dating from 1948. Legal provisions concerning mental health are also covered in other laws (e.g. on welfare, disability, general health legislation, etc.) (Ministry of Health, Myanmar, 2013).

Human rights and equity

Only 0.26 per cent of all admissions to the psychiatric inpatient units of general hospitals at state and regional levels and 1 per cent of all admissions to mental health hospitals are involuntary, although these figures do not include patients sent by their relatives without their consent (Ministry of Health, Myanmar and WHO, 2007).

The new draft Mental Health Law has been developed to accord with international and regional human rights instruments.

Aims of the mental health service

The mental health service seeks to promote mental health and to prevent mental disorders. Access to services is a priority. The objectives of the service are therefore as follows:

1. To implement strategies for promotion and prevention in mental health.
2. To reduce the treatment gap for mental disorders by 20 per cent (by the year 2020).
3. To develop policies based on human rights.
4. To provide evidence-based best practices for better care within the mental health service by collaborating with stakeholders, international medical communities, NGOs and INGOs.
5. To ensure preparedness for the mental health and psychosocial aspect of disasters.
6. To reduce the harmful use of alcohol.
7. To strengthen the health information system in relation to mental health issues.
8. To undertake research on mental health.

1. Strategies for promotion and prevention in mental health

Activities for promotion of mental health and prevention of mental disorder are pursued through:

a. A mental health literacy campaign.
b. Mental health first-aid training.
c. An anti-stigma and anti-discrimination campaign.
d. School mental health programmes.

These activities are being launched in a model township as a pilot programme.

2. The treatment gap

The treatment gap for the psychoses (facility-based) was calculated to be 95.8 per cent in 2012. A 20 per cent reduction in this gap is the aim, to leave the treatment gap nationwide at 75 per cent by the year 2020.

The strategy to achieve this is set out in the mental health reform plan, in the form of three simultaneous action programmes:

a. Upgrading the quality of care offered by the hospital-based mental health services.
b. Developing community-based mental health services.
c. Facilitating access to mental health services by consumers.

The following have already been implemented:

a. Facilitating access to services in rural areas by integrating mental health into the existing primary health care system.
b. Increasing the number of medical officers in mental health promotion and prevention services.
c. Providing comprehensive, integrated and collaborative services, offering best practice.
d. Enhancing school mental health services involved in promotion and prevention as well as dealing with the mental health problems of children and adolescents.
e. Launching an anti-stigma campaign and a mental health literacy campaign, and raising community awareness, to reduce the barriers to the utilization of community-based mental health services.

3. Human rights policies

A regional human rights review committee exists that has the authority to oversee regular inspections of mental health facilities, to review involuntary admissions and discharge procedures, to review complaints, to investigate processes and to impose sanctions. The committee consists of a legislator, administrative members, a police representative and doctors. It also reviews criminal cases, and patients sent from the courts under section 466 or 471 of the Criminal Code of the Union of Myanmar, and determines whether the criminal patients are of sound or unsound mind during their period in hospital. This committee meets in the hospital every three months. It is currently practised only at Yangon Mental Health Hospital which has a forensic unit.

Mental health hospitals have a quarterly review of their human rights protection of patients. An assessment of these reviews showed that only 50 per cent of all mental health hospital staff had had at least one day of training or other type of working session on the protection of patients' human rights in the previous year (Ministry of Health, Myanmar and WHO, 2007).

4. Evidence-based best practice

Evidence-based best practices are provided in collaboration with stakeholders, international medical communities, NGOs and INGOs.

Myanmar has been collaborating with following international medical organizations:

- AMT (ASEAN Mental Health Taskforce)
- MMP (Mekong Mental Health Partnership)
- AAMH (Australia Asia Mental Health)
- APCMHDP (Asia Pacific Mental Health Development Project)
- WHO

NGOs collaborating in mental health are:

- MMCWA (Myanmar Maternal and Child Welfare Association)
- MHS (Myanmar Mental Health Society)
- MANA (Myanmar Anti Narcotic Association)
- MMA (Myanmar Medical Association)
- MNS (Myanmar Nurses Association)

It is expected that collaborations with other national or international organizations will be developed in the near future.

5. Preparedness for disasters

Myanmar has painful experience of disasters. Mental health activities in the aftermath of disaster include:

a. Education on disasters in the psychiatry curriculum for medical and nursing students and in the postgraduate Master's degree course on mental health.
b. Training programmes in the integration of mental health services into the primary health care system.
c. Workshops on preparedness for the mental health and psychosocial aspects of disaster.
d. Collaboration with stakeholders, NGOs, international organizations and medical communities to implement mental health services after disasters.
e. Setting up a multi-sectorial approach in the implementation of mental health care programmes after disasters.

6. Harmful use of alcohol

A national workshop on policies and interventions to reduce the harmful use of alcohol was held in December 2012 and recommended the following:

a. Monitor taxes on the production and sale of alcohol.
b. Allocation of some tax revenue to a prevention and control programme for alcohol-related harm.
c. Declaration of drinking prohibition areas and periods and expansion of alcohol-free initiatives (e.g. alcohol-free grocery stores and restaurants).
d. Implement participatory and effective law-enforcement mechanisms on drunk driving.
e. Declaration of alcohol-free zones, avoidance of alcohol-sponsored sports, cultural and community events.
f. Enforce laws and regulations concerning the illicit production, sale and distribution of alcohol.
g. A public campaign on alcohol problem prevention.
h. Set up screening and treatment facilities and self-help groups, and support the role of the family in alcohol abstention.
i. Production of documents with key advocacy messages for policy-makers. Establish a committee for the prevention and control of harm from alcohol use at various levels, comprising representatives of relevant organizations, local authorities, religious groups, NGOs and volunteers, and determine the rules, regulations and functions of the committee.

7. The health information system

Data on six common mental disorders should be collected for the health management information system (HMIS). They are:

a.   Psychosis;
b.   Anxiety;
c.   Depression;
d.   Epilepsy;
e.   Intellectual disabilities (mental retardation);
f.   Alcohol dependence.

Basic health staff have already been trained in data collection but their skills still need to be strengthened.

8. Research on mental health

Research work is compulsory for postgraduate candidates as a partial fulfilment for the degree of Master of Medical Science (Mental Health). A prevalence study on mental disorders was done in 2004. Another study will be conducted in 2014. Epidemiological research has to be carried out. Collaborative research with international medical communities is to be conducted in the future.

Narcotic Drugs and Psychotropic Substances Law (1993)

This law relates to the control of drug abuse and sets out measures to be taken against those breaking the law. It was enacted to implement the provisions of the United Nations Convention Against Illicit Traffic in Narcotic Drugs and Psychotropic Substances. Other objectives are to cooperate with state parties to the United Nations Convention and international and regional organizations in respect of the prevention of the danger from narcotic drugs and psychotropic substances. Under this law, the Central Committee for Drug Abuse Control (CCADC), as well as 16 Working Committees and Sector and Regional Committees were formed to carry out the designated tasks in accordance with provisions of the law. The law also describes procedures relating to the registration, medication and deregistration of drug users.

National Health Plan (2011 to 2016)

Based on primary health care approaches, the Ministry of Health formulated People's Health Plans from 1978 to 1990, followed by the National Health Plans from 1991– 1992 to 2011–2016. These plans have been formulated within the framework of National Development Plans for the corresponding periods. Thus, the National Health Plan (2011–2016) was formulated in relation to the fifth five-year National Development Plan.

Psychiatric epidemiology

The WHO suggests that, for any country, 1 per cent of the total population will experience major mental disorders and 10 per cent minor mental disorders. On this basis, Myanmar, with a population of around 60 million, would be expected to have 0.6 million individuals with major mental disorders and 6.0 million with minor disorders, giving a total prevalence of 6.6 million.

Prevalence of mental disorders in Myanmar based on research

In 1976, a community survey carried out in Hle-gu (an urban area), in Bago division, found a total prevalence rate for all mental disorders of 86/1,000 (Pu *et al.*, 1976). In 1982, in a community survey carried out in Sein Panmyaning ward, Mayangone township (a suburban area), Yangon division, this figure was 56/1,000, the prevalence of psychoses was 5/1,000, neurotic and personality disorders 19/1,000, epilepsy 4/1,000 and mental retardation 4/1,000 (Win *et al.*, 1982). In 2004, a community survey carried out in Daw Pone township (a peri-urban area), Yangon division, revealed a point prevalence rate of all mental disorders of 85.6/1,000, psychoses 5.5/1,000, anxiety disorders 41/1,000, depressive disorder 5.7/1,000, epilepsy 3.5/1,000, mental retardation (moderate and severe) 5.3/1,000, alcohol dependence (abuse was excluded) 23/1,000 (7 per cent of males over 18), and dementia (moderate and severe) 1.8/1,000 (2.5 per cent of those aged over 65) (Myint *et al.*, 2004). In 2004, a community survey carried out in Pardagyi village (a rural area), Kyauktan township, Yangon region, revealed a point prevalence rate of all mental disorders of 77/1,000, psychoses 6/1,000, anxiety disorders 38/1,000, depressive disorder 5/1000, epilepsy 2/1,000, mental retardation (moderate and severe) 1/1,000, alcohol dependence (abuse was excluded) 23/1,000 (7.1 per cent of males over 18), and dementia (moderate and severe) 2/1,000 (3.5 per cent of those aged over 65) (*et al.*, 2004).

The calculated treatment gap for psychoses (facility-based) was 95.8 per cent in 2012. Myanmar's suicide rate in 2011 was 1.96 per 100,000 population.

Mental health workforce training and internship system: quality improvement for medical education

A postgraduate course for a Master's degree in Medical Science (Psychiatry) was launched in 1977 at the University of Medicine (1), Yangon. It was a two-year course in both theory and clinical training, covering psychiatry, general medicine, neurology and psychology. That course was, though, soon discontinued. A Diploma in Psychological Medicine (DPM) course was started in 1978 at the University of Medicine (1), Yangon. It was a one-and-a-half year course in both theory and clinical training, covering psychiatry, general medicine, neurology and psychology, as was the former course.

In accordance with Myanmar's National Health Plan and changing trends in psychiatric services, the diploma course was upgraded and the Master's course was re-launched in 2000 at the University of Medicine (1), Yangon. After postgraduate courses had been run twice, it was revised under the guidance of Academic Board of the Institute of Medicine (1), Yangon, and the Department of Medical Sciences. After that, the course was changed to a postgraduate programme, Master of Medical Science (Mental Health), to keep up with changing trends.

In the 2013 academic year, the curriculum and course structure of the Master's course was upgraded and it was extended from two years to three years. From 10 to 15 postgraduate candidates are trained annually.

For the training of nurses, there was a nine-month training programme for a Certificate in Psychiatric Nursing. That course was upgraded to Diploma in Psychiatric Nursing, which is a nine-month training programme at the University of Nursing.

Mental health systems

Formal mental health services started in Myanmar in 1948, when the country gained independence. In the early days, the mental health care system began in a hospital setting in

Yangon and then extended to Mandalay. In 1990, mental health care was included in the National Health Plan.

Attempts have been made to shift mental health care from hospital settings to community settings, to ensure effective care. The aim now is to integrate mental health into primary health care; the care and support of mentally ill patients will then be given by trained basic health staff, and psychological and social support will be given by families and the community. Mental health education is being provided through local NGOs, and NGOs are training basic health staff and community health workers (Kyaing, 2008).

Tables 24.1–24.6 give key data on Myanmar's mental health care infrastructure.

Table 24.1 Mental health workforce in Myanmar (2013)

Category of workforce	Number	Per million population
Psychiatrists	140	2.3
Public	90	
Private	50	
Postgraduate trainee doctors for mental health	50	—
Psychiatric nurses	156	2.6
Clinical psychologists	3	0.05
Psychiatric social workers	5	0.08
Occupational therapists trained in mental health	2	0.03
Specialists in psychosocial rehabilitation	—	—

Data obtained from Mental Health Project, Ministry of Health, 2013

Table 24.2 Mental health facilities in Myanmar (2013)

Facilities	Total no.
Mental health hospitals	2
General hospitals with mental health services	32
Beds in mental health hospitals	1,400
Beds for psychiatric cases in general hospitals	220

Data obtained from Mental Health Project, Ministry of Health, 2013

Table 24.3 Mental health financing in Myanmar

Expenditure	2010–11 (million Kyat)	2011–12 (million Kyat)
Mental health hospitals	13,807.62	15,036.82
National health expenditure	765,167.52	810,318.89

Data obtained from Department of Health Planning, Ministry of Health

Table 24.4 Persons with mental disorders treated in primary health care in Myanmar (January to September 2013)

Report status	83%
Number of persons suffering from psychosis	2,024
Number of persons suffering from anxiety disorders	1,472
Number of persons suffering from depressive disorder	1,175
Number of persons suffering from alcohol dependence	14,860
Number of persons suffering from epilepsy	961
Number of persons suffering from mental retardation	1,505
Total	21,997

Data obtained from HMIS, Ministry of Health, 2013

Table 24.5 Persons treated in mental health outpatient facilities in Myanmar (2013)

Number of persons treated in outpatient facilities of mental health hospitals	25,881
Number of persons treated in outpatient facilities of general hospitals	32,245
Total	58,126

Data obtained from Mental Health Project, Ministry of Health, 2013

Table 24.6 Persons treated in mental health inpatient facilities in Myanmar (2013)

Number of persons admitted to mental health hospitals	13,686
Number of persons admitted to general hospitals with psychiatric beds	1,067
Total	14,753

Data obtained from Mental Health Project, Ministry of Health, 2013

Historical perspective

The care of the 'insane'

The earliest history of services for the mentally ill in Myanmar goes back to 1886. The British authorities felt that a national facility was required; however, its function was merely containment. Sadly, the prime motivation for this was that the mentally ill caused a public nuisance. It was called 'the prison for the insane' and was built close to the City Prison in Rangoon (now known as Yangon). Initially with some 50 'inmates', by 1914 the numbers had risen to around 750 and yet more space was needed to accommodate the unfortunates.

Soon after the First World War, foundations were laid for a new purpose-built facility eight miles from Yangon in a village called Tadagalay. Tadagalay translates as 'a small bridge'. With this development, Tadagalay blossomed. The asylum was completed in 1928 with the first 250 residents arriving soon after, and the number steadily grew to about 1,000. Little is known of how these people were treated. It appears that the facility's purpose was containment for life, and it soon took on the name Tadagalay. Tadagalay became the local equivalent of 'Bedlam', not only in its function but also in its fame with the laity. The translated saying of 'you need to go to Tadagalay' means that one's head needs examining!

During the Second Word War, over half of the buildings of Tadagalay were destroyed, the site having been occupied by the Japanese army.

The concept of the 'insane' as mentally ill

Psychiatry as a branch of medicine (and with it the concept of the 'mentally ill patient') was introduced to Myanmar in 1945. The first department of psychiatry was established in temporary accommodation with provision for 45 patients. This was ten miles out of Rangoon, in a suburb called Insein, and in close proximity to a large prison. After about a year, Tadagalay once again became functional, and the patients at Insein were transferred back to Tadagalay. Soon after Burma gained independence, the name was changed from the prison for the insane to the Mental Hospital, marking a new and important phase in the history of psychiatry in Myanmar. Having achieved the status of a hospital, after 14 years the name was again changed, to the People's Psychiatric Hospital. However, among the populace, the name Tadagalay lives on. In 1967 it achieved the status of a specialist hospital, a few years later becoming the main teaching hospital for undergraduate psychiatry (Khin-Maung-Zaw, 1997).

The integration of mental health into the health care system

The integration of mental health services into the existing health care system is the main strategy to fulfil the objectives of the Mental Health Care Plan. Integration will increase the provision of mental health care for the whole country. Accordingly, a Mental Health Project was launched in 1990 sponsored by WHO and working under the guidance of the Ministry of Health, Myanmar.

Integrated mental health services are now practising alongside other medical specialties in hospital-based services at all general hospitals at state and regional levels.

The model townships for community-based mental health services (see below) aim to provide mental health services by integrating the services into grassroots primary health care, including rural health centres, local general practitioners (GPs) and the local community. The intention is to explore and evaluate gaps and challenges, and to construct a model which will be feasible, realistic, measurable and applicable. A model township in Yangon region has been developed and the model township programme will be expanded into two other areas.

At secondary care level, a satellite continuous care programme will be launched in Yangon region as a pilot project by mobile mental health teams from the Mental Health Hospital, Yangon. Four secondary care centres in Yangon region have been selected and the programme will be implemented in May 2014.

Mental health care delivery

There are hospital-based and community-based mental health services.

Hospital-based mental health services

Mental health services are available at the two mental health hospitals and in general hospitals. The two mental health hospitals are in Yangon in Mandalay. Yangon Mental Health Hospital is a 1,200-bed tertiary care teaching hospital with an outpatient department, general psychiatry units, mood disorder units, schizophrenia units, an alcohol de-addiction and research unit, a drug-dependency treatment and research unit, a forensic unit, a long-stay and rehabilitation unit, and a community mental health unit. In 2013, 18,922 patients attended the outpatient department and 11,289 patients were admitted. Mandalay Mental Health Hospital is a 200-bed tertiary care teaching hospital with a 100-bed general psychiatry unit and a 100-bed drug-dependency treatment unit. In 2013, 6,959 patients attended the outpatient department and 2,379 patients were admitted.

Mental health services are also delivered in general hospitals. There are 22 psychiatric units attached to all 300-bed general hospitals in all states and at all regional levels. Most have both in- and outpatient facilities, but eight have outpatient facilities only. Mental health services are led by consultant psychiatrists.

Community-based mental health services

Community-based mental health services are delivered at primary care level through the activities of the Mental Health Project, developing model townships for community-based mental health care services and the forthcoming satellite continuous care programmes.

The main aim of the Mental Health Project is to integrate mental health services into the primary health care system. The project was launched in 1990 under the guidance of the Ministry of Health and financially supported by the WHO. The intention is to provide care and support for mentally ill patients by trained basic health staff and psychological and social support by families and the community. Mental health education is being provided through local NGOs and trained basic health staff and community health workers. Some 700 medical officers and 1,400 basic health workers working at secondary and primary care level have been trained to deliver mental health services. Forty per cent of primary care centres now have manuals on the treatment of common mental disorders and at least one basic health worker has been trained to deliver mental health services. The model township programme was implemented in 2012 as a pilot project (see below). An outreach programme at Yangon Mental Health Hospital was started in 2004.

Medicines

Medicines have been provided by the Ministry of Health for patients attending mental health hospitals since the budget year 2012–13. Small amounts of drugs were periodically provided for primary care through the support of the WHO. Drugs used in model townships are provided through the financial support of well-wishers and donors. Administrative procedures for the import and distribution of drugs are controlled and regulated by the Department of Food and Drug Administration of the Ministry of Health. Antipsychotics (risperidone and olanzapine), antidepressants (amitriptyline and SSRIs), and sedatives and hypnotics (diazepam, lorazepam, clonazepam and alprazolam) are included in the National Essential Drug List.

Service delivery model

The mental health service delivery system is based on a primary health care approach.

Patterns of referral

The referral pattern for the mental health service is in accordance with the primary health care system.

Developing model townships for mental health

The objectives of this project are:

1. To promote the mental health status of the community.
2. To provide mental health services for people suffering from common mental disorders in their own community with their own resources.

Implementation of the project

The project has three phases.

Phase 1: capacity building for mental health facilities and access in the township:

1. Advocacy with partners.
2. Upgrading and strengthening the mental health facilities in the existing health system of the township.
3. Promoting access to mental health services for the local community of the township.
4. School mental health programmes.

Phase 2: working with the community:

1. A workshop aiming to build a bridge between providers and consumers. The participants will include local authorities, health personnel, school teachers, NGO members, community leaders, monks, traditional healers, patients and their families, and all interested persons. The outputs of this workshop should include suggestions for how patients will come to access mental health services.
2. Mental health promotion activities, with the collaboration and participation of the community.

Phase 3: monitoring and evaluation:

1. Monitoring (data collection and analysis in line with the activities of Phases 1 and 2):
2. Output data – numbers of persons trained at various levels, numbers of patients accessing mental health services, numbers of persons covered by campaigns, numbers of counselling centres developed in schools and the outputs of the workshop.
3. Outcome data – changes in awareness, knowledge, attitudes and practice of the local community for mental health and illnesses, and the treatment gap for common mental disorders.
4. Evaluation – will be done two years after implementation of the project. After recognizing the strengths and correcting the weaknesses of the project, it is hoped that a model that is suitable, feasible and applicable nationally will be developed.

Challenges

This project represents a great challenge:

1. Funding – there is no funding agency to support this project at the moment. Collaboration is being sought with national and international organizations for the components of the project but at present the project is being run by donations and a trust fund of the Mental Health Hospital, but this is not likely to be adequate for the whole project.

2. Technical expertise is hard to find for some of the training programmes, like youth counselling in school mental health programmes, and campaigning (e.g. the anti-stigma campaign).
3. Transportation of the mental health team to project areas can be difficult, as these areas are 30 to 40 km outside Yangon.

Present status and future plans

The objective is to construct a model at the primary care level for mental health promotion and services which is specific, measurable, feasible, applicable and realistic for Myanmar. This project is aiming to develop a continuous care programme run with local resources for the patients in their own community (ownership) and to promote the mental health status of the local community through their own efforts.

The project should expand to cover at least 80 per cent of the 330 townships of the whole country after a model has been constructed. Implementation will be done phase-by-phase, depending on resource development and the commitments of the leaders of the various sectors involved.

Outcomes achieved after implementation of Phase 1 of the model township programme

The model township programme in Kyauk-tan township is a pilot project. Kyauk-tan is located in Yangon region and one of the townships of the east Yangon district. It is 15 miles away from downtown Yangon city. The area is 325.76 square miles and its population is 162,931, of whom 27,573 live in urban areas and 135,358 in rural areas. The population density is 494.2 per square mile. It is composed of six wards, 47 village tracts and 91 villages.

The three-year project will run to 31 December 2015. It will be sustained as a continuous care programme of the Mental Health Hospital, Yangon, after completion of the project.

Tables 24.7–24.10 give data on the achievements of Phase 1.

Table 24.7 Situational analysis of mental health based on the health management information system (HMIS) report for the township for 2012

Disorders	HMIS data	Prevalence	Estimated data	Treatment gap (%)
Psychosis	3	6/1,000	977	99.7
Depression	1	5/1,000	814	99.9
Anxiety	0	38/1,000	6,191	100.0
Alcohol dependence	9	23/1,000	3,730	99.8
Epilepsy (major fit)	0	2/1,000	325	100.0
Mental retardation (moderate and severe)	1	1/1,000	163	99.4

Data obtained from a household survey done at Paragyi village, Kyauk-Tan Township, 2004 and from the report from the Township Health Department to the HMIS, 2012

Table 24.8 Situational analysis after implementation of Phase 1 (capacity building and access to mental health services): facilities for mental health services

Health facilities	Number	With access to mental health services before project	With access to mental health services after Phase 1
Township hospital	1	0	1
Station hospital	2	0	2
Rural health centre	7	0	7
Rural health sub-centre	36	0	36
MCH clinic	1	0	1
Private clinics	16	0	16

Data obtained from Mental Health Project, Ministry of Health, 2014

Table 24.9 Manpower trained for mental health services

Category of workforce	Before project	After implementation of Phase 1
Doctors		
Public	1	6
Private	0	25
Health assistants	2	9
Basic health staff, including nurses	2	70
Total	5	110

Data obtained from Mental Health Project, Ministry of Health, 2014

Table 24.10 Situational analysis of treatment gap after Phase 1

Disorders	No. of patients in 2012, before project	No. of patients in 2013, after Phase 1	Treatment gap in 2012, before project (%)	Treatment gap in 2013, after Phase 1 (%)
Psychosis	3	80	99.7	91.8
Depression	1	23	99.9	97.2
Anxiety	—	18	100	99.7
Alcohol dependence	9	76	99.8	98
Epilepsy (major fit)	—	26	100	92
Mental retardation (moderate and severe)	1	12	99.4	92.6
Total	14	235		

Data obtained from Mental Health Project, Ministry of Health, 2014

Output after Phase 1 (one year after implementation)

1. Facilities for access to mental health services have been raised from zero to 63 centres.
2. 110 doctors and basic health staff have been trained and certified for mental health work.

Outcome after Phase 1

The treatment gap has been reduced by 8 per cent for epilepsy, 7.9 per cent for psychosis, 6.8 per cent for mental retardation, 2.7 per cent for depression, 1.8 per cent for alcohol dependence, and 0.3 per cent for anxiety disorders.

Recommendations after Phase 1

1. Continuous supervision and medical education programmes for trained staff are needed to strengthen their capacities.
2. Provision of drugs and free drug supply, especially for those suffering from epilepsy and psychosis and those who cannot afford to buy drugs, are needed to reduce the financial barriers to long-term care.
3. Community empowerment with the anti-stigma programme in Phase 2 should facilitate a further reduction in the treatment gaps in the township.

Social/explanatory model(s) for mental illness

Stigma and myths

In Myanmar, many people still believe that mental illnesses are caused by evil spirits, witchcraft or because of not paying respect to the 37 *Nats* or supernatural spirits. If people become mentally ill or start behaving strangely, they are often sent to local healers or *Payawga sayas*. Many people still do not accept that mental illnesses are treatable. Many patients still remain untreated because of stigma and discrimination, misconceptions and unhealthy attitudes towards mental disorders.

Mental health and Myanmar society

Myanmar society is cohesive. Children, parents and elders are well looked after and valued. Patience, tolerance, goodwill, kindness and voluntarism are the elementary principles of Myanmar culture. Myanmar women are emotionally secure and have equal rights. Abuse is very uncommon. More than 90 per cent of the population are Buddhist and every village has at least one monastery. Monasteries and monks could play a substantial role in the promotion of mental health. Meditation has become popular even among the younger generation. These positive aspects of the culture naturally fulfil the basic requirements of social support for patients suffering from mental disorders (Myint and Tun, 2001).

Topics of interest specific to Myanmar

Strengths and weaknesses of the mental health system in Myanmar

The treatment gap for psychosis (facility-based) is 95.8 per cent. The scarcity of human resources, technical expertise and funding are obstacles to be overcome. Stigmatization, discrimination, lack of knowledge regarding mental health, and poverty are additional obstacles to the receipt of mental health services.

The inherent social cohesiveness, voluntarism and other positive aspects of Myanmar culture mean that patients with mental disorders have good social support.

Previously, mental health was a low priority for the health system. After changes in the political system, some progress has been made in the mental health care system, along with other sectors of the health system. Mental health has now become a medium priority for the health system.

This progress allows more opportunity for the development of human resources, collaboration with international medical communities and greater financial allocations for the mental health sector. In addition, changes in inpatient care at Yangon Mental Health Hospital, the commencement of hospital outreach programmes and community-based mental health services will give better access to mental health care.

References

Khin-Maung-Zaw (1997) 'Psychiatric services in Myanmar: A historical perspective', *Psychiatric Bulletin*, 21: 506–9.

Kyaing, N.N. (2008) Myanmar Country Paper for Revisiting Primary Health Care, Department of Health, Ministry of Health via WHO SEAR. http://s3.amazonaws.com/zanran_storage/www.searo.who.int/ContentPages/4814630.pdf accessed on 22 July 2014.

Ministry of Health, Myanmar (2013) 'Health in Myanmar, 2013', Ministry of Health, Nay Pyi Taw, the Republic of the Union of Myanmar.

Ministry of Health, Myanmar and WHO (2007) *WHO–AIMS Report on Mental Health System in Myanmar*, WHO, Yangon, and Ministry of Health, Nay Pyi Taw, Myanmar.

Myint, W.A. and Tun, N. (2001) 'Country report of Union of Myanmar for the development of community based neuropsychiatric services'. Presented at Second Conference of Myanmar Mental Health Society held on January 5th and 6th, 2005 at Myanmar Medical Association, Auditorium (A), Yangon, Myanmar.

Myint, W.A., Lwin, Z.S. and Oo, T. (2004) 'Prevalence study of common mental disorder in Daw Pone Township, Yangon Division, Union of Myanmar'. Presented at Second Conference of Myanmar Mental Health Society held on January 5th and 6th, 2005 at Myanmar Medical Association, Auditorium (A), Yangon, Myanmar.

Pu, T.N. *et al.* (1976) Psychiatric prevalence survey at Hle-gu area, Union of Myanmar. Presented at Second Conference of Myanmar Mental Health Society held on January 5th and 6th, 2005 at Myanmar Medical Association, Auditorium (A), Yangon, Myanmar.

WHO (2011) *Mental Health Atlas 2011*, Department of Mental Health and Substance Abuse, World Health Organization, Geneva.

Win, M.M., Pe, T.H., Aung, H. and Htay, H. (1982) 'Psychiatric prevalence study at Seinpanmyaing ward, Mayangon township, Myanmar'. Presented at Second Conference of Myanmar Mental Health Society held on January 5th and 6th, 2005 at Myanmar Medical Association, Auditorium (A), Yangon, Myanmar.

25

Psychiatry in Thailand

Pichet Udomratn and Manit Srisurapanont

Country location, population, religion

Thailand is an independent constitutional monarchy located in Southeast Asia and covers an area of about 513,115 square kilometers or 198,114 square miles. In 2012 its population was approximately 67.5 million. The population is mostly rural, concentrated in the rice-growing areas of the central, northeastern, and northern regions. Moreover, as Thailand continues to industrialize, its urban population (which is 45.7 percent of the total population) is growing.

Thailand's population is relatively homogeneous; however, this is changing due to immigration. Thailand is now home to more than 200,000 foreigners from countries that include but are not limited to the United Kingdom, other European countries, and the North American countries. Increasing numbers of migrants from Myanmar, Laos, and Cambodia as well as nations such as Nepal and India, along with those from the West and Japan pushed the total number of non-nationals residing in Thailand to around 3.5 million by the end of 2009. However, ethnic Thais make up the majority of the population with 75 percent of all inhabitants. Thai Chinese make up 14 percent, with the remaining 11 percent are made up of various other groups.

Thailand's highly successful government-sponsored family planning program has resulted in a dramatic decline in population growth from 3.1 percent in 1960 to around 0.4 percent today. In 1970, an average of 5.7 people lived in a Thai household (World Bank, 2001). At the time of the 2010 census, the figure was down to 3.2. Even though Thailand has one of the best social insurance systems in Asia, the increasing number of elderly people is a challenge for the country. In 2011, the percentage of persons who were 65 years and over was 9.2 percent of the total population while the percentages in the age groups of 0–14 years and 15–64 years were 19.9 percent and 70.9 percent, respectively. Life expectancy has also risen, which is a positive reflection of Thailand's efforts in executing public health policies. In 2011, life expectancy at birth for the total population was 73.6 years (71.2 years for males, 76.1 years for females).

Theravada Buddhism is the official religion of Thailand and is the religion of about 90 percent of its people. The government permits religious diversity and other major religions such as Islam, Christianity, and Hinduism make up the remaining 10 percent. However, there is much social tension especially in the southern provinces of Thailand. Spirit worship and animism are also widely practiced.

Mental health policy

The current mental health policy was formulated in 1995. Its main components are advocacy, health promotion, treatment, and rehabilitation, but it also includes sections on administration and technical development. The policy plan is to promote mental health and prevent mental health problems, to expand and develop treatment and rehabilitation services, to develop a management system to reform all aspects of mental health services, and to develop modern psychosocial and other technical knowledge in order to apply them fruitfully to Thailand's mental health situation (Udomratn, 2011:213).

Thailand recently approved the Mental Health Care Bill. It was initially drafted by the Department of Mental Health (DMH), Ministry of Public Health and then revised according to suggestions from service providers, caregivers, and ex-patients during a public hearing process before submitting it to parliament in 2005 (Udomratn, 2011:213–14). However, parliament was dissolved in February 2006 and it took two years to get a new parliament to approve the bill in February 2008. This bill, in essence, was similar to the legislation enacted in other countries, in that all persons in need of psychiatric treatment either will be able to access it voluntarily or will be brought to a hospital for evaluation and compulsory treatment.

Psychiatric epidemiology

In 2006, an extensive review of research papers published during 1992–2002 on the epidemiology and risk or related factors of major mental health problems and psychiatric disorders in Thailand was published (Udomratn, 2006). In 2004, the prevalence data on mental disorders in Thailand, from the first nation-wide survey conducted in 2003 by the Thai DMH, was released (Siriwanarangsan et al., 2004). It was a two-step cross-sectional community survey using AUDIT (Alcohol Use Disorders Identification Test) and MINI (Mini-International Neuropsychiatric Interview). There were 11,700 participants enrolled in the age range of 15–59 years old. All were selected for the two-stage cluster sampling technique. The top three prevalence rates (one-month prevalence) were alcohol use disorders (28.5 percent), major depressive disorder (3.2 percent), and generalized anxiety disorder (1.9 percent).

In 2008, the Thai DMH carried out a second nationwide survey using MINI version 5.0 with 17,140 participants who lived in households. The age range again was 15–59 years old. The top four prevalence rates in 2008 were rather similar to the 2004 survey but with lower prevalence rates: alcohol dependence (6.6 percent), alcohol abuse (4.2 percent), major depressive episode both current and recurrent (2.9 percent), and generalized anxiety disorder (0.9 percent) (Kittirattanapaiboon et al., 2013:6). Details of both surveys appear in Table 25.1. It was also found that the prevalence of psychiatric comorbidity (at least two psychiatric illnesses occurring in the same person) was 1.4 percent. Although comorbidity was uncommon, it increased the suicide risk, especially in women who had comorbid mood disorders and anxiety disorders (70.5 percent) compared with men who had similar comorbidities (25.9 percent). The most common disorders in women were the comorbidity of mood and anxiety disorders (14.7 percent) while those in men were the comorbidity of alcohol use disorders and mood disorders (3.4 percent).

As alcohol use disorders and mood disorders are found commonly in Thailand, more detailed data on both conditions should be helpful for both clinicians and policy-makers. A closer look at the patterns of alcohol dependence in Thai drinkers recently found that both

Table 25.1 Prevalence of mental disorders in Thailand from national surveys in 2003 and 2008

Mental disorders	2003				2008			
	Female	Male	Total prevalence	Estimated patients	Female	Male	Total prevalence	Estimated patients
Alcohol use disorders (alcohol dependence and alcohol abuse)	10	46.1	28.5	7,766,689				
Alcohol dependence					1.4	13.3	6.6	3,212,447
Alcohol abuse					0.6	9.2	4.2	2,060,125
Major depressive episode	4	2.5	3.2	871,744				
Current					2.7	1.6	2.2	1,081,076
Recurrent					0.9	0.4	0.7	327,882
Dysthymia	1.6	0.8	1.2	371,347	0.4	0.1	0.3	150,530
Manic episode	0.5	0.3	0.4	102,713				
Current					0.1	0.1	0.1	65,644
Past					0.5	0.9	0.5	314,560
Hypomanic episode	0.5	0.5	0.5	126,416				
Current					0.3	0.3	0.3	132,649
Past					0.8	1.4	1.0	501,123
Generalized anxiety disorder	2.4	1.4	1.9	503,030	1.2	0.6	0.9	447,567
Panic disorder	0.6	0.2	0.4	97,445	0.3	0.3	0.3	150,579
Agoraphobia	1.1	0.7	0.9	242,297	0.6	0.2	0.5	218,454
Psychotic disorders								
Lifetime	1.2	1.2	1.2	318,673	0.6	1.2	0.9	409,465
Current	0.6	0.6	0.6	160,653	0.3	0.8	0.5	246,830

Americans and Thais have gender bias on alcohol dependence criteria, indicated by different rates of alcohol dependence symptoms between men and women, but their patterns of bias may be different. While Thai women reported quit-control problems less often and reported drinking despite physical and mental problems more than Thai men, American women reported both withdrawal and larger or longer drinking less often than American men (Srisurapanont et al., 2012:176; Saha et al., 2006:936). Moreover, although Thai adolescents and adults reported similar rates of each alcohol dependence symptom, young adults in the US tended to report 'activities given up' less frequently and reported tolerance of drinking more often than the US adults (Harford et al., 2009:870; Saha et al., 2006:936; Srisurapanont et al., 2012:176). The criterion of time spent drinking may have the highest significance in discriminating between severe and mild alcohol dependence in both Americans and Thais. However, as the authors did not compare the Thai and US data directly, these findings still need further confirmation (Srisurapanont et al., 2012:177).

Regarding major depressive disorder (MDD), recently a group was formed called Mood Disorders Research: Asian and Australian Network (MD RAN), of which the authors were part. The aim of this group was to study and compare the symptomatic and clinical features of depression among MDD outpatients living in Australia and different countries in Asia. The first series of papers focused mainly on patients with MDD living in China, Korea, Malaysia, Singapore, Taiwan, and Thailand. The interesting results, which were related to MDD patients in Thailand, are as follows.

Using the Montgomery–Asberg Depression Rating Scale (MADRS) to find the common symptom presentations, it was found that among all symptoms and countries, the most severe symptom was reduced sleep in Thai patients (Sulaiman et al., 2014:5). Moreover, it was found that MDD outpatients in Thailand most often reported "feeling lonely", "feeling blue", and "worrying too much" but were the least likely to express suicidal thoughts. Thus, the suicide rate itself is rather low in Thailand when compared with East Asian countries like Korea or Japan.

When dividing the MDD patients from all six Asian countries based on this data into low and high suicidality groups (score of 6 or higher on the MINI suicidality module), it was found that only 10.7 percent of Thai patients were classified as a high suicidality group compared with 42.6 percent, 31.3 percent, and 21.9 percent of Korean, Taiwanese, and Chinese patients, respectively, who participated in this study (Lim et al., 2014:5).

Results from this set of data indicated that MDD in six Asian countries has more similarities than differences among the outpatient population. The between-country differences, while present and not due to chance, are small enough to enable the use of common clinical and self-report rating scales in studies involving Asians with MDD from various ethnic backgrounds.

Another set of data comes from findings of the Research on Asia Psychotropic Prescription (REAP). From this data set, the three most common symptoms of depressed Thai outpatients are persistent sadness, insomnia, and loss of interest (Chee et al., 2014, submitted for publication). These three common symptoms were similarly found in eight other countries in Asia, regardless of the region or the income level of the country. It seems that these three depressive symptoms are still the main findings by psychiatrists who make the diagnosis of depression in any country in Asia, including Thailand.

As affective disorder can occur seasonally, so-called seasonal affective disorder (SAD) has also been studied in Thailand (Srisurapanont and Intaprasert, 1999:97). Interestingly, of 112 respondents who completed the Seasonal Pattern Assessment Questionnaire (SPAQ), three men and three women (6.19 percent) had summer SAD and one man (1.03 percent) had winter

SAD. Moreover, two men and six women (8.25 percent) had subsyndromal summer SAD. Fifty-one respondents (51.5 percent) did not feel worse in any month. For the other 46 who felt worst in particular months, the number of responses was largest for April which is usually the hottest month in Thailand. The "feel worst" response was highly and significantly correlated with temperature but not duration of daylight and humidity (Srisurapanont and Intaprasert, 1999:98). The ratio of summer SAD prevalence rate to winter SAD prevalence rate in northern Thailand in this study (6:1 at the latitude of 19°N) was higher than that found at the latitude of 19°S (5:1) (Morrissey *et al.*, 1996:582). The significant correlation between the "feel worst" response and temperature but not duration of daylight appears to support the hypothesis that the tropical temperature but not daylight may be related to mood and behavior changes. As SPAQ was originally designed for the screening of winter SAD, a further study in Thailand is still needed to confirm the above results.

Mental health systems

In the past, the healthcare system in Thailand did not have a formal referral system so patients could go directly to any level of care they chose. In 2001, the Thai government introduced the policy of universal coverage (UC) under its "30 baht healthcare scheme" (30 baht is approximately US$1) and referral systems were strengthened. Under this scheme, people who have no health insurance or who are not civil servants or employees in the private sector in the social insurance security system must register with a hospital nearest to their residence. If they are ill, they can go to that hospital and pay the hospital only 30 baht per visit. This covers all kinds of treatments from medication to surgery. If doctors at the registered hospital cannot treat the patient for any reason, they will refer the patient to a larger hospital, which will in turn send the bill back to the first hospital for reimbursement. More recently, paying the 30 baht is no longer compulsory. The 30 baht fee is waived for those who cannot pay. Moreover, in emergency or accident cases, patients can go directly to any nearby hospital with only their national ID cards.

In 2013, a major health reform policy was implemented in Thailand. Healthcare authority was transferred to the Area Health Care Board (AHB) in each responsible area. The AHB manages health service plans, including comprehensive mental health services entirely in its area with the support of the psychiatric hospital located in that zone. Also, the District Health System (DHS) was set up to integrate healthcare with other health-related activities for the community, including prevention and promotion in mental health. The Thai DMH now focuses on monitoring the implementation of activities related to community mental health in order to close the mental health gap and improve the quality of mental health services.

Mental health services

Although the number of psychiatrists has increased from 387 in 2003 to 662 in 2013, the main problems of the mental healthcare system are still the same:

- The number of mental health workers is insufficient.
- General physicians and general practitioners are not confident in the assessment and management of psychiatric patients. Some mental disorders, especially depression, are under-diagnosed, whereas other diagnoses are made too often, such as anxiety disorders. Many patients receive anxiolytic or antidepressant medication in sub-therapeutic doses. Patients with a psychosis are an exception, as most are referred directly to a psychiatric hospital.

- The primary and secondary care services have little opportunity to care for psychiatric patients during the continuation and maintenance phases of their illnesses because of limited supplies of medications. District hospitals usually have only haloperidol for schizophrenia and amitriptyline or imipramine for depression. Although the Ministry of Public Health added fluoxetine (generic) and sertraline (generic) to the list of essential hospital drugs a few years ago, only the central hospitals and a few general hospitals are able to supply this. Atypical antipsychotics have also been supplied to psychiatric hospitals, university hospitals, and some central hospitals. Again, only risperidone (generic) and clozapine (generic) have been added to the essential hospital drugs list. However, other original psychotropic drugs can be prescribed on a case-by-case basis under certain conditions, or patients can pay for them from their own pockets. The shortage of psychiatric drugs at local hospitals, the long distances that patients have to travel to get treatment, and the high cost of travel (because of increasing fuel prices) are also problems for continuation of treatment.
- Patients and their families have a poor understanding of psychiatric disorders. In the case of psychoses, most have some knowledge about the symptoms but tend to believe that they were caused by stress, worry, or supernatural influences. This may result in patients discontinuing their treatment early.
- During the continuation and maintenance phases of treatment, even though some mental health teams in general hospitals can monitor symptoms, adjust the doses of drugs, and provide psychosocial intervention, often the patients and their families still prefer to see a psychiatrist, and this overloads many psychiatrists in tertiary care centers.

Social/explanatory models of mental illness

Many Thai laypersons believe that mental illnesses are caused by various sources, such as their having done something bad or inappropriate which angered their dead ancestors. So the dead ancestors punished them with mental disorders; this is the so-called "spirit possession syndrome". There is also the interaction between blood and "wind" (*lom*) in the body. According to traditional Thai beliefs, the human body is composed of four elements: earth, water, wind (*lom*), and fire. Moreover, menstrual blood is recognized as spoiled blood (*lead seai*). Many Thais, especially those with minimal education, explain their symptoms in terms of the blood (*lead*), especially in women, and wind (*lom*) in both men and women.

In a healthy state, many Thais believe that *lom* flows downward through the gastrointestinal tract to be expelled from the body and that it flows continuously downward along the arms and legs to exit the body through the hands and feet. *Lom* can also escape through the skin pores. In pathological states, the *lom* may move progressively upward in the body, or it may suddenly ascend directly to the head. If the downward flow of *lom* is blocked at the stomach or the limbs, it then moves upward in the body resulting in various serious problems. As it rises, the *lom* may hit the diaphragm, impairing inhalation and causing chest tightness or it may compress the heart to a much smaller and thinner shape causing it to function poorly and possibly rip as it makes abnormal motions. The *lom* may also enter the head, causing dizziness, blurry vision, faintness, and tinnitus, potentially bringing about syncope, paralysis, or even death.

Thai patients delay the decision to visit a psychiatrist for a long time. Besides the fear of being stigmatized, they initially try to help themselves according to their personal beliefs. If they believe that they did something bad, they will consult a "spirit doctor" (*morphi*). If the spirit doctor ascribes the illness to a transgression against a deceased ancestor, the spirit doctor will recommend as treatment addressing prayers to their ancestors and offering food to Buddhist monks, or a merit-making ceremony at the temple. Merit has a protective power and can be earned in many ways such as by giving a donation to monks or by doing some good deed.

If they believe the problem is caused by "wind" (*lom*), patients may initially use herbal medicine called "antiwind medicine" (*yaa lom*) to make wind come out of the body either by burping or passing wind.

In southern Thailand, many cases of panic disorder are initially thought to be suffering from *lom* syndromes either "wind" (*lom*) illness or "upsurge" (*wuup*) illness. More details of these syndromes can be found elsewhere (Udomratn and Hinton, 2009:183–204).

Topics of interest: how can Thailand successfully reduce the suicide rate?

The suicide rate has been a major public health concern in Thailand for some time. It dramatically increased from 4.0 per 100,000 in 1992 to 6.3 per 100,000 in 1994 and peaked at 8.6 per 100,000 in 1999 after the Asian economic crisis which initially started in Thailand in 1997 (Udomratn, 2006:23). The average suicide rate between 1998 and 2003 was 7.9 per 100,000, while during the 1988–1992 period the average suicide rate was only 6.5 per 100,000 (Lotrakul, 2006:91).

The male to female suicide ratio has increased steadily from 1.6:1 in 1988 to the highest ratio of 3.6:1 in 2000. The average ratio of male to female suicide rates for the 1998–2003 period was 3.4:1. Male suicide rates were higher than female suicide rates for all ages. The highest rate of male suicides occurred in those aged 25–29 years (21.9 per 100,000) followed by a small peak after the age of 60. Among females, suicide rates showed less variation with age (Lotrakul, 2006:91).

An increase in suicide rates between 1998 and 2000 was related to the Asian economic crisis of 1997. There was a sharp drop in the annual economic growth from 7 percent to −1.7 percent in 1997 and to −10.8 percent in 1998. During 1998, the Thai economy contracted by 10.2 percent. The crisis resulted in substantial declines in social welfare. More than a million Thais fell below the poverty line as a result of it. The unemployment rate increased from 2 percent of the total labor force in 1996 to 5 percent in 1998, and 5.3 percent in 1999. Suicide rates in 1999 were at their highest peak in Thai history ($n = 5,290$) (Wibulpolprasert, 2002:12).

There were so many suicide cases reported in newspapers and on television that the Ministry of Public Health (MOPH) made suicide reduction a priority requiring urgent action and the National Suicide Prevention Strategy (NSPS) was implemented by the Department of Mental Health by the year 2000. Decreasing the suicide rate became one of the key performance indicators (KPI) in the evaluation of the MOPH's effectiveness.

After the NSPS implementation the suicide rate dropped from 8.4 per 100,000 in 2000 to 7.1 per 100,000 in 2003, to 5.7 per 100,000 in 2006, and to 5.9 per 100,000 in 2010 (Table 25.2).

Activities under the NSPS

Many activities under the NSPS have been implemented:

1. A public education campaign on "suicide and mental disorders", especially major depression was conducted. It focused on making the public aware that serious mental illness (SMI) may lead to suicide but that it is a treatable condition involving biological factors, which can be successfully treated with the use of psychotropic medication. This educational

Table 25.2 Suicide rates (per 100,000) in Thailand by gender, 1988–2010

	1988	1989	1990	1991	1992	1993	1994	1995	1996	1997	1998	1999	2000	2001	2002	2003
Total	6.3	6.7	6.7	6.4	6.3	6.7	4.0	7.2	7.6	6.9	8.1	8.6	8.4	7.7	7.8	7.1
Males	7.8	8.7	8.8	8.6	8.3	9.1	5.6	10.6	11.3	10.7	12.6	13.3	13.2	11.9	12.0	11.0
Females	4.8	4.7	4.7	4.1	4.2	4.3	2.4	3.9	3.9	3.2	3.7	3.9	3.7	3.6	3.8	3.3
Male:female	1.6	1.9	1.9	2.1	2.0	2.1	2.3	2.7	2.7	3.3	3.5	3.4	3.6	3.3	3.2	3.3

	2004	2005	2006	2007	2008	2009	2010
Total	6.9	6.3	5.7	5.9	5.9	5.9	5.9
Males	10.5	9.9	9.2	9.4	9.3	9.3	9.2
Females	3.3	2.9	2.4	2.5	2.7	2.6	2.6
Male:female	3.1	3.4	3.8	3.7	3.4	3.4	3.6

campaign to increase the awareness that depression can be curable with medication contributed to modification of the conventional belief that depression is a disease of a weak personality.

2. Training was provided for general physicians with the aim of improving detection and offering appropriate treatment to those who suffer from mental disorders. Among other things, it consisted of instructions on how to differentiate depressive disorders from anxiety disorders, and then how to appropriately prescribe antidepressants.

3. The training of village health volunteers (VHVs) to use simple screening tests to detect high-risk groups for suicide, in order for these patients to be referred for early treatment by doctors, was another NSPS activity. It was also intended to train VHVs to perform periodic visits to the homes of patients who had been discharged from hospitals.

4. The final activity entailed monitoring the suicide rate closely every three months at all levels (provincial and district levels) and making data available so that a comparison of the outcomes of suicide prevention activities could be made. A color scheme was used to identify the severity of suicides in provinces. A high suicide rate of more than 14 per 100,000 was labeled in red. Those with fewer than 14 but more than 7 per 100,000 had a yellow label, and those with less than 7 per 100,000 were labeled in green.

Some challenges

Although the overall suicide rate in Thailand is not as high as in many other Asian countries like Sri Lanka, Japan, and Korea, it has a larger social effect than generally perceived because the highest proportion of suicide cases occurs among the most productive sector of the workforce. Still, some remaining challenges have been identified. In the northern regions of Thailand, especially in the provinces of Lamphun, Chiangmai, Chiangrai, and Phayao the suicide rate remains high even though the rate decreased from 2000 to 2006. One important factor associated with suicide was HIV infection which is also most prevalent in the north. In-depth investigations should be carried out. In particular, assessments should be conducted of suicide and HIV in male patients of reproductive age so that more specific interventions can be implemented. Reducing the suicide rate to a level lower than 5.7 per 100,000 may prove to be a difficult task because suicide is a multidimensional and complex issue. However, we remain hopeful of overcoming these challenges.

Conclusion

Psychiatry in Thailand, as in many developing countries, still has many problems in providing psychiatric services, including stigmas and traditional beliefs about mental disorders causing a delay in seeking help and/or frequent early discontinuation of treatment. Many strategic plans have been initiated by our DMH, such as increasing human resources, offering better quality of care at both community and tertiary care levels, and developing suitable screening tests and treatment programs for major psychiatric disorders. A better future can be expected for our patients and their families by the year 2020.

References

Chee, K.Y., Tripathi, A., Chong, M.Y., Xiang, Y.T., Sim, K. and Si, T.M. (2014) 'Country variations in depressive symptoms profile in Asian countries: findings of the research on Asia Psychotropic Prescription (REAP) studies' (submitted for publication).

Harford, T.C., Yi, H.Y., Faden, V.B. and Chen, C.M. (2009) 'The dimensionality of DSM-IV alcohol use disorders among adolescent and adult drinkers and symptom patterns by age, gender and race/ethnicity'. *Alcoholism, Clinical and Experimental Research*, 33:868–78.

Kittirattanapaiboon, P., Kongsuk, T., Pengjuntr, W., Leejongpermpoon, J., Chutha, W. and Kenbubpha, K. (2013). 'Epidemiology of psychiatric comorbidity in Thailand: a national study 2008'. *Journal of Mental Health of Thailand*, 21(1):1–14.

Lim, A.Y., Lee, A.R., Sulaiman, A.H., Si, T.M., Liu, C.Y. and Jeon, H.J. (2014) 'Clinical and sociodemographic correlates of suicidality in patients with major depressive disorder from six Asian countries'. *BMC Psychiatry*, 14:37. doi;10.1186/1471–244x-14–37

Lotrakul, M. (2006) 'Suicide in Thailand during the period 1998–2003'. *Psychiatry and Clinical Neurosciences*, 60:90–5.

Morrissey, S.A., Raggat, P.T.F., James, B. and Rogers, J. (1996) 'Seasonal affective disorder: some epidemiological findings from a tropical climate'. *Australia and New Zealand Journal of Psychiatry*, 30:579–86.

Saha, T.D., Chou, S.P. and Grant, B.F. (2006) 'Toward an alcohol use disorder continuum using item response theory: results from the National Epidemiologic Survey on Alcohol and Related Conditions'. *Psychological Medicine*, 36:931–41.

Siriwanarangsan, P., Kongsuk, T., Arunpongpaisan, S., Kittirattanapaiboon, P. and Charatsingha, A. (2004) 'Prevalence of mental disorders in Thailand: a national survey 2003'. *Journal of Mental Health of Thailand*, 12(3):177–88.

Srisurapanont, M. and Intaprasert, S. (1999) 'Seasonal variations in mood and behaviour: epidemiological findings in the north. *Journal of Affective Disorders*, 54:97–9.

Srisurapanont, M., Kittiratanapaiboon, P., Likhitsathian, S., Kongsuk, T., Suttajit, S. and Junsirimongkol, B. (2012) 'Patterns of alcohol dependence in Thai drinkers: a differential item functioning analysis of gender and age bias'. *Addictive Behaviors*, 37:173–8.

Sulaiman, A.H., Bautista, D., Liu, C.Y., Udomratn, P. and Bae, J.N. (2014) 'Differences in psychiatric symptoms among Asian patients with depression: a multi-country cross-sectional study'. *Psychiatry and Clinical Neurosciences*, 68:245–54.

Udomratn, P. (2006). 'Epidemiology of mental disorders in Thailand'. *ASEAN Journal of Psychiatry*, 7:22–5.

Udomratn, P. (2011). 'Thailand', in H. Ghodse (ed.) *International Perspectives on Mental Health*, London: RCPsych Publications.

Udomratn, P. and Hinton, D.E. (2009) 'Gendered panic in southern Thailand: "Lom" ("Wind") illness and "Wuup" ("Upsurge") illness', in D.E. Hinton and B.J. Good (eds) *Culture and Panic Disorder*, Stanford: Stanford University Press.

Wibulpolprasert, S., (2002) *Thailand Health Profile 1999–2000*. Bangkok: Bureau of Policy and Strategy, Ministry of Public Health.

World Bank (2001) *Thailand Economic Monitor 2001*. Bangkok: World Bank Thailand Office.

26

Psychiatry in Vietnam

Tran Thi Hong Thu

Country and people

Vietnam is a country occupying 331,700 square kilometres at the centre of South-East Asia. It is bordered by Laos and Cambodia to the west and the People's Republic of China to the north, and bounded by the Gulf of Thailand to the southwest and the East Sea (South China Sea) to the east. Vietnam's coastline is 3,260 kilometres long. Foreign visitors have called Vietnam the 'balcony on the Pacific'.

Vietnam has a population of 84 million and is the second most densely populated country in South-East Asia. Seventy-three per cent of the population live in rural areas and the population growth is 1.21 per cent per annum. The maternal mortality rate is 130/100,000 live births. The average income per capita is US$750, gross domestic product is US$638 per capita and the poverty rate was 16 per cent in 2006. Vietnam is a low-income-group country based on World Bank 2004 criteria but, due to extensive reforms in the past two decades, is on its way to becoming a middle-income country. The country's capital is Hanoi in the north, and the largest city is Ho Chi Minh City (HCMC) in the south. The pace of rural–urban migration is rapid. Lower fertility rates and improvements in healthcare are increasing life expectancy, and the resulting epidemiological transition from infectious diseases to non-communicable diseases will require a fundamental transformation of the healthcare system.

Mental health policies

In the past, medical care in Vietnam was free at all levels. However, after the adoption of the economic renovation policy in 1986, only part of patients' medical costs have been shouldered by hospitals, while private for-profit clinics have been permitted to open. The policies also encourage integrating mental health into primary health care services.

Mental disorders are increasingly being recognized as a major public health problem. The mental health policies are aligned with the national health policies. Vietnam's mental health policy was last revised in 1989,[1] and until 2004 it was actually put into practice effectively as a national plan of action for the treatment only of schizophrenia and epilepsy in hospitals. The main objective of the mental health programme is to provide services at community level.

Overall objectives up to 2010 were revised once more to cover all communes and to include depression in the project, though the focal point for the period 2006–2010 was schizophrenia. By June 2006, 3,323 communes were covered by this programme and in 2009 the management model for epilepsy and depression had been implemented in 53 communes. The activities of this model include mental health training of staff and health collaborators, as well as household surveys to identify people with depression and epilepsy, monthly delivery of medicines for patients, and monitoring and supporting patients through medication, and health education through village media.

In Vietnam the National Assembly approves and monitors policy, including mental health policy, and the Communist Party's Central Commission for Science and Education directs the development of health policy. The Department of Curative Medicine within the Ministry of Health (MOH) has responsibility for developing policies relating to mental health, including prevention policies, and the Health Strategy and Policy Institute, also within the MOH, promotes itself as providing an evidence base for policy formulation. Lastly, the National Committee for Population, Families and Children (referred to as the National Committee) is a government body that deals with all sectors that have an impact on families and children. In terms of international agencies, the WHO and international universities have provided regular support.

There are no specific legal rights for the mentally ill, but the National Institute of Mental Health (of the United States) together with the MOH's Department of Policy are in the process of devising them. There are no alcohol policies, nor any policies to counter discrimination. A national mental health human rights review body does not exist, but there is legislation to protect the human rights of patients. All hospitals have at least one review/inspection of their human rights protection of patients each year.

About 1 per cent of all admissions to mental hospitals are involuntary and 1 per cent of patients were restrained or secluded at least once within the last year in community-based psychiatric services, in comparison with 2–5 per cent of patients in mental hospitals.[1] Inequity of access to mental health services for other minority users (e.g. linguistic, ethnic, religious minorities) is a moderate issue in Vietnam.

Within the governmental sector, it seems that the concept of prevention of mental disorders has not been recognized. There is no link between the public mental health services and other sectors in this respect, and no documents are available for the public on the prevention of mental disorders. Alcohol abuse is a relatively large burden in Vietnam, as indicated by its 5.3 per cent prevalence rate. Policies to reduce alcohol abuse, such as restrictions and increased taxation could be effective in reducing this burden (Table 26.1).

In MOH statistics, patients in mental hospitals in Vietnam are categorized in three diagnostic groups: those with schizophrenia, schizotypal and delusional disorders (60 per cent), those with mood disorders (25 per cent), and those with neurotic, stress-related and somatoform disorders (15 per cent). Diagnoses for patients in outpatient facilities are unknown. There are 33 psychiatric hospitals, 25 psychiatric departments in general hospitals and 24 mental health units in social diseases centres in Vietnam.

The government pays for the control and medication only of epilepsy and schizophrenia, while medication and treatment for other mental illnesses is paid for by patients, out-of-pocket. However, within the MOH National Target Programme on mental health, psychiatric medicines are provided free of charge. The government spends approximately US$2 million per year on mental health (compared to US$46 million allocated in Thailand, and no allocation in Laos in 2004), while some additional financing comes from international donors. For example, the WHO had by 2007 funded mental health in Vietnam with a total of US$80,000. About 50 per cent

Table 26.1 Results of a clinical epidemiological survey on some common mental disorders in Vietnam[1]

Illness	Rate (%)
Schizophrenia	0.47
Epilepsy	0.35
Age-related memory loss	0.88
Depression	2.8
Anxiety	2.6
Behaviour disorder in youths and teenagers	0.9
Alcohol abuse	5.3
Drug addiction	0.3
Total	13.6

of the population have free access to essential psychotropic medicines. For those who pay out-of-pocket, the cost of antipsychotic medication is 33 per cent of one day's minimum wage in the local currency and the cost of antidepressant medication is 13 per cent of one day's minimum wage in the local currency. Some severe mental disorders are covered by social policy schemes.

There are no regular national programmes for information on or the promotion of mental health, though public education and awareness campaigns have targeted the general population as well as health care providers, leaders and politicians. Public programmes, including information panels, booklets distributed to patients and their families, and talks on national TV and radio have been organized by the central mental hospital. However, this has mainly focused on psychotic disorders within the context of the Community-Based Mental Health Project. According to decision 49/2003 Nghị Định-Chính Phủ (NĐ-CP) of the Prime Minister, the MOH, with 14 departments, has the task of controlling and managing health care services in the whole country. There are 78 organizations/units directly belonging to the MOH.

In Vietnam, using evidence to present mental illness as a 'new problem' seems to have had some resonance in terms of shaping policy. Changes to policy, though, are unlikely to come from political pressure but are more likely to result from a long-term engagement between researchers and policy-makers, which has in fact already begun.

Mental health systems

Vietnam is one of the few countries to adopt community-based rehabilitation (CBR) as a means of delivering rehabilitation to all its citizens. Two per cent of the training for medical doctors is devoted to mental health, in comparison with 1 per cent for nurses and none for non-doctor/non-nurse primary health care workers. Furthermore, 22 per cent of primary health care doctors have received at least two days of refresher training in mental health. Other than doctors or nurses, primary health care workers are not allowed to prescribe psychotropic medications under any circumstances. The majority (51–80 per cent) of primary health care clinics have at least one psychotropic medication in each of the therapeutic categories (antipsychotic, antidepressant, mood stabilizer, anxiolytic and antiepileptic). Psychotropic drugs are widely available in mental hospitals and outpatient mental health facilities.

Table 26.2 Human resources in mental health in Vietnam (rate per 100.000 population)[2]

Human resources	No.	Per 100,000
Psychiatrists	286	0.35
Other medical doctors, not specialized in psychiatry	730	0.90
Nurses	1,700	2.10
Psychologists	50	0.06
Social workers	125	0.15
Occupational therapists	4	0.00
Other health or mental health workers (including auxiliary staff, non-doctor/non-physician primary health care workers, health assistants, medical assistants, professional and paraprofessional counsellors)	650	0.80

The community mental health programme has been carried out in 63 provinces, controlling and managing three mental disorders: schizophrenia, epilepsy and depression. Altogether there were 7,700 community mental health projects by the year 2010 providing a national coverage of around 69 per cent.

The national and regional mental health authorities are involved in the planning, management and coordination, and the monitoring and quality assessment of mental health services. Mental health services are organized in terms of catchment/service areas. The major provider of psychiatric services is the government. It is also largely responsible for the planning of human resources and training of staff. The practice of psychiatry has been moving away from the custodial and institutional care of patients to community services and facilities. However, in Vietnam a large number of beds are still retained due to the difficulty of discharging patients. There are no community residential facilities available in Vietnam. Although mental health services in Vietnam have considerably improved over the last decade, mainly in terms of accessibility, the demand for community-based care and the illness burden remain high. This is a drain on resources and reduces the staff-to-patient ratio (Table 26.2).

Social capital

There is little published evidence about the extent and nature of mental health problems in Vietnam. There is a conflict between the punitive and the therapeutic approach to offending behaviour that results from mental disorder. Changing lifestyles associated with economic restructuring in recent times, and the associated stress, mean that anxiety and depression are common. A number of studies have shown that combining medication with locally feasible psychological interventions can be effective and cost-effective among the poorest people in a low-income country, and produce significant reductions in total health care costs.

No official consumer or family associations exist for the mentally ill, though recently a group of families with autistic children in Hanoi started to work together, exemplifying a trend of establishing civil organizations in the field of mental health.

The medical management of mental illness in Vietnam only involves medication, and there is no family education or psychotherapy. Only doctors are allowed to prescribe psychotropic medication. The psychologists who work in hospitals perform clinical testing.

Traditional medicine is used for neurasthenia and dissociative disorders, and treatment consists mainly of acupuncture, massage and herbal medicines. Patients with schizophrenia, personality disorders, paranoia or suicidal thoughts are not treated with traditional medicine.

One of the most pressing tasks in Vietnam now is probably to assess the level of the mental health burden on society, and in different geographic and sociodemographic groups, so as to be able to plan public health programmes and mental health services.

Networks of key stakeholders (that is, of researchers and policy-makers) have been established and are active. Although the idea of local NGOs undertaking research is a new phenomenon in Vietnam, these NGOs do understand the need for early engagement with policy-makers.

If criteria for evaluating policy recommendations are applied to the emerging policy described above, the main gaps identified are the lack of knowledge about the feasibility and cost of any intervention. Thus there is a need for intervention studies that examine the cost-effectiveness of interventions. The main challenge is policy implementation rather than formulation. Although mental health policy in developing countries is rarely driven by evidence we should not be naive about the process in developed countries either.

Trends and issues

Evidence on the burden of mental illness in Vietnam is limited. Nonetheless, the process of developing policy has been influenced by the evidence, because links between stakeholders were established at an early stage.

The strengths of the mental health system in Vietnam are:[2]

- There is legislation to protect the human rights of patients.
- There are efforts to promote equity of access to mental health services.
- Essential psychotropic medicines are available in all hospital facilities.
- The mental health sector has formal links with other relevant sectors (health, education, criminal justice, etc.).
- Mental health providers interact with primary care staff.
- A mental health policy, plan and legislation exist (although they need updating).

The weaknesses include:[2]

- The network of mental health facilities is not yet complete.
- The mental health system provides more services in mental hospitals than in the community.
- Despite mental health legislation to protect human rights, practical implementation of the legislation is weak.
- Insufficient training is provided to primary care staff.
- Family and consumer associations do not exist.
- The mental health information system does not work well.

To sum up, mental health care in Vietnam is still characterized by unclear policy with barriers and low priority to mental health services, especially within the governmental sector. The aim should be to promote mental health, to provide a person-focused service that is comprehensive, accessible and cost-effective, and to pursue continuous learning and research. There are four key issues:

1. The provision of locally feasible and effective non-pharmaceutical interventions;
2. Health insurance coverage for treatments, including pharmaceuticals for common mental disorders;
3. Replacement of care in large tertiary hospitals with less stigmatizing forms of service provision; and
4. Increased commitment to preventive measures for mental illness, including increased mental health information provision to the general public.

Topics of interest

The Vietnamese mental health system is challenged by a lack of human resources. When compared with other Asian countries in the region, the proportion of physicians working in the mental health field in Vietnam is about average, but the proportion of psychiatrists is below that in countries such as China and Thailand. This is the result of insufficient training of psychiatrists. Hence, the largest challenge for Vietnamese mental health care is to attract mental health workers. However, training of primary care staff, e.g. psychiatric nurses, is limited and complicated by the absence of psychiatric/mental health topics in the nursing curriculum and the lack of psychiatric nursing textbooks and periodicals in Vietnamese.[3] Therefore, more emphasis should be put on increasing the capacity of the mental health services and on human resource development. In that process, more representative epidemiological data and intervention research is needed.

References

1. WHO, *WHO–AIMS report on mental health system in Vietnam*, 2006. Available from: www.who. int/mental_health/evidence/who_aims_report_viet_nam.pdf (accessed March 2014).
2. Jacob KS, Sharan P, Mirza J, Garrido-Cumbrera M, Seerat S, Mari JJ, Sreenivas V and Saxena S, Mental health systems in countries: Where are we now? *The Lancet* 2007, 370:1061–77
3. Goren, S., Looking for child psychiatric nursing – Vietnam 2005. *JCAPN* 2007, 20(3):156—62

Index

Page numbers in *italics* refer to figures. Page numbers in **bold** refer to tables.

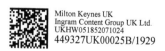